Health and Medicine through History

Health and Medicine through History

From Ancient Practices to 21st-Century Innovations

VOLUME 1: Antiquity through the 18th Century

Ruth Clifford Engs, Editor

GREENWOOD
An Imprint of ABC-CLIO, LLC
Santa Barbara, California • Denver, Colorado

Library of Congress Cataloging-in-Publication Data

Names: Engs, Ruth Clifford, editor.
Title: Health and medicine through history : from ancient practices to 21st-century innovations / Ruth Clifford Engs, editor.
Description: Santa Barbara, CA : Greenwood, [2019] | Includes bibliographical references and index.
Identifiers: LCCN 2018055964 (print) | LCCN 2018056496 (ebook) | ISBN 9781440858925 (eBook) | ISBN 9781440858918 (set : alk. paper) | ISBN 9781440858932 (volume 1 : alk. paper) | ISBN 9781440858949 (volume 2 : alk. paper) | ISBN 9781440858956 (volume 3 : alk. paper)
Subjects: | MESH: History of Medicine
Classification: LCC R131 (ebook) | LCC R131 (print) | NLM WZ 40 | DDC 610—dc23
LC record available at https://lccn.loc.gov/2018055964

ISBN: 978-1-4408-5891-8 (set)
978-1-4408-5893-2 (vol. 1)
978-1-4408-5894-9 (vol. 2)
978-1-4408-5895-6 (vol. 3)
978-1-4408-5892-5 (ebook)

23 22 21 20 19 1 2 3 4 5

This book is also available as an eBook.

Greenwood
An Imprint of ABC-CLIO, LLC

ABC-CLIO, LLC
147 Castilian Drive
Santa Barbara, California 93117
www.abc-clio.com

This book is printed on acid-free paper ∞

Manufactured in the United States of America

For Jeff Graf and Jeff Franz

Contents

Acknowledgments

No reference book of this nature springs solely from the mind of the author. Numerous individuals helped with finding references, suggesting details for content, and offering suggestions for the flow of the work. I am deeply indebted to my editor Maxine Taylor at ABC-CLIO who brainstormed many ideas and offered constructive comments on the whole work. Robin Tutt did an outstanding job of reworking various primary sources including graphs, charts, and quotations, and Bridget Austiguy-Preschel was a most thorough production editor.

I am most beholden to medical, academic, and other professionals who reviewed various parts of the manuscript for which they had considerable knowledge and offered suggestions and comments. Any errors are mine. These experts include Gellisse Bagnall, Christopher D. Beck, Leila Dabbagh, William D. Engs, Shirin Hassan, Jain Liu, Khalid Khan, Mark O'Keefe, and Michael Wenzler.

Both the Lilly and Wells Libraries of Indiana University, Bloomington, along with their librarians were also helpful in suggesting material for many aspects of this publication. I want to profoundly thank Jeffrey Graf, reference librarian extraordinary, who has helped me over many years with finding or suggesting material. As usual, much love and appreciation go to my husband, Jeffrey Franz, for allowing me the space and time to write.

Introduction

Concerns about health and disease and their treatment have been common since before recorded history in all civilizations across all continents. For example, early evidence of surgery, such as trepanation—drilling a hole in the scull or removing a small bit of it—to relieve illness and treat head wounds and other maladies have been found as early as 7000 B.C.E. Cure and healing in many areas of the world were often tied up with religious beliefs. However, some health and medical practices and beliefs have gone in cycles in terms of advancements. Ancient practices have been lost in dark ages as civilizations declined but were rediscovered in later centuries. For example, sanitation, sewage disposal, and access to clean water were found in the ancient civilizations of Mohenjo Daro and Harappa of the Indus Valley of India from around 2500 B.C.E. These practices would have curtailed many diseases but were lost when these civilizations declined. They were reinvented by the classical Greek and Roman civilizations, only to be lost again in the early Middle Ages of Western civilization. It was not until the late 19th and early 20th centuries C.E. that adequate sanitation and clean water again emerged, which dramatically decreased various water- and food-borne disease globally over the 20th century C.E. and into the 21st century C.E.

Over the centuries, the beliefs and practices concerning health and medicine have radically changed. Sometimes advances have been repressed by religious, political, or even medical groups for decades. These have included, for instance, autopsies to determine cause of death, eating limes to prevent scurvy, and washing hands to prevent the spread of infectious disease. Some treatments that were common in antiquity but were discounted in more recent times have again been instituted, such as the Roman practice of setting compound arm and leg fractures and using hot water and wine to disinfect the wound. In the 19th century C.E., shattered limbs were often amputated, and it was not until World War I that fractures were set again along with the use of antiseptics to prevent infections. Over the centuries, on the whole, advances in preventative treatment and rehabilitation have expanded, and our knowledge has greatly increased on many subjects. The use of the scientific method emerged in the 17th century C.E. However, evidence-based medicine—based upon scientific methods rather than cures passed down through apprenticeships and oral and other traditions—emerged in the mid-19th century C.E. but did not reach full acceptance until the 20th century C.E.

Volume 1 of this book discusses health and medicine from antiquity to the middle ages and the 15th through the 18th centuries C.E. Volume 2 looks at the 19th and 20th centuries C.E. and the first two decades of the 21st century C.E. Both volumes have the same standardized set of chapter outlines. This makes it easy for the reader to compare a particular topic, such as surgery, over the span of history. Each time period in this work has an extensive bibliography and a short glossary. For Volume 2, which contains the 20th century C.E. and beyond section, since many resources are now found on scholarly, governmental, archival, and academic Internet sites, most of the references include a website for ease of location. Volume 3 contains data and primary documents that include graphs, illustrations, tables, and excerpts from various sources from the beginning of recorded history.

This work is aimed at a variety of students. These include those studying health, medicine, history, comparative religions, and environmental and military sciences. This work will help them to discover conditions, beliefs, practices, and changes within a given period of time, in addition to tracing topics over time. The book is from an international perspective, so traditional healing practices from various health systems are covered. Since it examines different cultures and nations, comparisons can also be made cross-nationally and regionally for most topics. In addition, practices and statistics of different regions of the world are discussed. This work is also aimed at the general reader who is interested in these subjects, and it will serve as a handy reference work for libraries.

Ruth Clifford Engs
School of Public Health
Indiana University
Bloomington, IN

PART I

Antiquity through the Middle Ages

William H. York

1

Key Factors in Health and Wellness

HEALTH AND DISEASE IN HISTORY

In early hunter and gatherer societies, with small, scattered populations, humans were unlikely to have been exposed to numerous contagious bacterial and viral diseases that require large, dense populations to spread (such as smallpox). Furthermore, the nomadic lifestyle of these early societies would have minimized the possibility of contact with water polluted by human waste and piles of refuse and garbage that might attract disease-carrying insects. Finally, prior to the period of widespread domestication of animals, these peoples were less likely to contract diseases passed on by close contact with dogs, pigs, birds, and cattle, not to mention the mice and rats drawn to human dwellings. This is not to say that early humans lived without disease; indeed, they still faced a number of diseases caused by eating animals or passed on by worms and lice. The limited population sizes, however, would have limited incidences of infection and death from infectious diseases. As humans began to live together in larger, permanent settlements starting around 10,000 B.C.E., they encountered a whole new range of diseases of civilization. Living in cities brought humans into closer, regular contact with pathogens and parasites that were spread by contact with domesticated animals or through poor sanitation and fouled water supplies. The larger and denser populations also made it easier for infectious diseases to spread, allowing some (like smallpox and measles) that had previously caused little trouble to emerge and thrive. Furthermore, archaeological evidence indicates that as humans started to live in permanent settlements and rely on agriculture and domesticated animals for food, their diets became less varied and focused on a limited number of staple crops, leading to malnutrition from not getting appropriate nutrients. The changed diets would only further enable the spread of diseases due to weakened immunities. Clearly, the move to civilization brought a trade-off—on the one hand, it may have allowed for increased security, but on the other, it led to an increase in disease. In this context, the need for an effective means of treating disease became even more crucial once humans started to congregate in cities.

Faced with these conditions, humans in the earliest civilizations began to develop theories about health and disease and to recognize different professionals in society who were deemed proficient in the craft of healing. This book is about the early medical beliefs and practices in civilizations from around the world from their earliest origins in antiquity until roughly 1500 C.E. We will focus on the medical traditions in seven different premodern societies: Mesopotamia (ca. 3000–500 B.C.E.), Egypt (ca. 3000–300 B.C.E.), Greece and Rome (ca. 1200 B.C.E.–500 C.E.), India (ca. 2000 B.C.E.–1400 C.E.), China (ca. 2000 B.C.E.–1400 C.E.), the Islamic World (600–1400 C.E.), and the European Middle Ages (ca. 500–1450 C.E.). The broad geographic scope will allow us to recognize the distinct beliefs and practices and how they developed in relation to the cultural beliefs of each individual civilization. At the same time, however, when viewed together, they display the commonality of approaches human societies have taken toward a shared interest in preserving health and curing disease.

Some of the explanations for disease, theories about the body, methods of treatment, and kinds of practitioners we will consider in this book may bear little relation to the medical beliefs and practices with which we ourselves are familiar with in the 21st century. Indeed, one might feel tempted by the strangeness of some of the medical systems to dismiss them as superstitious, irrational, and even dangerous. Or, we might choose to recognize only those beliefs and practices that appear to suggest the origins of our own modern, scientific medical ideas. In following either of those temptations, however, we would fail to recognize the complexities of medical decisions faced by our predecessors in the earliest human civilizations and the innovative means by which they sought to address them. Furthermore, although some of the medical traditions examined in this book have fallen into disuse, others (the Indian and Chinese medical traditions) are still regularly practiced and continue to develop around the world today. Increasingly in the West, many people are turning to so-called alternative medical beliefs, which are often based on the ancient traditions we will examine here. We must, therefore, recognize that the medical theories and procedures valued in any given society are determined as much by cultural beliefs as by any objective measure of the efficacy of the treatments. As such, the ability to view these medical traditions together should remind us that healing is a social activity, and the decisions a society makes about how to treat the sick, injured, and disabled are reflective of its most sacred beliefs and cultural values.

HEALTH, DISEASE, AND THE BODY

In the Hippocratic text *Epidemics I*, the author states that "the art [of medicine] has three factors: the disease, the patient, the physician. The physician is the servant of the art. The patient must cooperate with the physician in combating the disease" (Jones 1984, 165). We will consider the roles of physicians and patients in later chapters, but we should examine definitions of disease and health here. Indeed, explanations for what constitutes disease vary over time and cultural context, as do the meanings associated with being diagnosed with having a particular condition. In many cases, the definitions are closely linked with conceptions about the functioning of the body, and hence, it is necessary to consider theories about the body's anatomy and physiology when seeking to understand beliefs about the causes and processes of disease. Therefore, before we examine the development of the different healing practices and the health care practitioners associated with each, it will be useful first to examine the theoretical explanations for what constitutes disease and how it works in the body according to the different medical traditions.

Disease Theory in the Ancient Near East: Mesopotamia and Egypt

Mesopotamian healers had little theoretical knowledge of anatomy or physiology. They identified the heart as the site of intelligence, the liver as the source of anger, and the kidneys as the foundation of strength. Furthermore, they also recognized that various parts of the body (e.g., the chest or the guts) could become inflamed, but there was no systematic explanation for the disease process in the body. Rather, the Mesopotamian medical tradition held that disease was caused by gods, demons, evil spirits, or magic. Accordingly, treatment in the Mesopotamian tradition was mostly directed toward combating those external causes of sickness through appropriate rituals, incantations, and sacrifices. The demonic or magical explanation for the cause of disease could imply that the sick person was in some way at fault for the illness, receiving the curse as a punishment for some offense they had committed. Belief in the religious and magical causes of disease also necessitated that those responsible for treating disease should be priests and magicians, who could perform the necessary rituals to exorcise the offending spirit from the body. Likewise, the preservation of health required that the individual seek to maintain an appropriate state of spiritual purity by following the appropriate practices to pacify the demons or supernatural beings who might cause disease. We shall look more closely at the role of religious and magical healing in Mesopotamian society in a later chapter. For now, it suffices to note that the Mesopotamian belief system did not require a detailed understanding of the body or the causes of disease within the body.

In the Egyptian tradition, we find a blend of religious/magical explanations with naturalistic explanations for disease. The naturalistic understanding of disease causation explained how disease worked within the body as a natural (not magical) process. Egyptian physicians believed that the body was filled with a network of vessels or channels, called *metu,* which included blood vessels, ducts, tendons, and muscles. The *metu* were believed to originate in the heart from which they extended to different parts of the body so that the heart could "speak" through them. The various *metu* were believed ultimately to unite again at the anus, thus making them ideal channels by which a variety of substances—including blood, air, mucus, urine, semen, feces, various disease-bearing entities, and good or evil spirits—could be transported through the body. The large number of remedies aimed at strengthening or softening the *metu,* which could become mute or even die, indicate just how important these vessels were to the Egyptian understanding of the body and disease.

In addition to carrying useful materials through the body, the *metu* were believed to be the channels through which *wekhedu* traveled. Although scholars continue to debate the meaning of the term *wekhedu* (suggestions include "pain" or "purulency"), the best translation is likely "morbid (disease-causing) principle." In theory, *wekhedu* originated in the anus (although it was distinct from feces) and spread through the *metu* to the rest of the body, where it caused abscesses, pain, and a variety of different kinds of diseases. Based on the recognition of the fact that the bowels were the first part of the body to putrefy after death, Egyptian theorists believed that the bowels were the source of putrefaction and hence *wekhedu* in the body. Thus, many remedies were designed for the care of the anus, to help expel *wekhedu* by means of regular medicinal purges and enemas.

Disease Theory in the Western Medical Tradition: Greece, Rome, the Islamic World, and Medieval Europe

The earliest Greek medical writings are the books of the Hippocratic Corpus, the roughly sixty texts written between about 420 and 350 B.C.E. and ascribed to Hippocrates of Cos, a doctor famed for teaching medicine in the fifth century B.C.E. The authors of these books sought to provide a naturalistic explanation for health and disease in terms of the physiological functioning of the body. The Hippocratic theories, which originated in the fifth and fourth centuries B.C.E. and were subsequently modified and clarified by later Greek authors, most importantly Aristotle (384–322 B.C.E.) and Galen (129–ca. 216 C.E.), provided the essential philosophy for understanding the mechanisms of disease in Western Europe into the 18th century. Furthermore, the Hippocratic theories were also adopted by early Arabic medical authors and hence provided the foundation for Islamic medical theory as well. Arabic and European physicians continued to refine and augment the theoretical model they inherited from the Greeks over the course of more than 1,000 years. In this section, we shall examine the core elements of this system, which came to be referred to as humoralism.

In their efforts to understand and explain the natural order of the cosmos without attributing natural events to the actions of gods, Greek pre-Socratic philosophers sought to identify the primary constituents out of which the universe was composed. Numerous competing answers existed for this question, and it was not until a much later period that the theoretical model proposed by Empedocles (ca. 490–430 B.C.E.) became predominant. According to Empedocles, all matter in the universe was believed to be composed of a specific combination of the four basic elementary substances (fire, air, water, and earth). The elemental theory sought to explain the process of change in the universe in terms of the strife between opposed pairs of elements (air-earth, fire-water) and the attraction between other elements (e.g., air has properties in common with fire and water).

In the same period, authors of the Hippocratic medical texts considered the essential building blocks of the body, and they too proposed a number of competing answers. Various Hippocratic texts suggest that the body included one or more essential fluids called *chymoi*, which is usually translated as "humors." In the second century C.E., the famous Greek physician Galen of Pergamum emphasized the theory proposed in the Hippocratic text *On the Nature of Man* that the body contained four humors: blood, phlegm, bile (often called yellow bile or choler), and black bile (or melancholy). Blood, bile, and phlegm were observed being excreted in times of illness or injury and correlate to fluids we recognize today. Modern scholars continue to debate what bodily fluid black bile might be associated with, but it was supposed to be visible in vomit and excreta. These humors were believed to combine in the body to regulate its proper functioning; even the blood found in the veins was considered to consist of a mixture of humoral blood with the three other humors so that one might be able to separate out the other humors from venous blood.

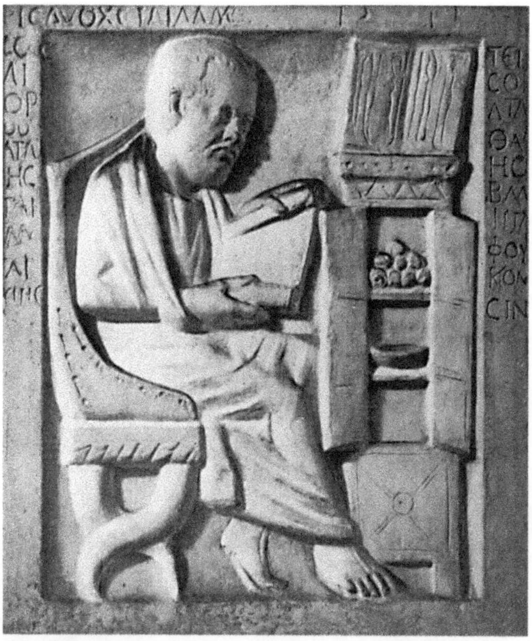

This bas-relief from a Roman sarcophagus shows a doctor reading a scroll before a cabinet that contains other scrolls and a bowl. The doctor's surgical instruments rest on top of the cabinet, ca. 100 C.E. The image emphasizes both the doctor's theoretical learning from books and his practical skills in surgery. (Hulton Archive/Getty Images)

Galen also credited Hippocrates with the concept of the four opposing qualities (hot, cold, wet, and dry), although this concept is normally attributed to Aristotle. Galen's efforts presented a unified system for drawing connections between the body (microcosm) and the greater universe (macrocosm). In this system, each of the humors was likened to one of the four elements, and furthermore, each element/humor was described as manifesting two of the basic qualities so that, for example, blood was linked to the element air, and both were described as being hot and wet, while phlegm was linked with the element water, and they were cold and wet (see figure 1.1). The explanatory power of this scheme extended further to identify each humor with the four seasons; the four winds; the four ages of man (childhood, youth, adulthood, and old age); and later with different heavenly bodies and signs of the zodiac; and among Christian scholars, with the four Evangelists. In this way, the actions of the humors in the body could be understood in terms of macrocosmic influences whereby seasonal changes and other environmental conditions might cause an elevation in certain humors (e.g., blood became more prevalent in the spring) possibly leading to disease.

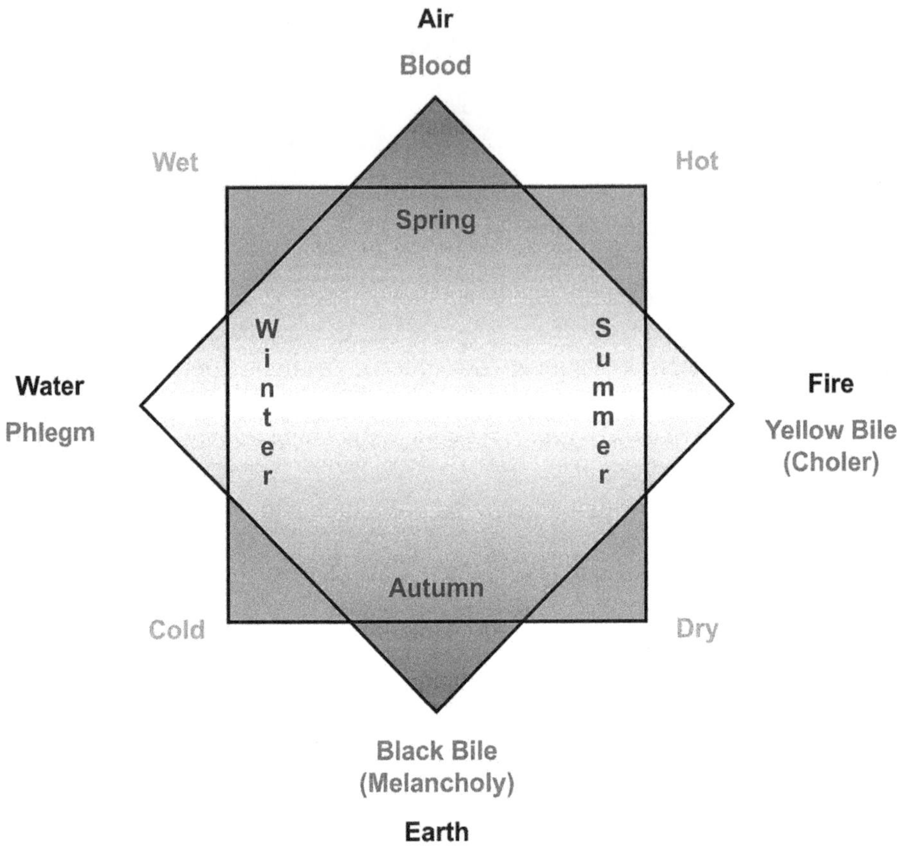

Figure 1.1 The humoral system.

One of the most fundamental ideas in the Hippocratic Corpus is the notion that health requires balance, while disease results from imbalance in the body. According to the humoral theory, imbalance was normally conceived of as an excess of one or more humors, and it might be systemic (affecting the entire body) or localized (in a specific part of the body), depending on the disease. Fevers were viewed as diseases of the whole body, while diseases like catarrh (a respiratory infection accompanied by a cough) and podagra (gout, an infection in the feet) resulted from an excess of one humor in a specific area of the body (in the chest and feet, respectively). During the Middle Ages, each person was thought to have his or her own individual healthy balance of humors, referred to as one's temperament or complexion, in which it was possible for one of the humors to predominate. For example, a person whose healthy balance of humors contained a little more blood than the other humors would be referred to as being sanguine, one with a little more yellow bile was choleric, one with more phlegm was phlegmatic, and one in whom black bile dominated was melancholic. The different temperamental types might be more prone to different kinds of diseases and may require slightly modified forms of treatment. The exact nature of the imbalance might be diagnosed by careful observation of a number of signs or symptoms, but following Galen, doctors specifically examined the pulse and the urine. Treatment of disease would aim at restoring balance in the body by purging excess humors (e.g., through bloodletting or inducing vomiting) or countering the excess with pharmaceutical remedies.

Numerous factors might influence an individual's humoral balance, and physicians emphasized that health could be restored through the careful adjustment of those factors. Beginning with Galen, medical scholars emphasized the importance of the six "nonnaturals," environmental, physiological, and psychological conditions that affected health and over which the individual would have some control. The nonnaturals are the surrounding air, exercise and rest, sleep and waking, food and drink, retention and excretion, and the "accidents of the soul." The environmental influence of the surrounding air would include exposure to any areas of stagnant, putrescent, or foul-smelling airs found near swamps, crypts, or other places with close proximity to decaying matter. The other nonnaturals existed in a state of balance in which the individual would be expected to adjust his levels of activity (including coitus) and rest as well as diet and excretion. Likewise, the individual should control the "accidents of the soul," which included the passions and emotions, to maintain an appropriate mental balance. If these conditions were not sufficiently regulated, then shifts in the humoral balance would lead the body to succumb to a contra-natural (against nature), or diseased, state. Thus, in his *Isagoge (Introduction to Medicine)*, the Eastern Christian physician Hunayn ibn Ishaq (d. ca. 873 or 877), known as Johannitius in the West, wrote about the need to consider the effect of the foods people ate on their humors, noting that "foods are of two kinds: good food is that which brings about a good humor, and bad food is that which brings about an evil humor." For example, he indicated that fresh bread and lamb produce healthy blood, mustard and garlic beget yellow bile, cabbage and the meat of old goats make black bile, while pork produces phlegm (Cholmeley 1912, 145–146). Furthermore, seasonal shifts and weather changes might cause the body's humoral balance to shift in response, meaning that the individual would need to monitor her diet and regimen continually with regard to other environmental conditions. In addition to regulating diet and exercise, individuals could take other prophylactic measures in response to seasonal influences on the body; for example, people would be sure to receive a preventative bloodletting in the spring (the season when blood, the hot and wet humor, would rise) to guard against diseases caused by excess blood.

Disease Theory in Indian Ayurvedic Medicine

From an early stage, Indian Ayurvedic medicine developed a highly complex theoretical understanding of the body and how it related to the origin and progress of disease. The central belief of Ayurvedic disease theory revolves around the concept of the three *doshas*, or humors, which are responsible for the proper functioning of the body: *vata* (wind or air), *pitta* (bile or fire), and *kapha* (phlegm or water). Although the *doshas* are found throughout the body, each one is believed to have a primary seat within a particular part of the body where it tends to congregate and have the greatest influence: *vata* (colon, large intestines), *pitta* (small intestines), *kapha* (lungs, chest). Learned Indian doctors, like Greek medical philosophers, believed in a correspondence between the human body (microcosm) and the universe (macrocosm) and regarded each of the *doshas* as being composed of two of the five constituent elements of the cosmos (ether, air, fire, water, earth). Thus, according to a system of correspondence, the body's internal *doshas* are linked to the macrocosm so that *vata* is believed to be composed of ether and air, *pitta* is composed of fire and water, and *kapha* is composed of water and earth. Furthermore, the balance in the body of the quantity and quality of the *doshas* can be affected by numerous macrocosmic and microcosmic factors, including the food eaten, the level of physical activity, the climate, and the age and emotional state of the individual.

In addition to the *doshas*, there are other components of the body that are regarded as significant in the disease process, especially the *dhatus*, the *ojas*, and the *malas*. The *dhatus*, the seven basic structural constituents (tissues and fluids) of the body, evolve in sequence from the most gross to the more compact and refined, with each forming and nourishing the following one in turn. *Rasa* (plasma or chyle), the largest material substance, produces *rakta* (blood), followed by *mamsa* (muscle and flesh), *meda* (fat), *asthi* (bone), *majjan* (marrow and nerve tissue), which forms the most refined of the *dhatus, shukra* (semen). In addition to the *dhatus*, another product of the process of nutrition and digestion is *ojas*, which is perhaps best identified as an essence of vitality or energy. *Ojas* can be depleted by anxiety, anger, depression, hunger, pain, and excessive physical exercise, leading to ill health. In addition to the fundamental elements of the *dhatus* and *ojas*, the body also produces three main waste products, *malas*, as a result of the process of digestion: feces, urine, and sweat. The maintenance of health requires that the *malas* be effectively eliminated from the body, but they also play an essential role in the body. For example, feces is important for helping to separate waste from nutritive materials, while sweat is believed to be valuable for regulating the body's temperature and moistening the skin. Disproportions of the *dhatus* and *malas* manifested various signs in the body. For example, the loss of lymph chyle would lead to pain about the region of the heart, heart palpitations, and thirst; loss of blood would be marked by a roughness of the skin, a craving for acidic foods or drinks, and "loose and flabby" veins; the loss or scanty formation of fecal matter would cause a sensation of pain in the sides and around the heart, accompanied by gas and a rumbling sound in the intestines and in the region of the liver.

In Ayurvedic medicine, the process through which the *dhatus* and *malas* are produced is regulated by the *agni*, or fire. *Agni*, imbued with a transformative power, is a digestive force by which one substance absorbs and assimilates nutrients and is changed into another. Traditional Ayurvedic medical texts recognize several forms of *agni*, each responsible for different transformative actions, including processing the five elements in foods so that they can be absorbed by the body, directing the metabolic process for the creation of the *dhatus* and *malas*, and even, on the psychological level, assisting transformations in thought and feeling. The other essential components of the digestive process are the *srotas*, an interconnected network of channels or tubes in the body through which *doshas*, nutrients, and waste materials are transported to the *dhatus* and organs. Each system of *srotas* is associated with a different organ or part of the body, and hence a disruption in an organ would produce ill effects throughout its network of *srotas*.

Ayurveda recognizes health as a state of harmony when the *doshas* exist in the optimal quality and quantity in the appropriate areas and when the *agni* and the *srotas* together maintain proper digestion and allow for the proper distribution of nutrients to the body for the production of *dhatus* and ensure the timely removal of *malas*. Most important, the maintenance of health requires that the *doshas* remain in a proper state of equilibrium, existing in the normal quantity in the appropriate parts of the body without becoming irritated or inflamed. However, diet, lifestyle, and psychological stress (in addition to age and seasonal changes) can all adversely affect the state of the *doshas* and thus compromise an individual's health. The disruption of the *doshas* can, in turn, impair the *agni* and the digestive process, which could lead to blockages in the *srotas* and compromise timely removal of *malas* and the proper functioning of the *dhatus* and other organs. Furthermore, when the *agni* is impaired, the body is more prone to producing *ama*, a kind of toxic waste substance resulting from inefficient digestion that can cause disease. Finally, the proper level of *ojas* in the body also plays an important part in health, and when digestion is disrupted, this level decreases, further weakening the body's vitality and ability to resist disease. An Ayurvedic physician, therefore, needs to consider a complex series of interlocking factors relating to the body when attempting to diagnose the cause of a patient's illness.

Ayurvedic medicine emphasizes the idea that health not only entails a physical condition but also requires mental and spiritual wholeness and integration. The proper preservation of health, therefore, necessitates that the individual not only maintain a harmonious balance of physiological functioning but also achieve a state of consciousness in which his or her emotional state and cognitive awareness are also in alignment with the body. This holistic view of health attends to far more than physical and mental conditions and also seeks to consider the spiritual and social interconnectedness of the individual. In this way, Ayurvedic medicine has several points of commonality with other practices like yoga, which encourages meditation and active poses aimed at bringing body, mind, and spirit into harmony with one another.

Disease Theory in Traditional Chinese Medicine

The body in traditional Chinese medicine is conceived as interacting with the universe according to an intricate theory of systematic correspondences. This theoretical system originated during the Han dynasty (206 B.C.E.–220 C.E.) and was first expressed in the *Huangdi Neijing (The Yellow Emperor's Classic of Internal Medicine)*. Within this philosophy, the fundamental concept for Chinese medicine is the theory of yin and yang. Yin-yang theory conceives the universe as being composed of a series of paired opposing aspects, such as male and female, light and dark, sun and moon, summer and winter, or heaven and earth. In addition to creating opposition, the aspects of yin and yang are also considered to be united and interdependent, for neither can exist without the other, each contains elements

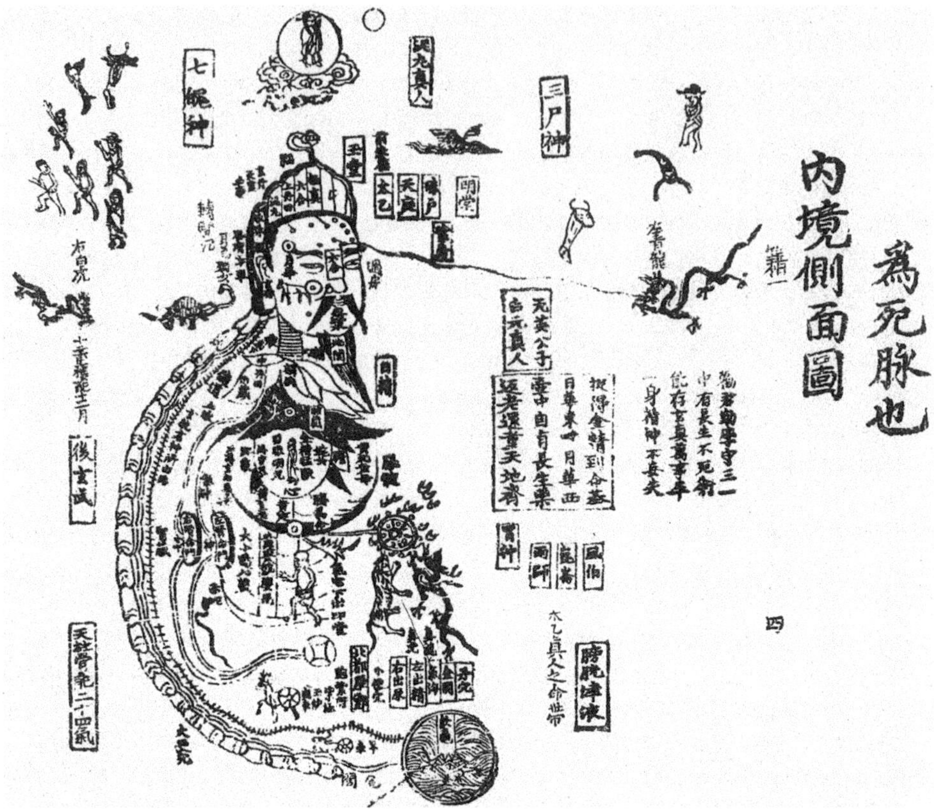

This 15th-century Chinese woodblock illustration depicts the internal topography or landscape of the human body. Such illustrations reflect Taoist medico-alchemical concepts of the body, the relationship between the microcosm and the macrocosm, and the quest to prolong life and attain immortality. (Wellcome Collection)

of the other, and they can in fact transform into one another. The body, then, functions in a state of dynamic ebb-and-flow equilibrium, whereby yin and yang flourish together and vivify each other to maintain health. When this fluctuating state of equilibrium becomes disturbed, depending on whether there is an excess or deficiency in either yin or yang, different illnesses will occur. This concept is expressed in the *Huangdi Neijing* where the physician Ch'i Po explains,

> When Yang is stronger the body is hot, the pores are closed and the people begin to pant; they become boisterous and coarse and whether one looks up or down no perspiration appears. People become feverish (hot), their gums are dry and give trouble, the stomach is affected and people die of constipation. When yang is stronger people can endure winter but they cannot endure summer.
>
> When yin is stronger the body is cold and perspiration appears regularly all over the body. People see their fate clearly; they tremble with fear and get chilled. When they are chilled their spirits become rebellious. Their full stomachs can no longer digest and they die. When yin is stronger people can endure summer but they cannot endure winter.
>
> Thus, yin and yang alternate, their victories vary and so does the character of their diseases. (Veith 1972, 115–121)

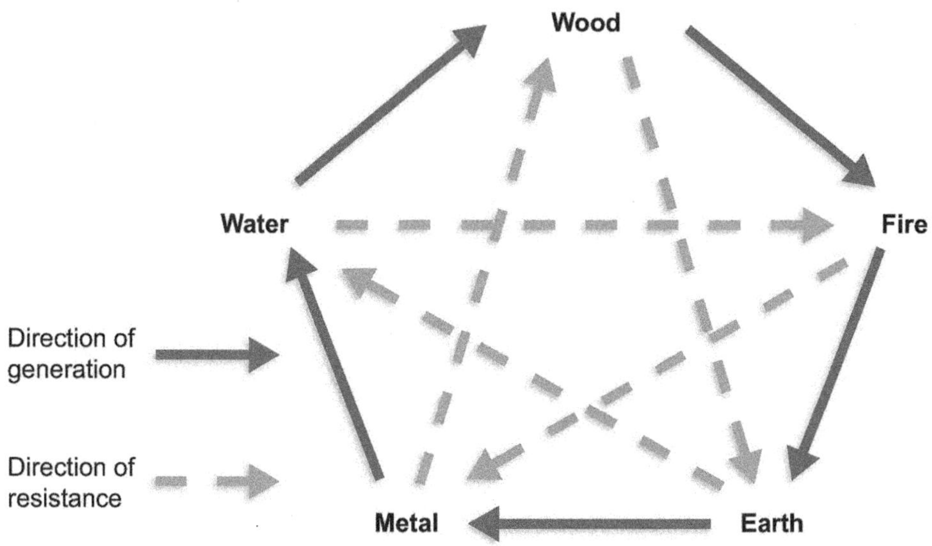

Figure 1.2 The *wu xing,* or five phases.

The system of correspondences uniting the body with the cosmos is also based on the theory of the *wu xing* (the "five phases" or "five elements"). This theory explains that everything in the universe is composed of the motion and change of the five elements (wood, fire, earth, metal, and water). The motions or phases of the elements allow each to create another in a cycle with water generating wood, wood generating fire, fire generating earth, earth generating metal, and, finally, metal generating water. At the same time, each element is restrained or opposed by another, so that water is contained by earth, while fire is extinguished by water (figure 1.2).

The elements of the *wu xing* are also understood as existing within a series of systematic correspondences to provide a holistic understanding of the relationship between man and nature. Some of these correspondences are shown in table 1.1.

According to these correspondences, each of the organs relates to a different element so that an illness in one organ can be expressed in terms of the five elements. Likewise, the systematic correspondences indicate points for treatment that can restore the harmonious balance of the cycle of relationships in the body that is necessary for the maintenance of health. So, for example, an individual with a flushed face and rapid pulse might be diagnosed as having excess heart fire, so the doctor might seek to nourish the kidneys (water) in order to restrain the heart and resist the excess fire through the use of medicines or other means. Or, a patient with a deficiency of the kidneys might be treated with medicines to promote the kidneys directly or, better yet, with medicines to strengthen the lungs, which in turn serve to nourish the kidneys according to the cycle of the five elements.

The yin-yang and *wu xing* theories have many similarities, and they are applied together in the process of diagnosing and treating patients. Both rely on an understanding of the need to maintain a balance in the body and explain how a doctor

Table 1.1 The systematic correspondences of man and nature

Element	Season	Direction	*Zang* Organ	Six *fu* Organs	Sense organs	Emotion
Wood	Spring	East	Liver	Gallbladder	Eyes	Anger
Fire	Summer	South	Heart	Small intestine and the "three burning spaces"	Tongue	Joy
Earth	Late summer	Middle	Spleen	Stomach	Mouth	Thought
Metal	Autumn	West	Lungs	Large intestine	Nose	Sorrow
Water	Winter	North	Kidneys	Urinary bladder	Ear	Fear

would need to go about either purging or nourishing different aspects of the body in order to restore a healthy equilibrium in sick patients. These theoretical systems also overlay the more anatomical understanding of the body's organs. Traditional Chinese medicine divides the body's internal organs into the five yin organs (*zang*, or viscera) and the six yang organs (*fu*, or bowels) according to their physiological functions. *Zang* organs (liver, heart, spleen, lungs, and kidneys) are responsible for generating and storing, while the *fu* organs (gallbladder, small intestine, stomach, large intestine, urinary bladder, and the "three burning spaces") have the power of eliminating wastes from the body. The *zang* and *fu* organs also fit within the *wu xing* theory, with each organ corresponding to a specific phase or element, thus further tying them into the theoretical model for understanding health and illness (see table 1.1).

Chinese medical theory also distinguishes certain vital fluids that flow through the body, the most important being qi ("chee") and blood. The concept of qi originated as early as the Spring and Autumn and the Warring States periods (770–221 B.C.E.). Initially, qi seems to have had the meaning of a "vapor" or "breath" associated with life but was increasingly recognized as the vital principle (sometimes translated as "energy") that flows through the body. Different types of qi (classified according to their composition, the organ in the body with which they are associated, and their physiological function) are responsible for promoting growth; nourishing, warming, and stimulating the organs; and protecting against external influences by regulating the openings of the body through which excretion and secretion of fluids occur. Blood, the other fundamental fluid in the body, serves to nourish and moisten the body. It is primarily composed of nutritional qi, and it is also regulated by the qi. Both qi and blood are supposed to flow through meridians or pathways, which connect all of the organs and limbs of the body. The harmonious movement of these fluids, especially qi, is deemed necessary for health; obstructions or stagnation leading to accumulation of either fluid in a part of the body leads to disease.

According to this theoretical system, individuals must maintain the harmonious functioning of their bodies by regulating their diet, physical activity, and their emotional state. Extremes in any of these areas would lead to an unhealthy imbalance in the yin-yang, *wu xing*, or the flow of qi. In addition to individual behavior, a number of external factors might also cause disease. Traditional Chinese medicine categorizes the environmental or climactic factors that contribute to disease as the "six excesses" (wind, cold, summer heat, dampness, dryness, and fire). In normal conditions, the environmental factors (referred to as the "six qi") are not harmful and are even important for normal health, but when the climate changes rapidly, or in abnormal or extreme conditions, they are called the "six excesses" that can invade the body to cause illness. Thus, as with the Hippocratic and Ayurvedic traditions, Chinese medical theory recognizes the close interaction between the body (microcosm) and the universe (macrocosm).

HEALTH AND SOCIAL WELL-BEING

Reflecting on her good fortune in her old age, Adad-guppi, the mother of the Babylonian king Nabonidus (556–539 B.C.E.), thanked the moon-god for her long and comfortable life:

> He [Sin, the moon-god] added (to my life) many days (and) years of happiness and kept me alive . . . one hundred and four happy years (spent) in that piety which Sin, the king of all gods, has planted in my heart. My eyesight was good (to the end of my life), my hearing excellent, my hands and feet were sound, my words well chosen, food and drink agreed with me, my health was fine and my mind happy. I saw my great-great-grandchildren, up to the fourth generation, in good health and (thus) had my fill of old age. (Oppenheim 1969, 561)

Adad-guppi's testimony indicates that she did not see her health as only a biological state but understood it in the context of her relationship to her god, her family, and her own emotions. This broader concept of health would necessitate the balancing of one's body, as well as one's emotions, and spiritual and social connectedness.

Although the premodern healing traditions we have reviewed developed concepts to identify and classify specific diseases, they mostly viewed health as existing on a continuum, requiring careful efforts to maintain equilibrium in the body. Within these systems, health was not merely the absence of disease, and people did not consider medical advice only when they were sick. Rather, the individual needed continually to be aware of environmental factors as well as the influence of diet and regimen on his current bodily state and take appropriate actions to regulate his activities accordingly in order to safeguard his health. Furthermore, these systems expected that people consider their emotions and their relations to gods, family, and society. Disease processes in the body would certainly play a factor in determining individual well-being, and physicians would have a role in helping to restore health, but the more holistic concepts of health considered here place great emphasis on the part played by individuals in balancing aspects of their physical, mental, and spiritual lives. In later chapters, we will consider these important aspects of health and well-being.

2

Education and Training

A wide variety of medical practitioners coexisted in most premodern societies. Anyone could peddle cures or offer treatments part-time, in addition to performing his other occupational duties, but others might seek to make a living solely by offering medical care. In most cases, practitioners were trained through some form of apprenticeship or acquired their knowledge through practice. Over time, a written medical tradition developed in many premodern societies, suggesting that the body of knowledge associated with the theory and practice of medicine was deemed sufficiently complex and extensive to merit being recorded in texts. Not all healers would necessarily be literate or have access to the written medical tradition, but those whose medical education was complemented by their access to the medical books might distinguish themselves by claiming to have a more sophisticated understanding of health and disease. As a result, a hierarchy of medical practitioners developed in many cultures in which those physicians, whose education included having access to the learned and increasingly theoretical textual medical tradition, were elevated above the majority of other doctors and health care providers, trained solely through apprenticeship or experience in practice. For this reason, it is crucial to examine the rise of written medical traditions in the different cultures we are considering in order to understand the impact learned medicine had on the methods of medical education and the knowledge healers might be expected to possess.

MEDICAL LEARNING IN THE ANCIENT NEAR EAST

Mesopotamia

Surviving sources on Mesopotamian medicine (ca. 3000–300 B.C.E.) are mostly written in the cuneiform ("wedge-shaped") writing system, inscribed on clay tablets that were baked for preservation. In total, we have fewer than 1,000 tablets or fragments of tablets on medical subjects, and modern scholars must often assemble the fragments as though piecing together a jigsaw puzzle. Because many of the medical texts survive in multiple copies, scholars can see that they underwent constant changes as they were edited, compiled with other texts and copied through the years, suggesting that the Mesopotamian authors continued to modify them based on their own experiences in practice.

The vast majority of surviving tablets come from a single trove, the library of Ashurbanipal (669–629 B.C.E.), the last great king of Assyria, which was destroyed when the invading Medes and Chaldeans invaded the royal city of Nineveh in 612 B.C.E. Ashurbanipal boasted that he had assembled a collection of texts on the three paths to healing: through the use of drugs, operating with the brass knife, and through the prescriptions of the sorcerers. Thus, although they represent sources from a single find, it is clear that Ashurbanipal felt his collection represented a fairly complete coverage of the medical writings of his day and it included copies of much older texts, some perhaps extending back to originals first produced in the third millennium B.C.E.

Most of the surviving medical texts are lists of prescriptions, including both herbal remedies and healing incantations. Others offer collections of case histories arranged under headings that might give some indication of the condition to be treated (e.g., "if the hand of a ghost seizes on a man . . ." or "if a woman gives birth to a child with . . ." or "if a man is affected in the lungs . . ."), which would be followed by suggested remedies. In addition to these shorter texts, one finds a few longer, more sophisticated medical works, such as the *Treatise of Medical Diagnoses and Prognoses*, which consists of forty tablets organized around the recognition of certain signs that should be observed when determining the cause of the illness and foretelling its future course in the patient. This text opens with a discussion of the omens that might be observed on the way to the sick person's home, followed by a list of the signs (from head to foot) the doctor should watch for in the patient's body. Later sections cover the daily progress of several conditions with the intent of providing a prognosis, and the methods of treating specific conditions (whether by incantations or herbal remedies), with a final section specifically devoted to the diseases of women and pregnancy.

The sources reveal that there were three main kinds of healers in Mesopotamian societies: the *baru* ("seer"), trained in the art of divination; the *ashipu* ("exorcist"), a priest who treated sick people as one of his many religious duties; and the *asu* ("physician"), a priest devoted to treating the sick with charms, drugs, and surgical cures. Rather than competing with each other for patients, it seems that each of these healers served a particular function in the healing process, and they would work together to bring about the cure of the patient. This point is clearly made in one letter written to the king in which a sick official requests that the king "appoint at my side an *ashipu* [exorcist] and an *asu* [physician] . . . may they perform the ceremonies on my behalf" (Sigerist 1951, 431). The *asu*, however, was most specifically dedicated to the treatment of the sick. In a hymn praising Gula, one of the primary healing deities, the goddess describes herself as an *asu*, providing some sense of the range of activities with which the *asu* might be associated:

I am a physician, I can heal,
I carry around all [healing] herbs, I drive away disease,

I gird myself with the leather bag containing health-giving incantations.
I carry around texts which bring recovery,
I give cures to mankind.
My pure dressing alleviates the wound,
My soft bandage relieves the sick. (Lambert 1967, 121)

We should first note that the *asu* was known for his textual learning. Beyond that, the *asu* was also associated with a variety of therapeutic devices including herbal cures, incantations, and wound dressings. From other sources, such as the Code of Hammurabi, a listing of 282 laws engraved on a stone block in the first half of the 18th century B.C.E., we know that the *asu* was also the healer responsible for providing a variety of surgical operations. Thus, textual learning and practical experience together define the *asu*'s education.

As members of the priestly classes, the *ashipu* and the *asu* would have been among the most well-educated people in Mesopotamian society and would have trained within the major temples, where they would have learned the skills necessary for reading and writing the cuneiform script. In this context, their medical training probably required the study of the written sources of learned medicine, and having access to that written tradition no doubt served as a significant distinguishing feature of these health care providers, establishing their credentials as learned men. Some evidence suggests that medical learning was protected as a form of secret knowledge that was not to be spread widely outside this community of medical scholars. For example, several texts end with instructions such as, "May he who knows instruct him who knows. And may he who knows not, not read this" and "He who does not keep the secret will not remain in health." Such efforts to control access to medical learning reinforce the idea that the written learned tradition of medicine was a central component of the identity of these healing classes. Although there is no evidence of formal apprenticeship programs for the *baru*, *ashipu*, or *asu*, it is possible that part of their training would involve developing their skills through practice under the guidance of an experienced teacher. The efforts to control access to written medical learning and the fact that practical medical training through apprenticeship receives little attention in the texts suggest that access to the written medical sources was considered the central component of the identity of these health care professionals.

Egypt

Our knowledge of ancient Egyptian medicine (covering the period from ca. 3150–332 B.C.E.) is based largely on roughly a dozen important medical papyri produced between 1900 B.C.E. and 300 B.C.E. These papyri, usually written in the hieratic script (similar to the hieroglyphic writing system), if translated and printed, would comprise just over 200 pages of text today and likely represent only a small fraction of the medical works produced in ancient Egypt, which have otherwise been lost through the ravages of time. The earliest of these papyri, the Kahun papyrus, produced around 1825 B.C.E., is a fragmented and relatively short document that focuses exclusively on diseases of women. The Ebers papyrus (ca. 1500 B.C.E.), a compendium of several shorter medical treatises, seemingly arranged at random, is by far the longest medical papyrus. It includes several remedies for specific medical conditions, including eye diseases, urinary difficulties, dental concerns, crocodile bites, and other conditions that are more difficult to define such as *wekhedu* (which could either mean "pain" or refer to a substance thought to cause putrefaction and decomposition within the body).

The written sources indicate at least three categories of people were involved in healing in ancient Egypt: priests, magicians, and *swnw* (typically pronounced "sewnew" and translated as either "physician" or "doctor"). Although it is now clear that priests did not restrict their healing to merely saying prayers and *swnw* were equally likely to prescribe magical cures, it does appear that the *swnw* were known mostly for their naturalistic medical theories concerning the body and disease, the application of physical treatments, and the preparation of pharmaceutical remedies. The phrase "placing of the hands" is commonly associated with *swnw* in the medical papyri, perhaps indicating that they were specifically known for hands-on diagnosis and treatment. Many *swnw* were identified as focusing on particular areas of practice (e.g., doctors of the abdomen or doctors of the eyes), suggesting a high degree of medical specialization.

The Edwin Smith surgical papyrus (ca. 1550 B.C.E.), the oldest surviving surgical text in the world and second longest of the Egyptian medical papyri, provides perhaps the best sense of the practice of a *swnw*. Unlike most other medical papyri that simply present a compilation of remedies, it is organized as an instruction book listing a number of different medical cases with helpful advice on how the *swnw* would arrive at a diagnosis and determine treatment. It presents each case in four parts: the title or concise description of the condition, the examination of the patient and the symptoms, the diagnosis and prognosis, and the treatment. The diagnosis is typically followed by one of three prognoses, indicating the *swnw*'s opinion as to the outcome: "An ailment which I will treat," "An ailment with which I will contend," or "An ailment not to be treated." One entry (likely describing a case of tetanus) reads as follows:

> *Title*: Instructions for a gaping wound in his head, extending to the bone, penetrating the *tepau* of his skull.
>
> *First Examination*: . . . You should then probe his wound though he shudders greatly. You should then cause him to lift his face. It is painful for him to open his mouth. His heart beats too slowly (or weakly) for speech. You observe his saliva falling from his lips but not falling completely. He discharges blood from his two nostrils and from his two ears. He suffers stiffness in his neck. He does not find he can look at his two shoulders and his breast.
>
> *First diagnosis and prognosis*: You shall say concerning him . . . the cord of his mandible is contracted; he discharges blood from his two nostrils and from his two ears; and he suffers stiffness in his neck—an ailment with which I will contend.
>
> *First treatment*: As soon as you find that man, the cord of his mandibles and his jaws are contracted, you should cause one to make for him something hot until he is comfortable and his mouth opens. You should then bind it with oil and honey until you know he has reached a decisive point.

> *Second examination*: If you find in that man that his flesh has developed heat under the wound, which is in the *tepau* of his skull. That man, he has developed toothache under that wound. You put your hand on him and you find his brow is wet with sweat. The muscles of his neck are taut, his face is flushed. . . . The odor of . . . his head is like the excrement of small cattle. His mouth is bound, his two eyebrows drawn, his face is as if he was weeping.
>
> *Second diagnosis and prognosis*: You shall then say concerning him . . . he has developed toothache; his mouth is bound; he suffers stiffness of his neck—an ailment not to be treated. (Nunn 1996, 181–182)

The medical papyri were undoubtedly used for teaching purposes, but this would require that the *swnw* be literate. Those young and literate *swnw*, who possessed a copy of a medical papyrus, would have been able to use them in their studies, while the less fortunate might have had access to written medical knowledge through the *per ankh* (House of Life), a scriptorium where books were compiled. Otherwise, medical practice appears to have been taught from father to son through a system of apprenticeship. Numerous funeral stela, gravestones, indicate that sons followed the professions of their fathers in ancient Egypt, and one Greek historian considering Egyptian healers suggested that medicine was the one profession where children were required to follow in their parents' footsteps. Therefore, though it is likely that the *swnw* was often a member of the learned, literate class who would have access to the written medical texts, some *swnw* may have only been trained through apprenticeship, learning the craft of medicine by practicing with their fathers.

MEDICAL LEARNING IN THE ANCIENT GREEK AND ROMAN WORLD

Hippocratic Medicine

The Hippocratic Corpus, which is a collection of about 60 medical texts written between 420 and 350 B.C.E. and attributed to Hippocrates of Cos, represent the earliest Greek writings on medical subjects. Although it is likely that some of these texts were written by the historical Hippocrates, scholars continue to debate which ones might have genuinely been written by him. It is clear that the texts of the Hippocratic Corpus were written in different Greek dialects and often present contradictory theoretical opinions and cures and thus the same individual could not have written them all. They are united, however, by a shared interest in establishing a naturalistic, rational system for explaining disease and cures, without reference to divine or magical interventions. Furthermore, they identify those healers who followed this more naturalistic approach to medicine as *iatroi* (sing. *iatros*), or doctors.

The books of the Hippocratic Corpus attempt to do many different things. Some seek to justify a particular theoretical viewpoint regarding the practice of medicine (e.g., *On Ancient Medicine* and *The Art of Medicine*) or offer a theoretical explanation for the humoral causes of disease in the body (e.g., *On the Nature of Man*). By contrast, other texts focus more on providing detailed observations of the symptoms and course of diseases in patients (e.g., *Epidemics*), explain the practice of diagnosis and prognosis (e.g., *On Prognosis*), offer advice for how to regulate diet and regimen to maintain health (e.g., *A Regimen for Health*), or discuss certain kinds of surgical operations (e.g., *On Head Wounds* and *On Joints*). Still other texts offer opinions on how an *iatros* should behave or appear to have been aimed at teaching (e.g., the *Oath* and the *Aphorisms*). Therefore, although the Hippocratic Corpus shares a naturalistic approach to disease and healing, the works offer a diverse array of opinions on the kinds of knowledge necessary for practice.

The *iatroi*, who followed the doctrines in the newly forming written medical tradition, would practice alongside an array of religious healers, midwives, bone-setters, and folk practitioners. But the *iatroi* were a diverse group themselves, whose writings suggest some significant theoretical and practical differences, making it impossible to generalize about the expected requirements for training and practice. Indeed, there were no medical regulations, and those who sought to practice medicine were not required to undergo any examinations or to adhere to a specific set of expectations. Even the *Oath*, perhaps the most famous Hippocratic text, represents only one opinion as to the minimum expectations for the behavior of medical practitioners, and it is not reflected in other books from the Corpus. In general, a Hippocratic *iatros* likely practiced as an itinerant healer, traveling from town to town, offering his services for a fee, in competition with a diverse range of other healers. In this context, it appears that perhaps the main skill the *iatros* could offer to distinguish himself from others was his claim to a theoretical understanding of the disease process combined with an ability to diagnose a particular illness and offer an accurate prognosis for its course (abilities emphasized in several texts from the Corpus) that would convince a potential client of his abilities.

Most *iatroi* were probably trained through a system of apprenticeship where fathers would teach their craft to their sons or train those from outside the family for a fee. The *Oath* gives some indication of the expectations of an apprentice, who was expected to swear to follow his teacher as he would his father and "to give a share of precepts and oral instruction and all the other learning to my sons and to the sons of him who has instructed me and to pupils who have signed the covenant and have taken an oath according to the medical law, but to no one else" (Edelstein 1967, 6). No reference is made to the necessity of having access to a written tradition, but students would be expected to learn certain precepts through oral instruction. In some cases, the precepts were likely presented as we find them in the *Aphorisms*, as a series of brief, memorable statements that offered guidance for diagnosis, prognosis, and treatment. For example, the first aphorism emphasizes the many things the *iatros* should take into consideration when practicing his craft: "Life is short, the art long; opportunity is elusive, experiment is dangerous and judgment is difficult. It is not enough for the physician to do what is necessary, but the patient and the attendants must do their part as well, and circumstances must be favorable" (Chadwick and Mann 1950, 206). Later aphorisms offer more direct advice, relating that the elderly can handle fasting better than the young; that fluid diets are especially beneficial in cases of fever; or that pregnant women should not be given drugs after the seventh month of gestation.

Galen and the Hippocratic Tradition

As the body of written medical knowledge grew, many came to believe that a physician should be well versed in the theoretical principles it conveyed. One of those who held that physicians should be trained through reading texts was Galen of Pergamum (129–ca. 216 C.E.). He was born to a wealthy family in the Greek-speaking part of the Roman Empire and received a typical upper-class education, which emphasized the importance of philosophical learning. Fairly early in his life, he decided to pursue a career in medicine and went to study in Alexandria, Egypt, the most famous center of medical learning in his day, where he studied the texts of learned Greek medicine. He returned to Pergamum, where he served as doctor to gladiators for several years before heading to Rome to further his career and enhance his reputation. Galen regularly engaged in public (often heated) disputations with rival doctors in Rome, earning their animosity, but he also achieved several successful cures and soon could claim a clientele drawn from the highest levels of Roman society. By 168, he became doctor to the emperor and held this position with successive emperors until his death. Galen's meteoric rise is testimony to his skills as a healer but also to the growing success of the learned Greek tradition within the Roman world.

In addition to his successful medical practice, Galen also wrote extensively on medicine and over 350 works confirmed as written by him survive today, more than from any other writer on medicine from antiquity. He wrote extensively on the theories and methods of diagnosis through the pulse and other signs and on how to link these observations to knowledge about the underlying physiological and pathological processes of the body. In order to make these connections, he emphasized the need for physicians to understand human anatomy and the functioning of the different structures in the body. He wrote extensive commentaries on the books of the Hippocratic Corpus, smoothing over their contradictions, emphasizing certain points and de-emphasizing others. In the process, Galen explained the Hippocratic Corpus so as to make it appear as a unified whole, and it was his interpretation that would guide later people's understanding of those texts into the 20th century. Together, Galen's medical writings drew upon the texts of the learned Greek tradition and reformed them into a cohesive, systematic, philosophical tradition that would shape medical learning in the West for several centuries. Furthermore, Galen wrote about the various therapeutic methods (including diet, drug lore, bloodletting, and other forms of surgery) and the theories that would govern their application in practice. Taken together, Galen's medical writings explored the entire range of learned medicine available in his day and impressed his stamp upon it.

In his works, Galen also established very high expectations for the range of knowledge a doctor should command, declaring that both textual learning and experience in practice were essential for the ideal physician. He argued that the ideal physician should be highly educated and learned in Greek philosophy (including the works of Aristotle, Plato, and the Stoic philosophers) as well as the written medical tradition, since he maintained that philosophic reasoning should guide the practice of the healer at the bedside. At the same time, Galen believed the physician needed to be an attentive observer who could learn through experience how to diagnose a patient's illness based on a wide variety of symptoms and know which remedies were especially appropriate in different cases. Although many Romans were doubtful of the value of text-based medical knowledge (favoring traditional, empirical remedies), Galen helped to shape the written medical tradition that would define learned medical practice in the later Islamic and European worlds.

MEDICAL LEARNING IN INDIA: THE WRITTEN TRADITION OF AYURVEDA

The Origin of the Ayurvedic Medical Texts

Ayurveda (literally "knowledge for longevity") has its roots in the oral traditions passed on by practicing healers from the Vedic period (ca. 1500–500 B.C.E.), including the rational or naturalistic medical knowledge of the sramanas, wandering ascetics who pursued knowledge of the natural world for its own sake, and the magical healing of the *bhishaj*, healers known for their incantations and spells aimed at curing specific ailments and also for making amulets and talismans from plants and other substances that could ward off demons and malign spells in order to bring about a cure. The transition of these oral traditions into written form came about mostly as a result of the work of Buddhist monks. Shortly after the rise of Buddhism in the sixth century B.C.E., Buddhist ascetics (monks and nuns) began to organize into monastic communities called *sanghas*. These communities encouraged wanderers to visit and engage in debates over a variety of subjects, including medicine. The *sanghas* quickly became centers for medical learning, where Buddhist monks, starting in the mid-fifth century B.C.E., began to collect, organize, and write down the content of the oral tradition, creating the central texts of Ayurvedic medicine. As a result, it is difficult to know exactly when the earliest texts of the Ayurveda were first composed in written form, although estimates for the different texts suggest dates between 1000 and 500 B.C.E., and even then, the texts continued to be revised and added to until the fourth or fifth century C.E., making it difficult to speak of dates of composition with much certainty.

The earliest of the Ayurvedic texts, the *Caraka Samhita*, appears to have been written down around the second century C.E., although it compiles a number of seemingly disparate materials that were much older. It consists of 120 chapters divided into eight parts including sections on the theoretical classification of diseases, pharmacology, anatomy, and embryology. It also includes more practically oriented sections on diagnosis, prognosis, and therapy for specific diseases. In general, it reflects the more naturalistic medical tradition of the sramanas, but it also contains some magical and religious therapies, indicating that it draws upon multiple sources of Vedic medicine. The other early Ayurvedic text, the *Susruta Samhita*, like the *Caraka*, includes passages that reflect a much earlier origin, but it appears to have been written down in its current form around the fourth

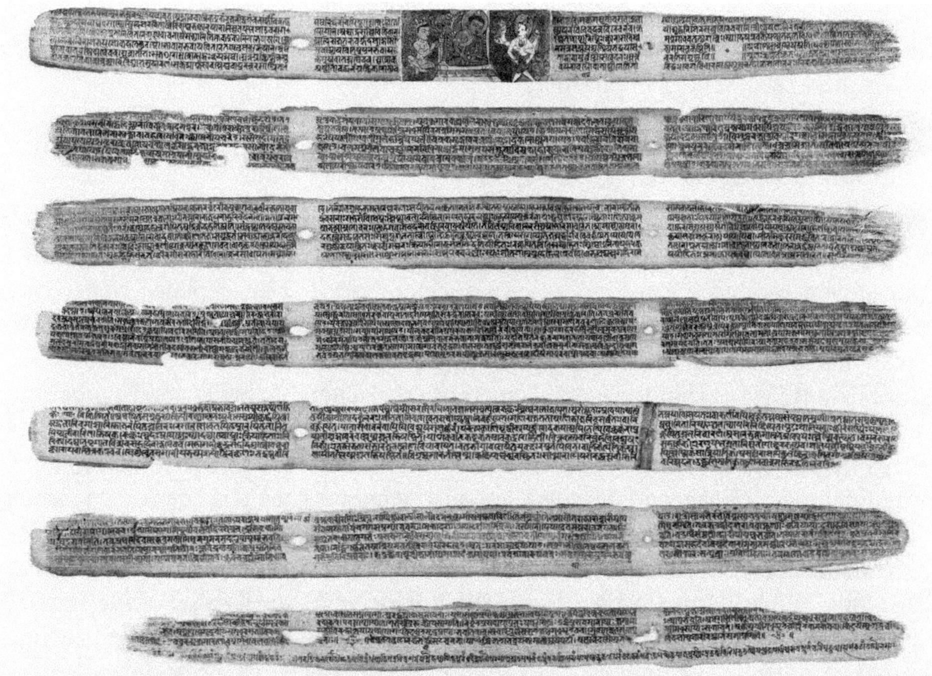

These passages from a copy of the *Susruta Samhita*, one of the foundational texts of Ayurvedic medicine, are written on palm leaves. This version was produced in the 18th or 19th century, reflecting the longstanding value of this medical book. (Science History Images/Alamy Stock Photo)

century C.E. The *Susruta* is divided into six large sections and covers similar material to the *Caraka* (theories of pathology, embryology, and pharmacy, as well as discussions of various methods of diagnosis, prognosis, and treatment, and some explanations for managing diseases ascribed to demonic attacks). Unlike the *Caraka*, however, the *Susruta* also provides extensive coverage of the theory and practice of surgery and discusses methods of surgical training.

Since the *Caraka* and *Susruta* draw upon a number of earlier sources, they are not clearly organized and sometimes include conflicting material. Later, in the fifth century C.E., the *Astangahrdaya (The Heart of Medicine),* ascribed to Vagbhata, was composed with the intention of synthesizing the disordered and conflicting material found in the previous texts to create a systematic presentation of the principles of Ayurvedic medicine. Indeed, it would eclipse the *Caraka* and *Susruta* to become the most widely translated and circulated Ayurvedic text and the core text for Ayurvedic medical education into the 19th century. Together, the *Caraka*, the *Susruta*, and *The Heart of Medicine* are known as the *Brihat Trayi* ("greater triad") to distinguish them from the later three medical texts known together as the *Laghu Trayi* ("lesser triad"): the *Madhava Nidana* (composed between 700 and 1100 C.E.), the *Sarangadhara Samhita* (14th century C.E.), and the *Bhavaprakasha* (16th century C.E.). The *Laghu Trayi* and other medical works from the 8th through 16th centuries reveal the growing consolidation of Ayurvedic medicine and devote increasing attention to the classification of diseases, to new methods of diagnosis (including pulse lore), to descriptions of newly discovered sexually transmitted diseases (including syphilis), and to the growing use of metal and mineral substances in pharmacy.

Medical Education

Medical education in the Vedic period was based in an oral tradition; teachers would sing the hymns or recite the verses from the Vedas or medical collections and the student would be expected to learn them by heart. This explains why written versions of these works were sometimes not produced until centuries after the oral "text" had been in circulation and also why they existed in mostly verse form. The *Caraka* and *Susruta* both reflect this method of teaching, being framed explicitly as accounts of a teacher passing along his knowledge to a single student. To this end, they offer advice for teachers on elocution, how to recite the words of the verses and traditional lore clearly and properly, and also admonish the teacher to provide useful commentary upon the materials to help the student's comprehension and memorization. Students were expected to hone their theoretical knowledge by regularly engaging in discussions by means of which they could clarify their understanding of the materials and develop their eloquence. The true doctor, by these accounts, would be a man of learning eager to seek out new knowledge for its own sake.

Medical students did not only learn theoretical precepts. The author of the *Susruta* declared that "he who is only trained in theory, but is not experienced in practice knows not what he should do when he has a patient and behaves as foolishly as a youth upon a battlefield. On the other hand, a physician who is educated practically, but not in theory, will not earn the respect of better men" (Kutumbiah 1962, xlix). Therefore, students were also expected to assist their teacher in the treatment of patients, to help in the preparation of medicaments, and to practice their skills with the tools of the trade. Indeed, the *Susruta* suggests that students practice their surgical skills by working on pieces of wood, dried gourds, fruit, and dead animals.

From the fifth century B.C.E. onward, the Buddhist *sanghas* began to play an increasingly important role in medical education serving as centers where wandering ascetics interested in pursuing an education in the arts, sciences, traditional Brahmanism, and also medicine might gather to engage in intellectual debate. The role of Buddhist monasteries as centers for education was expanded toward the end of the Gupta dynasty (mid-sixth century C.E.) when the *mahavihara* ("greater monasteries") started to develop a core curriculum. A Chinese Buddhist pilgrim visiting the *mahavihara* at Nalanda in the early seventh century C.E. noted that it drew students from all over and that they would study core subjects including the five sciences (*vidya*) and the major works of Buddhist philosophy. Medicine was one of the five sciences, and therefore, all students would study the texts of the classical Ayurvedic tradition alongside the other important Vedic texts. As a result, by the end of the seventh century C.E., Ayurvedic medicine was established as a central component of the curriculum as one of the five sciences taught in Buddhist monasteries and as Buddhism spread to other parts of Asia, the Ayurvedic medical system spread with it.

MEDICAL LEARNING IN CHINA

Foundations of Traditional Chinese Medicine

The most renowned early text of the Chinese medical tradition, the *Huangdi Neijing* (*The Yellow Emperor's Classic of Internal Medicine*), was likely written by several authors, bringing together earlier medical materials, including writings on demonic and magical medicine, and coalesced into its final form during the Han dynasty (206 B.C.E.–220 C.E.), probably just prior to the first century C.E. The *Huangdi Neijing* consists of two parts, the *Suwen (The Basic Questions)* and the *Lingshu (The Divine Pivot)*. The *Suwen* is presented as a dialogue between the Yellow Emperor, Huangdi, and his ministers and provides the fundamental theories concerning anatomy, physiology, and methods of diagnosis and treatment. It includes discussions of medical concepts of yin and yang, the circulation of qi in the body, the theory of the correspondence of the "five phases" (*wu xing*), and theories about the organs and their functions. The *Lingshu*, by contrast, is more narrowly focused on acupuncture and moxibustion therapy as a means of regulating the flow of qi through the body's twelve meridians. The *Huangdi Neijing*, therefore, represents a move toward providing a naturalistic theoretical system for understanding health and disease (in contrast to the belief in magical, demonic medicine prevalent in earlier periods) and it would quickly become the foundational text for traditional Chinese medicine.

Numerous texts from this early period, including the *Huangdi Neijing* and the *Nanjing (Classic on Difficult Medical Problems)*, reveal the development of the theory and practice of acupuncture as a form of treatment. Other texts, like those by Zhang Zhongjing (150–219 C.E.), one of the most famous physicians from the later Han dynasty, were especially concerned with the methods of diagnosis and how to match treatment to the theoretical explanations for disease. In his two texts, the *Shang-hanlun* (*On Cold-Induced Diseases*) and *Jingui Yaolue (Synopsis of the Golden Bookcase)*, Zhang focused his attention on the classification of diseases according to which of the meridians or viscera they affected and placed heavy emphasis on linking the observed symptoms to the underlying part of the body being affected. In this way, he sought to unite clinical observation with the theoretical understanding and the theory of systematic correspondence of anatomy and physiology. Zhang's text and others also reveal the development of a detailed theory of drug therapy, explaining how medicines should be prescribed according to the theory of systematic correspondence to treat the specific causes of the disease in the body. Thus, the foundation for the theoretical precepts of traditional Chinese medicine was largely laid by the end of the third century C.E.

The Rise of Formal Medical Education

The *Huangdi Neijing* offers insight into the methods of medical education up through the Han dynasty. In this work, the medical master, Huang Di, the legendary Yellow Emperor, is depicted teaching the theory and practice of medicine to a small group of students. The Yellow Emperor emphasizes the importance of referring to the classical medical texts as a basis for instruction, but also expects students to acquire empirical knowledge by assisting their masters in the treatment of patients. Following this model, individual physicians would take on apprentices and train them in the art of medicine through a discussion of key texts and practice at the bedside. Although education was done on an individual basis, records from the Zhou dynasty (1045–256 B.C.E.) reveal the early existence of state-administered medical examinations for physicians, although it is not clear how effectively they were enforced. However, there is no indication that they were tied to state-administered medical education.

The move toward governmental supervision over medical education was most pronounced in the Tang dynasty (618–907 C.E.). Medicine had previously become one of the subjects taught at the Imperial Academy, which oversaw the education of civil servants, but under the Tang, the Imperial Bureau of Medicine was established and divided the teaching of medicine into four sections: internal medicine, acupuncture, massage (which included the treatment of wounds), and incantations. Furthermore, a separate department within the Bureau was made responsible for maintaining botanical gardens and teaching the subject of pharmacology. From the beginning, students studied the classical medical texts and more organized summaries, including the *Huangdi Neijing*, the works of Zhang Zhongjing, and the *Zhenjiu Jiayijing* (*The ABC of Acupuncture and Moxibustion*), the central text on the practice of acupuncture.

Chinese medical education underwent further profound changes starting in the 11th century C.E. with the rise of technologies for woodblock printing, which allowed for the wider diffusion of medical learning. Under the Song dynasty (960–1279 C.E.), the Bureau for the Re-editing of Medical Books was created in 1057 for the purpose of collecting, editing, and printing the important medical texts from the preceding 1,000 years. The first books printed by this bureau (in order) were the *Suwen* from the *Huangdi Neijing*, the *Shang-hanlun* and the *Jingui Yaolue* by Zhang Zhongjing, and the *Zhenjiu Jiayijing.* At the same time that medical texts were being brought to a wider audience through printing, the Imperial Bureau of Medicine supervised the establishment of medical schools in each of the prefectures in China and reformed the medical curriculum and examination system. Medical education revolved around the study of the previously named texts, alongside the *Nanjing*, the *Zhubing Yuanhoulun* (*Treatise on the Causes and Symptoms of Maladies*) by Chao Yuanfang (fl. sixth–seventh century C.E.), and the pharmacology text by Sun Simiao (581–682), the *Qianjin Yaofang (Prescriptions of the Thousand Ounces of Gold).*

Students in the medical schools during the Song dynasty and later would be tested both orally and clinically, and in both cases, they were expected to be able to display their knowledge of the theoretical medical system and use it to justify their treatments. Exam scores were ranked, and those who scored in the highest rank would be given official appointments as teachers and asked to write medical books; those in the second rank would be given licenses to practice, while students with lower scores were told to study further and take the exam again or to pursue careers in a different profession. Teachers were also examined each year based upon the success rate of their students, and in the Yuan dynasty (1271–1368 C.E.), two decrees were passed for punishing incompetent or lazy teachers who failed to ensure that their students attend lectures regularly and study the prescribed texts.

In many ways, the greater consolidation of medical education also encouraged the development of medical specialization. Increasingly, from the Tang dynasty forward, a number of more narrowly focused medical treatises were produced indicating the increased interest in medical specialties such as pediatrics, gynecology, and obstetrics. The move toward medical specialization in turn led to a fragmentation of Chinese medicine into four main schools of thought during the Yuan dynasty, each of which emphasized different factors in the cause of disease and advocated different methods of treatment. For example, the Hejian school, inaugurated by Liu Wan-su (1110–1200) maintained that disease was largely caused by the elements of fire and heat in the body and therefore founded the "school of cooling" which employed "cold" and bitter medicines to counteract unhealthy heat in the body according to the theoretical framework of systemic correspondences. By contrast, Chang Ts'ung-cheng (1156–1228), founder of a competing school of thought, focused his attention on harmful influences from outside the body as the cause of disease; therefore, Chang aimed at expelling the harmful agents from the body by using a variety of emetics and purgatives to induce sweating, sneezing, salivation, vomiting, and other forms of purgation. Despite their differing opinions on disease causation and treatment, the leaders of each of these schools turned to the same range of ancient medical texts to support their positions. In this way, they testify to the fact that the major elements of traditional Chinese medicine had been established by the classical texts from the previous periods, but they also reveal that Chinese medicine was an extremely dynamic system that continued to evolve and develop in response to new theories and observations in practice.

Those physicians trained in the schools supervised by the Imperial Bureau of Medicine represented a minority of all health care providers in Chinese society, however. They were the elite among medical practitioners and were mostly involved only in treating wealthy patients at court, although some may also have provided charitable medical assistance to the general public at times as well. The majority of people would still seek medical assistance from wise women, itinerant drug sellers, magical or religious healers, or other forms of healers who continued to learn their craft through apprenticeship or in practice, with little or no exposure to the texts of learned medicine.

MEDICAL LEARNING IN THE ISLAMIC WORLD

Translation and the Written Tradition of Islamic Medicine

The rise of Islam in the seventh century and its rapid spread from Arabia and the Near East across North Africa and into Spain brought the Arabic-speaking world into increased contact with outside cultures and new ideas. Cultural exchange as a result of trade with the Byzantine Empire, the Persian Empire, and indirectly with places as far-flung as India and China allowed for rapid influx of new learning back to the Islamic world. Under the patronage of the caliphs in

Baghdad, scholars in the late eighth and increasingly in the ninth centuries translated texts from a variety of languages (Syriac, Pahlavi, Sanskrit, and especially Greek) into Arabic. Although the translation effort made available works from many medical traditions, including texts of Ayurvedic medicine, translations of Greek texts were by far the most numerous. Hunayn ibn Ishaq (d. ca. 873 or 877), a Nestorian Christian in southern Iraq known later in the Latin West as Johannitius, was one of the leading figures in this translation movement; he and his circle of colleagues were responsible for translating 129 Galenic medical works into Arabic. As a result, the ninth century stands as a formative period for Islamic medicine that was largely shaped by Greek medical philosophy, and most especially Galen's approach to medicine. The Greek system provided a rationalist foundation to Islamic medicine that would transform the Arab medical beliefs and come to characterize the Islamic physician.

By the 10th century, Islamic scholars shifted their attention from translation efforts to producing new medical scholarship of their own. Some of these early works provided detailed observations on specific diseases and their cures, including Hunayn's *Ten Treatises on the Eye* and *On Smallpox and Measles* by Abu Bakr Muhammad ibn Zakariya al-Razi (d. ca. 925, known as Rhazes in the Latin West). Islamic scholars also wrote more far-reaching, comprehensive medical compendia that covered a wide array of theoretical and practical issues in medicine and attempted to organize the vast materials found in their Greek sources. *The Book for Al-Mansur* (later translated into Latin as the *Liber medicinalis ad almansorem*), written by al-Razi and dedicated to a local Iranian prince, is one example of these compendia. In this text, he divided medicine into "theory" and "practice" and drew upon the Greek tradition to discuss the wide range of knowledge deemed valuable for a learned physician. *The Book for Al-Mansur* was divided into 10 books: the first 6 books covered theoretical subjects including anatomy, physiology, general pathology, and pharmacy, while the last four books covered the practical subjects of diagnosis and therapy (including surgery), with book 9 devoted to discussions of specific diseases arranged from head to foot. Similarly, Abu al-Qasim al-Zahrawi (fl. ca. 1000, known as Albucasis in the Latin West), who worked in Cordoba, Spain, wrote another compendium, *The Arrangement of Medical Knowledge for One Who Is Not Able to Compile a Book for Himself*, drawing upon the Greek authorities. Although he relied heavily on the Greek texts, al-Zahrawi often added to it with testimony from his own personal experience, especially in sections where he covers subjects that received little attention in other sources, such as midwifery. The surgical chapters also reflect his personal innovation, and they included numerous illustrations of surgical instruments, in themselves a new addition to the surgical literature. Perhaps the most widely influential of these Islamic medical compendia was the *Canon of Medicine* by Ibn Sina (d. 1037, known as Avicenna in the Latin West). Ibn-Sina's *Canon* attempted to situate medicine within the system of Aristotelian natural philosophy. Unlike the previous compendia by al-Razi, al-Zahrawi, and others, Ibn Sina organized his massive text into five books covering the major tenets of theoretical medicine and emphasizing the distinction between diseases specific to one part of the body and more generalized conditions. He also explained specific forms of treatment for different diseases (including bloodletting, cautery, and surgery) and provided a theoretical discussion of medicinal substance and how to mix compound medicines. The careful and logical arrangement of these materials provided a systematic organization and elaboration to the Greek medical theories, and the *Canon* quickly became one of the preeminent texts of Islamic medicine. Based on this text, Ibn Sina would be recognized in the Latin West as one of the three foremost medical authorities, alongside Galen and Hippocrates.

Practitioners and Their Training

The rapid expansion of Arabic medical literature in the Islamic world led to the development of a new kind of medical practitioner, the physician, who would be knowledgeable in the theories presented in the learned written tradition. By the 10th century, many scholars wrote about the need to examine and license physicians before they would be allowed to practice. Although these regulations were mainly applied in the large urban centers, and were likely to have been largely unsuccessful at excluding those who did not meet minimum standards from practice, they do indicate a growing belief that a physician should be familiar with the learned written sources and able to discuss the theories presented in them when considering problems of diagnosis and treatment. Although physicians were also expected to have experience with bonesetting, reducing dislocations, cautery, cutting with the knife, and other manual procedures, the emphasis placed on their theoretical knowledge shows that their identity was largely founded on their familiarity with the written medical tradition.

Physicians might come by their knowledge of the written medical tradition in a variety of ways. Some, like Ibn Sina, claimed to have been self-taught by studying the authoritative medical texts for themselves. More often, physicians likely learned their trade through apprenticeship, either with a family member or another practicing physician. By far the most important space for acquiring a medical education, however, was the hospital. According to Ali ibn al-Abbas al-Majusi (fl. ca. 983, known as Haly Abbas in the Latin West), in his medical compendium, the *Complete Book of the Medical Arts*:

> One of the requirements for the student of this art is that he should be in attendance at the hospitals and the places of the sick; that he consult extensively with the most skilled teachers among the physicians about the patients' situations and circumstances; and that he examine frequently the conditions of the patients and the symptoms apparent in them, calling to mind what he has read about these conditions and what they indicate of good and ill. If he does this, he will reach a high degree of perfection in this art. (Pormann and Savage-Smith 2007, 81)

Based on al-Majusi's description, we see that physicians were expected to be able to readily incorporate their theoretical, textual training into practice at the patient's bedside. Islamic hospitals thus offered an ideal setting in which to study medicine because they brought together learned physicians able to teach the textual tradition and the opportunity to observe a variety of diseases and gain experience with the various means of therapeutics when interacting with the patients.

Although the learned physicians were well regarded for their medical expertise, they represented a small minority of all medical practitioners in the Islamic world. Physicians were more likely to practice in the aristocratic courts, in the hospitals, and in the homes of wealthy patients. However, a wide range of less respectable healers offered their medical services in the marketplace. These lower-status healers were often itinerant, offering a range of specialized services as bonesetters, oculists, or sellers of various remedies, and likely had little, if any, training in the theoretical medical tradition. Judging from the large number of vitriolic attacks against women healers found in the texts of Islamic physicians, it appears that women were especially active as healers in the marketplace, treating not only women and children but also men. One physician even speaks with amazement about the patient who "acquiesces to whatever extravagant measure [the woman healer] might order, consumes whatever she prepares for him, and listens to what she says and obeys her commands more than he obeys the physician. He believes that this woman, despite her lack of intelligence, is more knowledgeable and of sounder opinion than the physician" (Pormann and Savage-Smith 2007, 103). Clearly, this physician believed that his textual training should convey a greater respect and distinguish him from the women healers. This example makes clear, however, that patients would seek out a wide variety of learned and nonlearned healers and the limited numbers of learned physicians meant that most people, especially in rural settings, would only be able to turn to the self-taught empiric healers for medical treatment.

MEDICAL LEARNING IN MEDIEVAL EUROPE

Translation and the Rise of Universities

As with the Islamic tradition, learned medicine in medieval Europe was built upon the written texts from the Greek medical tradition. For much of the early Middle Ages, the majority of those texts were not available in Latin, the language of learning in the West, and few knew how to read Greek. However, the 11th and 12th centuries witnessed a dramatic increase in trade and cultural exchange between Western Europe, the Greek East, and the Arab world so that from about 1080 onward, scholars were able to translate both Greek and Arabic medical texts into Latin. The rapid influx of previously unavailable medical scholarship containing a more theoretically sophisticated medical system greatly expanded the amount of learned medical literature available and strengthened the philosophical component of medical knowledge.

The sudden profusion of new medical learning in Latin sparked profound changes in the study and practice of medicine in the West. Since the late 10th century, Salerno, in southern Italy, had been recognized as a center of medical practice, not book learning. Over the course of the 12th century, however, the Salernitan practitioners were ideally located to take advantage of the newly translated medical literature, and they began to incorporate it into their teaching to provide a more theoretical, academic medical education. By the mid-12th century, the Salernitan masters had identified a collection of texts, referred to as the *Articella*, which would form the core of the medical curriculum. The *Articella* consisted of five main texts (Johannitius's *Isagoge*, Hippocrates's *Aphorisms* and *Prognosis*, and two short Byzantine treatises on the methods of diagnosis, Theophilus's *On Urines* and Philaretus's *On Pulses*), which were soon supplemented in the curriculum by Galen's *Art of Healing* (known as the *Tegni* or *Microtegni* in the Middle Ages in order to distinguish it from Galen's *Therapeutic Method*, known as the *Megategni*) and Hippocrates's *On Regimen in Acute Diseases*. The Salernitan master, Bartholomaeus of Salerno (fl. ca. 1175), wrote a series of commentaries on the *Articella* and the *Tegni*, which he used as the basis of his teaching. Far from simply reiterating the basic points of the texts, Bartholomaeus sought to use them as a starting point from which he could explore larger theoretical issues in medicine, incorporating Aristotelian and Arabic philosophical learning so as to explain the place of medicine in relation to the larger subject of natural philosophy. As a result, by comparison with the more practically oriented texts previously available in Latin, which focused largely on providing remedies for specific diseases, the new Salernitan medical texts were more concerned with providing theoretical explanations for the underlying causes of disease and justifications for the efficacy of those remedies.

The translations not only encouraged new approaches to medical learning in Salerno but sparked the rise of the first universities across Europe as people sought to assimilate the newly available scholarship on a wide range of subjects, including medicine. Several centers gained a reputation as informal sites of learning in the 12th century, but over time some developed into a more formalized academic community and institution of instruction known as a *studium generale* or university, which received the right to design curriculum and rules for conferring degrees. By the beginning of the 13th century, Salerno had been eclipsed as a center for medical learning by university medical schools, the greatest being the universities in Montpellier, Paris, Bologna, and Padua. Other universities had medical faculties, but they were often small and had very few medical students, finding it difficult to compete with the larger medical schools. Universities drew students from all over Europe, brought together by the common language of instruction, Latin. Jews, however, were excluded from earning degrees, although in some universities, like Montpellier, they could attend lectures if they paid the appropriate fees. Women were denied access to university education entirely.

The curriculum was remarkably similar in the many university medical schools across Europe. Students would first study the seven liberal arts, which were divided into the *trivium* (grammar, logic, and rhetoric) and the *quadrivium* (arithmetic, geometry, astronomy, and music) in order to receive a bachelor's degree. In addition to these subjects, students would also learn about the natural sciences, based on the works of Aristotle. Following these preliminary studies, a student could opt to pursue an advanced degree in one of the liberal arts or in one of the higher disciplines of theology, law (canon/ecclesiastical law or civil law), or medicine. The medical doctorate, which conferred the *licencia ubique docendi* (license to teach in any university), required at least 10 years of study and was very expensive, so many students would instead pursue a bachelor of medicine degree,

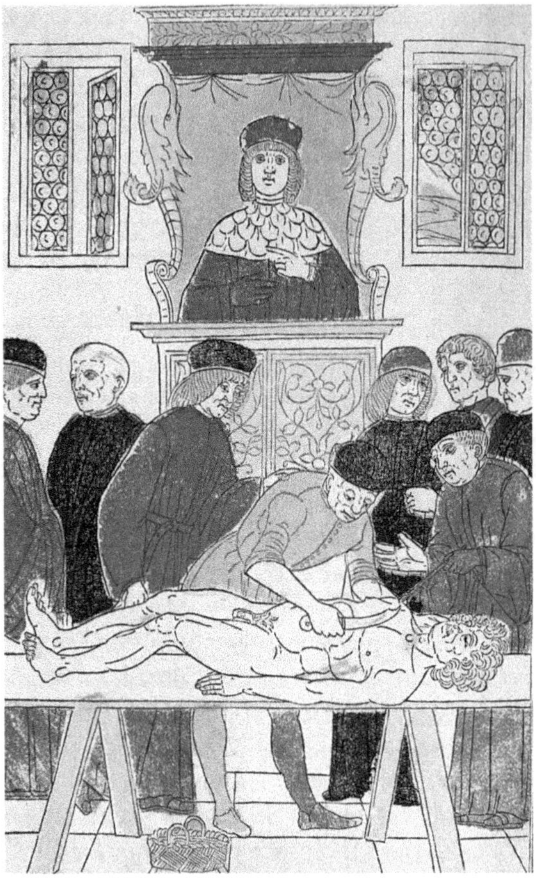

This image is from the title page of the *Fasciculo di medicina* by Johannes de Ketham (1493). It depicts an anatomy lecture in which a medical student (seated in the high chair) reads from a copy of a learned text on anatomy, while a surgeon performs the less-exalted task of dissecting the body. The professor of medicine (the elderly gentleman to the right with the stick for pointing) would offer additional comments and explanations to expand upon the details described in the text. Students (in their long academic gowns) gather around the body to hear the lecture and discuss the lesson. (Harris Brisbane Dick Fund, 1938/The Metropolitan Museum of Art)

conferring the right to practice, which still required several years of study beyond work in the liberal arts.

Following the example set in the *Isagoge* and the *Pantegni*, the medical curriculum was divided into the areas of *theoria* (theory) and *practica* (practice). Under *theoria*, students would study the philosophy of medicine, physiology (including anatomy), and principles of pathology to understand the causes of disease. Courses on *practica* covered the methods of diagnosis and treatment. Lectures were based upon specific books, most often the books of the *Articella*, and selections from Avicenna's *Canon*, supplemented by short works by Galen and other Greek and Arabic medical authors. University professors would read passages from the selected texts and then provide commentaries and explanations on the passage, typically with reference to other books on medicine. The method of teaching by commentary was reflected in the most popular learned genre of medical writing from this period, the "commentary" on a specific text. Although providing a commentary on a single text might seem reductive, in practice it allowed the lecturer to show his wide knowledge of the written medical tradition as he considered particular *questiones* (questions), or issues under theoretical dispute (e.g., "Can a child raised only by mutes learn to talk?," "Should purgation be done only with drugs in cases of leprosy?," "Is it appropriate to use phlebotomy in cases of strong pain?," or "Do women emit semen, and if so is it necessary for conception?"), which were of significance for elucidating theoretical problems or for actual practice.

The heavy emphasis in the universities on reading and interpreting the books of the ancient medical authorities in the medical schools was intended to provide students with certain, true knowledge, supported by logical argumentation, as opposed to knowledge gleaned through experience in practice, which was considered anecdotal and prone to misinterpretation by the practitioners. This does not mean that university medical students did not receive any practical training. Indeed, they were often required by university statutes to attend a practicing physician and thus gain some experience at the bedside to supplement their theoretical learning. Nonetheless, the distinguishing mark of a university-trained physician would be his theoretical training and command of the written texts of the Greek and Arabic medical authorities; a student who had received a university medical education could claim to understand the humoral theory of health and disease as explained by the Greek authorities and its implications for therapeutic practice. By contrast with non-university-trained healers, therefore, a university physician would claim that his treatments were supported by rational, theoretical medicine, and not simply by empirical practice.

The Hierarchy of Medical Practitioners and the Nonlearned Tradition of Medieval Medicine

In Latin, the term *medicus* ("doctor") could be used to refer to anyone who practiced medicine or surgery, but with the rise of university medicine the term *physicus* ("physician") was increasingly used to distinguish a medical practitioner trained at university (and thus familiar with natural philosophy and the theoretical basis of medicine) from other doctors not trained in the written tradition. Throughout the Middle Ages, the *physicus* remained comparatively rare and most people would receive treatment from a range of different kinds of healers arrayed in a kind of hierarchy of prestige.

Those healers below the level of the *physicus* on the medical hierarchy typically learned their craft through some form of apprenticeship or on-the-job training. Next, in terms of prestige to the *physicus*, came the skilled *chirurgicus* ("surgeon"), who performed a wide range of surgical procedures including lancing boils, setting bones, conducting lithotomies (a surgical method for removing bladder stones), or even executing difficult operations to reduce hernias. Like the *physicus*, skilled surgeons were also comparatively rare so that the majority of healers fell into a range of less prestigious occupations. Barber-surgeons, as their name implies, would provide a shave and a haircut, but they also put their sharp knives to use performing minor dental and surgical procedures, such as pulling teeth or letting blood. Apothecaries collected a wide range of spices and herbs and would mix them to produce healing drugs for a fee. At the very bottom of the medical hierarchy, composing the majority of all medical practitioners, one would find a variety of healers who specialized in one kind of procedure (e.g., treating eye diseases, cutting for bladder stones, or setting bones), sold simple herbal remedies, or offered magical or religious healing. Midwives, who were supposed to focus on the treatment of women and children, would also fall into the bottom rung of the medical hierarchy. Despite the fact that physicians commanded more prestige (and higher fees), patients regularly sought aid from all varieties of healers.

While the learned Latin medical tradition remained primarily under the control of the university-trained physicians, who could read the Latin texts, increasingly some of these medical texts were translated into the vernacular languages of Europe. Vernacular translations of recipe books existed in the 13th century, but in the late 14th and early 15th centuries, an increasing number of theoretical medical texts were translated into vernacular languages making them available to a wider medical audience. Soon it was not uncommon for learned surgeons, apothecaries, and other healers, who would not know Latin, to have access to the tradition of learned medicine written in their own language. Thus, the dissemination of Greek and Arabic theoretical medicine continued to a wider range of healers (surgeons, apothecaries, and others), at once signifying the respect given to elite medical science and ensuring its enduring value.

3

Religion and Medicine

Faith systems help to explain humanity's place in the cosmos and offer guidance on how an individual can lead a life in harmony with the universe. From this perspective, illness is a state in which the individual fails to attend to his or her physical, mental, or spiritual well-being and hence falls out of alignment with the universe. Religious explanations often ascribed the onset of illness to the influence of gods or other supernatural forces, inflicted either on a whim or as a punishment for sin. Such beliefs necessitated that any cure attend not only to the physical condition but also to the underlying spiritual cause. Therefore, whereas "medicine" is concerned with health in the more limited sense of physical condition, religion has historically taken a more holistic approach that also considers a patient's mental and spiritual well-being. The overlapping interest between religion and medicine in the preservation and restoration of health explains why healers in traditional societies would be equally likely to offer religious, magical, and naturalistic cures.

FAITH, MAGIC, AND HEALING IN MESOPOTAMIA AND EGYPT

Gods and the Causes of Disease

In ancient Mesopotamia and Egypt, numerous gods were associated with healing. The goddess Gula, "the great one," was one of the most important healing gods in Mesopotamia, as was the goddess Ninisina, a fertility goddess who was also described as a midwife. Similarly, in Egypt, several gods and goddesses were recognized for their general healing powers (especially Osiris, Isis, and Sekhmet), while others offered more specialized medical care (e.g., Serqet offered protection against scorpion stings and the bites of venomous animals, while Bes and Taweret were known for assisting in pregnancy and childbirth). The sick wrote prayers requesting the aid of these deities or wore protective amulets shaped in their likenesses. Indeed, many clay votive offerings to Gula survive, shaped like sick people clutching their afflicted body parts or in the shape of dogs, her divine symbol.

The gods were not always beneficent but were also known for their role in causing disease. Both the Mesopotamians and the Egyptians believed diseases could be caused by outside malign influences including gods, demons, ghosts, and other supernatural forces. Egyptian medical texts speak of *aaa*, which appears to be a poisonous substance (sometimes the seminal discharge of an incubus) introduced into the body through magical means, and cures are offered for "driving out the *aaa* of a god or goddess," as well as others that refer to the *aaa* of a dead man or woman. Mesopotamian records also express the belief that disease might arise as a punishment for individual sin or for breaking taboos, although it might not always be clear which sin was being punished, as one prayer makes clear:

> Loosen my disgrace, the guilt of my wickedness; remove my disease; drive away my sickness; a sin I know (or) know not I have committed; on account of a sin of my father (or) my grandfather, a sin of my mother (or) my grandmother, on account of a sin of an elder brother (or) an elder sister, on account of a sin of my family of my kinsfolk (or) of my clan . . . the wrath of god and goddess have pressed upon me. (Sigerist 1951, 445)

Wicked sorcerers or other humans might even use incantations or curses to encourage the gods to inflict disease on their enemies. For example, the Code of Hammurabi, written ca. 1750 B.C.E., concludes by warning that should any subsequent ruler destroy these codes, he would suffer numerous curses:

> May Ninkarrak [a form of Gula, goddess of healing], the daughter of Anum, my advocate in Ekur, inflict upon him in his body a grievous malady, an evil disease, a serious injury which never heals, whose nature no physician knows, which he cannot allay with bandages, which like a deadly bite cannot be rooted out, and may he continue to lament (the loss of) his vigor until his life comes to an end! (Meek 1969, 180)

When examining a patient, therefore, the doctor would first need to determine the origin of the condition (i.e., what the patient had done and which being was responsible for the affliction) before being able to determine a course of treatment, which would typically require some form of ritual intervention, to thwart evil incantations or to purify the afflicted in order to placate the gods.

Religious Healing in Ancient Mesopotamia

Herodotus, a Greek historian writing in the fifth century B.C.E., indicated that the Babylonians in Mesopotamia had no physicians or specialized medical personnel; sick people went to the marketplace where passers-by would offer advice on the nature of the illness and suggest treatment. Although the medical system in Mesopotamia may not have resembled the Greek system that Herodotus knew, it is clear that the Mesopotamians did have an established system of medical treatment and a variety of different kinds of specialists involved in the health care process. One significant difference that may have led to Herodotus's misunderstanding is that in Mesopotamia, religion, magic, and science were all united in an inseparable learned system in which naturalistic and religious explanations for diseases coexisted, and cures, whether herbal remedies or charms, were all believed to be imbued with magical or spiritual healing properties. As a result, healers in the Mesopotamian world were typically members of the priestly classes, unlike the *iatroi* Herodotus knew in the Greek world.

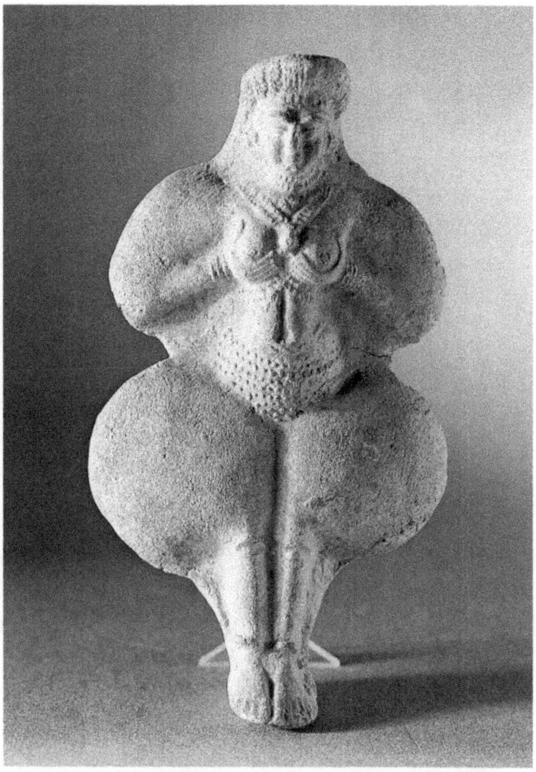

This terracotta Mesopotamian fertility figure (ca. 14th–12th century B.C.E.) was discovered in present-day Shush, Iran. Figures like these were kept by women in ancient Mesopotamia to aid in fertility and to offer protection during pregnancy and childbirth. (G. Dagli Orti/De Agostini/Getty Images)

Two priestly classes in particular had duties as medical practitioners: the *baru* ("diviner") and the *ashipu* ("exorcist"). Most *baru* appear to have worked directly for the kings, local lords, or the army, thus holding high social status. In addition to their normal duties as diviners, they would be called upon to provide an initial diagnosis of disease by examining omens from the gods and interpreting signs. For example, the *baru* believed that if he should see a black dog or a black pig on his way to the patient's home, then that sick person would die, but if he should see a white pig, then the patient would survive. The *baru* would also examine sheep entrails, in which they believed the gods "wrote" messages, to divine the cause of illness. Numerous handbooks survive that list the various discolorations and markings in the entrails that the *baru* would observe, along with a description of their significance. They also made use of clay models of sheep livers that indicated specific points of interest on the liver and provided brief annotations about their significance to aid in divination. Beyond having a role in making the initial diagnosis to identify the cause of the disease, however, it appears that the *baru* was not involved in treatment.

The *ashipu* was a priest who performed purification rituals or exorcisms to cleanse temples and other spaces in preparation for religious ceremonies. Most of their activities, therefore, had nothing to do with treating illness. They were also adept at interpreting the various omens that could aid in prognosis and diagnosis, however, and unlike the *baru*, the *ashipu* could perform the rituals necessary to purify a sick person by driving out the evil spirits causing the disease and then reconciling her or him with the gods. They also provided patients with various healing incantations. For example, a cure for an eye affliction required that the healer take threads of red and white wool and tie seven knots in each, and then placing the red thread over the injured eye and the white thread over the healthy eye, he should recite a charm such as this one: "O clear eye, O doubly clear eye, O eye of clear sight! O painful eye, O doubly painful eye, O eye of painful sight! A pair they are one eye, yet a mountain is set as a bar between them . . . (on) their surface a knot is tied, (on) their under parts a wall is built" (Thompson 1924, 31). The *ashipu* was also capable of offering herbal drugs that could be taken while reciting a healing charm, as with this remedy for the disease caused by "hand of a ghost":

> If a man has been seized by a ghost and the *ashipu* is unable to get it to withdraw, you crush together the following [a list of unidentifiable plants follows], you rub him with oil, you wrap up (the herbal mixture) in a piece of leather and put it around his neck. If "hand of a ghost" is persistent in a man's body and cannot be gotten rid of, to expel it you take (various minerals) and carob seeds, you char them over coals, you pulverize them, you mix with cedar resin; you recite (the following) incantation seven times. (Biggs 2005, 12–15)

In many respects, therefore, the *ashipu* would offer the same kinds of healing services as the *asu* (doctor), indicating that little distinction was made between religious and naturalistic healing in Mesopotamian society.

Magical Cures in Egypt

There is ample evidence that a variety of magicians and priests, distinct from the *swnw*, practiced medicine in ancient Egypt. Many, like the *sau* magicians, made protective charms and amulets that could be used to protect against disease or during pregnancy. The *wab* priests of Sekhmet, the lion-headed goddess, were also recognized as important healers, although they played a slightly inferior role to the *swnw*. Sekhmet was believed to bring pestilence and famine, and thus her priests played an important role in healing since people needed to appease her to prevent disease. These individuals practiced comfortably alongside the *swnw*, and indeed the *swnw* often also had the title of magician, suggesting that he combined both roles in his own practice.

The *swnw* also regularly incorporated magical healing into his repertoire, and several incantations or spells that can be used for healing are listed alongside herbal remedies in the medical papyri. For example, the Ebers papyrus offers this incantation against *wekhedu*:

> I trample Busiris; I throw down Mendes; I ascend to the sky to see what is done therein. Nothing will be done in Abydos until the driving out of the [evil] influence of a god, a goddess, male *wekhedu* , female *wekhedut*, and so on, and the influence and all evil things that are in this my body, in this my flesh and in these my limbs. . . . I will not say: I will not repeat: Perish as you came into being! Words to be said four times and spat out over the site of the disease. Really effective: a million times. (Nunn 1996, 105)

Therefore, as was the case in Mesopotamia, Egyptian healers were prepared to offer a combination of religious, magical, and naturalistic cures.

RELIGIOUS AND NATURALISTIC MEDICINE IN ANCIENT GREECE

Homer's *Iliad* (written during the eighth century B.C.E.) describes the god Apollo spreading plague among the Achaeans encamped before the walls of Troy by firing disease arrows at them until "the corpse-fires burned on, night and day, no end in sight. Nine days the arrows of god swept through the army" (Fagles 1990, 79). In response, the Achaeans consulted a soothsayer to determine how they had offended Apollo and what they would need to do to propitiate him and end the plague. Following the soothsayer's advice, they purified themselves and made appropriate sacrifices to placate Apollo, and only then did the plague cease.

The gods were also known for curing disease, and Greek patients who sought religious healing could invoke a wide range of gods, including Apollo who was the leading healing deity in the Greek pantheon. Increasingly from the third century B.C.E. onward, Asclepius, who was recognized for his healing abilities in Homer's *Iliad*, eclipsed Apollo as the primary healing god, and his cult spread throughout the Mediterranean region. In early myths, Asclepius was said to be the mortal son of Apollo and a mortal mother, known for his knowledge of drugs and incantations for use in healing, but over time, he came to be recognized as a god in his own right and the Greeks built several temples dedicated to him. Sick people could travel to one of his temples and undergo purification rites before being allowed to enter the *abaton*, or sacred dormitory, where they would sleep for the night. They believed that Asclepius would appear in their dreams and either cure them or offer advice on how they could procure a treatment. After recovery, many supplicants left inscriptions thanking the god for his divine cure, like the one left by Ambrosia of Athens, who had been blind in one eye:

> She came as a suppliant to the god. As she walked about in the Temple she laughed at some of the cures as incredible and impossible, that the lame and the blind should be healed by merely seeing a dream. In her sleep she had a vision. It seemed to her that the god stood by her and said that he would cure her, but that in payment he would ask her to dedicate to the Temple a silver pig as memorial of her ignorance. After saying this, he cut the diseased eyeball and poured in some drug. When day came she walked out sound. (Edelstein and Edelstein 1998, 230)

In another inscription, we learn that Asclepius revealed this remedy to a man who had suffered a cough for two years: "Italian wine flavored with pepper to drink; then again starch with hot water, then powder of holy ashes and some holy water, then an egg and pine-resin, then again moist pitch, then iris with honey, then a quince and a wild purslane to be boiled together" (Edelstein and Edelstein 1998, 252). The prescription, which mixes holy substances with more ordinary ingredients, suggests that religious and naturalistic healing continued to comfortably coexist in the Greek world. By the end of the first century B.C.E., the cult of Asclepius was so widespread that, of all the pagan gods, he was the only serious competitor to Christ as a healing god.

By contrast to the evidence from the Homeric period and the religious healing offered in the temples to Asclepius, the Hippocratic authors in the fifth and fourth centuries B.C.E. sought to provide naturalistic explanations for disease and hence naturalistic cures. The most obvious expression of this idea is found in *On the Sacred Disease*, which discusses the condition of epilepsy. The early Greeks believed that this disease was caused by divine visitation—hence the name "sacred disease"—and the cure consisted of undergoing a process of ritual purification and reciting healing incantations. The author of *On the Sacred Disease*, however, vigorously counters the perception that the "sacred disease" is caused by the gods, declaring that charlatans and faith healers invoke a divine cause for the ailment merely to account for their failure to cure it. Rather, he explains the disease within the naturalistic framework of the nascent humoral theories, declaring that epilepsy is caused by excess phlegm on the brain, and offers a number of empirical proofs and anatomical explanations for the disease. As to the cure, the author declares,

> This disease styled "sacred" comes from the same causes as others, from the things that come to and go from the body, from cold, sun, and from the changing restlessness of winds. . . . Whoever knows how to cause in men by regimen moist or dry, hot or cold, he can cure this disease also, if he distinguish the seasons for useful treatment, without having recourse to purifications and magic. (Jones 1923, 183)

The Hippocratic authors did not necessarily deny the value of religious cures, but they did seek to separate naturalistic and religious healing and to mark the *iatros* as one who offered natural, not magical or religious, remedies for disease.

MEDICINE AND RELIGION IN INDIA AND CHINA

Magic and Medicine in Early Indian and Chinese Civilizations

The earliest medical beliefs in India and China bear a strong resemblance to those of ancient Mesopotamia and Egypt. The four sacred scriptures of the Hindu religion that were written during the Vedic period in India (ca. 1500–500 B.C.E.), the *Rigveda*, the *Yajurveda* , the *Samaveda*, and the *Atharvaveda*, described the religious rituals to be performed by the Brahmans, or priestly class. One of these texts, the *Atharvaveda*, is less concerned with the rituals of sacrifice and prayer and more focused on materialistic and naturalistic matters, containing a number of magical incantations aimed at providing protection against demons, witchcraft, and natural disasters. It describes a number of illnesses caused by demons, poisoning, or accidents, and reveals several incantations and magical charms aimed at protecting against those diseases, and also for ensuring fertility and a successful pregnancy, promoting hair growth, or generally guaranteeing a long life. In this tradition, the *bhishaj*, professionals who combined the craft medical knowledge of artisans with the intellectual learning of priests, would be expected to know the appropriate incantations and spells to cure specific ailments and also how to produce amulets and talismans from plants and other substances that could ward off demons and malign spells in order to bring about a cure. In its earliest origins, therefore, Vedic medicine was based in a system of healing magic and Ayurvedic medicine was profoundly shaped by this tradition.

During roughly the same period in China, in the time of the Zhou dynasty (1045–256 B.C.E.), disease was also conceived of as having divine or supernatural causes. Chinese demonic medicine was based on the belief that demons or other evil spirits would inflict illness on individuals. The earliest surviving Chinese medical texts, discovered in the Mawangdui gravesites, which date to about 168 B.C.E., including the *Wu-shih-erh ping fang (Fifty-Two Prescriptions against Fifty-Two Ailments)*, reveals a belief in the demonic cause of disease and provides a variety of magical spells and talismans to ward them off. The *wu*, shaman-like practitioners who offered the curing incantations and talismans, would also sometimes use herbs and other medicinal substances as remedies to treat demon-related illnesses. These beliefs bear a striking resemblance to the magical medicine of the Vedic period in India.

Confucianism and Taoism in Chinese Medical Thought

The life of Confucius (551–479 B.C.E.) and the spread of Confucian philosophy coincided with the political and social chaos of the late Zhou dynasty and Warring States (ca. 475–221 B.C.E.) periods. Confucian thought was oriented around the question of how to organize social life in order to maintain political harmony and end warfare. As it gained adherents, Confucianism also influenced the early development of traditional Chinese medicine, in particular offering a metaphorical way of thinking of the body as a well-ordered state, as can be seen in the *Huangdi Neijing* (*The Yellow Emperor's Classic of Internal Medicine*):

> The heart is the sovereign of all organs and represents the consciousness of one's being. It is responsible for intelligence, wisdom, and spiritual transformation. The lung is the advisor. It helps the heart in regulating the body's *qi*. The liver is like the general, courageous and smart. The gallbladder is like a judge for its power of discernment. The pericardium is like the court jester who makes the king laugh, bringing forth joy. The stomach and spleen are like warehouses where one stores all the food and essences. . . . [So the] *zang* and *fu* organs must work together harmoniously, just like a kingdom. . . . It is in this way that one's life is preserved and perpetuated, just as a country becomes prosperous when all its people are fulfilling their duties. If the spirit is disturbed and unclear, the other organs will not function properly. This creates damage. The pathways and roads along which the *qi* flows will become blocked and health will suffer. The citizens of the kingdom will also suffer. These are the relationships of a kingdom. (Ni 1995, 34)

In this way, the maintenance of health required that the individual regulate all aspects of his life and body, just as a king would manage a peaceful and ordered state. By extension, disease was envisioned metaphorically as political or social breakdown that would disrupt the flow of communication and commerce.

The teachings of Taoism, founded by the philosopher Lao-Tzu (sixth century B.C.E.), also spread in China in response to the political and social disruption during the Warring States period and had a similar influence on the direction of traditional Chinese medicine. Whereas Confucianism emphasized the goal of creating political and social order among humans, Taoism was more concerned with teaching how man should conform to "the Way" and live in harmony with nature.

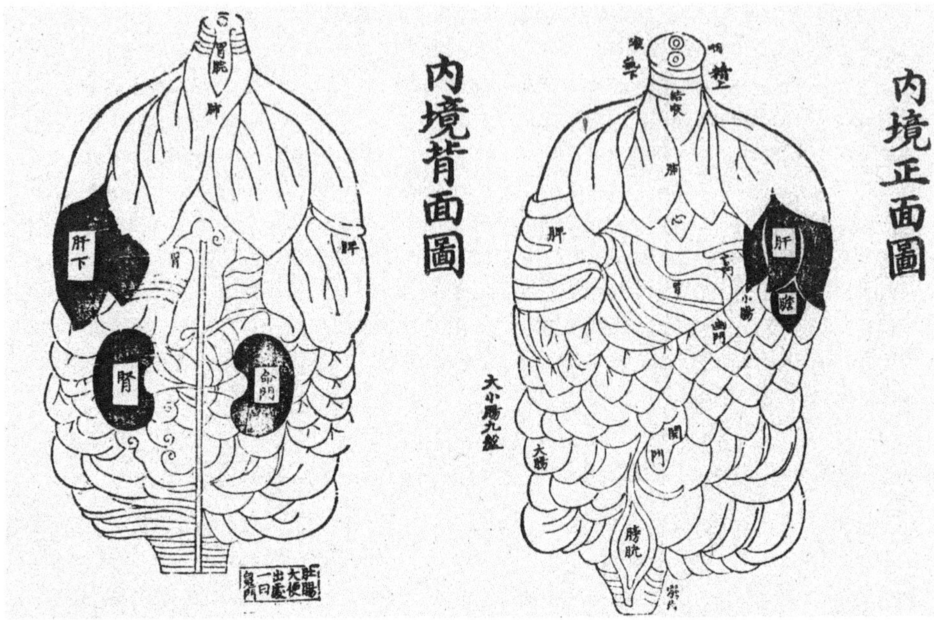

This 15th-century woodblock illustration is based on a medical text from the Song dynasty in China. It depicts the internal organs of the body from the front (left) and back (right). (Wellcome Collection)

For some, the pursuit of harmony with nature was equated with the pursuit of longevity. The *Huangdi Neijing* refers to the "Perfect Ones" of antiquity who had achieved these goals:

> In the past, people practiced the Tao, the Way of Life. They understood the principle of balance, of *yin* and *yang*, as represented by the transformation of the energies of the universe. Thus, they formulated practices such as Dao-in, an exercise combining stretching, massaging, and breathing to promote energy flow, and meditation to help maintain and harmonize themselves with the universe. They ate a balanced diet at regular times, arose and retired at regular hours, avoided overstressing their bodies and minds, and refrained from overindulgence of all kinds. They maintained well-being of body and mind; thus, it is not surprising that they lived over one hundred years. (Ni 1995, 1)

As is evident in this passage, Taoism envisioned a holistic approach to health that emphasized exercise, meditation, and diet as a means to maintain health. Although Taoism did not deny the role of demons in causing disease or the use of magic as cures, its emphasis on nature encouraged naturalistic explanations for illness and the continued development of pharmacological knowledge and herb lore as another means of curing disease.

In this way, the early writings in traditional Chinese medicine are founded upon diverse systems of belief. Confucianism and Taoism together offered a philosophical structure for the early development of medical theories. Both systems drew upon the cosmological theory of systematic correspondence, the theory of *yin* and *yang*, and the doctrine of *wu xing* ("five phases"). They offered a philosophical framework within which to understand the functioning of the human body as it related to society and the wider cosmos, which overlay the earlier beliefs of demonic medicine. Furthermore, they also emphasized a system of health care that defined health as more than simply physical well-being but more broadly as the state of harmonious balance between body, soul, society, and the cosmos.

Buddhism in Indian Medicine

From the fourth century B.C.E. onward, Buddhist ascetics (monks and nuns), who gathered in monastic communities called *sanghas*, took on the role of healing the sick within their community and sometimes even traveled to heal others in the surrounding areas. Many of these monks pursued knowledge about medical theory and practice, learning the medical beliefs of the *bhishaj*, and they played a significant role in collecting, editing, and writing down the content of the oral tradition of magico-religious Vedic medicine.

At the same time, however, they were also greatly influenced by the empirical medical learning passed on by ascetic wanderers from North India called sramanas. The sramanas were generally known for their empirical and rational approach to disease and treatment, placing less emphasis on magical healing than the Vedic tradition. Unlike the Brahman healers, they held no taboos about touching dead bodies and encouraged ascetics to learn anatomy by dissecting animals and observing decomposing human bodies. Furthermore, the early sramanic texts offer more naturalistic herbal remedies and medicinal foods as cures, with less emphasis on magical cures than in Vedic medicine. As a result, the early Ayurvedic texts that were finally written down by Buddhist monks (including the *Caraka* and the *Susruta*) unite the empirical and rational approaches of the sramanas with the magico-religious healing of the Hindu Vedic tradition (Zysk 1998).

The Buddha was frequently referred to as the "king of physicians" for his emphasis on helping the suffering. Indeed, his spiritual contemplation began with witnessing disease, old age, and death in the natural world, and he taught that healers should consider the eightfold causes of disease: an imbalance in one of the three *doshas*, changes of the seasons, engaging in unusual or excessive activities (sitting or standing too long), emotional stresses (being assaulted by a robber or arrested as an adulterer), or the result of previous actions (karma). The recognition of the theory of the three *doshas* and other naturalistic and physical causes of disease (seasons and excessive activity) reaffirms the rational approach to healing present in the Buddhist tradition that influenced Ayurvedic medicine. However, the Buddha's classification of disease placed equal emphasis on the physical, mental, and spiritual causes of suffering. Mental suffering, which typically arose from the emotions of greed, anger, or ignorance, required that patients seek a cure through meditation and spiritual contemplation. Nonmonastic Buddhist texts also reflect a comingling with indigenous magico-religious healing traditions. For example, in Tibetan Buddhist medicine, magical healing became an integral part of the ascetic's healing arsenal; they would offer protective charms, rituals, and mantras that could ward off supernatural causes of disease and purify the individual to reverse the effects of karma. As Buddhism spread, the more magico-religious form of Buddhist medicine as well as the empirico-rational monastic medicine explicated in the *Ayurveda* were both exported to neighboring countries in Central Asia.

FAITH HEALING IN THE ISLAMIC AND CHRISTIAN TRADITIONS

Prophetic Medicine in the Islamic World

With the spread of Islam from the seventh century onward, Muslim scholars compiled treatises purporting to reveal the "Medicine of the Prophet" as an alternative form of healing for pious Muslims, who opposed the Greek medical philosophy, which often made use of medicinal substances that were forbidden by Islamic law. These texts included collections of quotations on sickness and therapeutics drawn from the Quran and the hadith, sayings attributed to the Prophet Muhammad (d. 632). Specific conditions, including fevers, leprosy, plague, nosebleeds, and headaches are all addressed in the Prophetic Medicine manuals, as are other more esoteric calamities such as the "Evil Eye," a condition that some authors felt the need to defend as real.

The treatment provided in the Prophetic Medicine treatises was generally fairly minimal. Surgery was barely mentioned, aside from circumcision. Cautery, bloodletting, cupping, the regulation of diet and regimen, and the use of drugs formed the core of the naturalistic treatments offered. Simple drugs were favored over compound medicines, honey being perhaps the most commonly prescribed medicinal substance. In addition, these treatises present several prayers and incantations that could be used in aid of a cure. One such incantation was offered in a cure for treating colic:

> Write for him [the patient] the opening surah of the Quran, the surah "Purity," and the two surahs for seeking protection [the last two surahs of the Quran, "Dawn" and "People"]. Then write underneath: "I take refuge in the presence of God, the Great, and in His might, which is unceasing, and in His power, which nothing can resist, from the evil of this pain, and the evil within it." Then swallow with rainwater on an empty stomach. You will be cured of it, God the exalted permitting. (Pormann and Savage-Smith 2007, 150)

The emphasis here is on the belief that God will provide a cure. Talismans and amulets were also often used to ward off epidemics and other diseases or to alleviate the suffering of women during a difficult childbirth.

Although several physicians trained in Greek humoral medicine questioned the efficacy of using amulets, talismans, and other magico-religious healing techniques, there was often considerable overlap between these two healing systems. Some Prophetic Medicine manuals drew upon the medical learning available in texts based on the Greek tradition and even sought to reconcile the two traditions, emphasizing that although God would provide the cure for disease, humans still needed to discover it and apply it correctly. At the same time, physicians were not always ready to rule out the efficacy of magical or occult cures. Some even included various amulets and other magical cures alongside herbal remedies in their medical texts; one physician recommends placing a lock of hair from a dead person on a painful tooth to alleviate the pain or placing the hair under the head of a sleeping person to help him sleep longer. In this way, Prophetic Medicine managed to coexist with the philosophical Greek medical tradition in the Islamic world.

Magical and Miracle Cures in Medieval European Medicine

In the ancient world, Christianity was widely recognized as a healing religion. Christ was regularly described by the early church fathers as *Christus medicus* ("Christ the doctor") and as a result, Christianity competed for followers with other religions devoted to healing gods, like the cult of Asclepius. The New Testament describes a number of miracle cures provided by Jesus, and evidence throughout the course of the fourth century C.E. suggests that Christians increasingly attested to witnessing miraculous healing and sought divine aid to restore health. This does not mean that Christians eschewed secular medicine or that they did not visit physicians trained in the Greek tradition. In the 11th century C.E., Bishop Fulbert of Chartres described the relations between religious and secular healing in a hymn:

> As Christians we know that there are two kinds of medicine, one of earthly things, the other of heavenly things. They differ in both origin and efficacy. Through long experience, earthly doctors learn the powers of herbs and the like, which alter the condition of human bodies. But there has never been a doctor so experienced in this art that he has not found some illnesses difficult to cure and others absolutely incurable. . . . The author of heavenly medicine, however, is Christ, who could heal the sick with a command and raise the dead from the grave. (Park 1992, 64)

Fulbert's account indicates that he saw the two healing systems as complementary but noted the limitation of secular medicine in the case of certain intractable conditions in comparison to the extraordinary possibilities of heavenly medicine.

People seeking miracle cures in the Middle Ages would typically turn to the cult of saints. Supplicants could pray to a particular saint, or in many cases, go on a pilgrimage to visit the shrines of saints where they could receive a miraculous cure by touching the saints' relics, drinking the waters in which they had been dipped, or sleeping near the saint's tomb. Monks associated with the shrines kept records of the miracle cures performed by their saints, like these:

> A man crippled from birth got about by dragging himself along with hand-trestles. His thumb, too, was bent back, the nail nearly through the palm. While huddled at Godric's tomb crying and moaning he straightened his legs and began to extend them. During this many heard a crackling noise of bones and ligaments stretching. At dawn he arose and walked up to present the trestles as an offering; his hand was healed, only a red spot remaining in the palm.
>
> Matilda, a young girl, felt a swelling and pain in her right breast and then there was a discharge from nine openings in the afflicted part. After human medicines failed, she vowed some wax to William of Norwich and applied it to her breast; relief followed when she removed the wax. She went to the cathedral to offer the wax, and baring her breast applied it to the tomb, after which the disorder was completely cured. (Finucane 1977, 91, 105)

The monks' lists of cures offer insight into the variety of conditions for which people sought divine healing. Among adults, the most common cures were for cripples and paralytics, followed by cures for the deaf, mute and blind, and then cures for the mad or possessed. Other conditions receiving miracle cures included wounds, sterility, tumors, and various skin conditions (such as leprosy). This list suggests that most supplicants sought heavenly healing for chronic conditions that were not otherwise susceptible to treatment by secular medicine and in general they undertook the expensive pilgrimage to a shrine only after the doctors had failed to bring about a cure.

Although all saints might be called upon for miracle cures, certain saints were renowned for curing specific diseases. Saint Sebastian and Saint Roch were associated with the plague, for example, while Saint Lazarus was associated with leprosy, Saint Agatha with breast cancer, Saint Mathurin with mental illnesses, and Saint Maur with gout. In an unusual case in southern France, some people venerated a greyhound (known for its loyal service protecting a child) as a "saint," and they brought their sick children to the shrine of "Saint Guinefort" for healing. On the other hand, other saints were recognized for their more general healing abilities, including Saint Job (renowned for being afflicted with a number of diseases) and Saints Cosmas and Damian (brothers who had been physicians in life and were recognized as the patron saints of doctors). The sick could offer intercessory prayers requesting heavenly healing to any of these saints in lieu of going on an actual pilgrimage; in many cases, they might promise to go on a pilgrimage to the shrine of the saint after the cure had been performed.

Starting in the 12th and 13th centuries, physicians trained in the Greek humoral tradition in the universities began to grow increasingly skeptical of magical and religious folk medicine. Nonetheless, many scholastics continued to include magical cures using amulets and charms in their medical writings for a number of reasons. Sometimes physicians cynically suggested that they only included magico-religious cures to provide patients with what they expected or because they thought these cures could still have a positive psychological effect on patients. Other physicians argued that even though they could not provide rational explanations for the efficacy of magical incantations and amulets, they might still function according to some unknown occult property—just as they could not explain the power of the magnet to attract iron shavings, for example. Magico-religious elements appear frequently in certain circumstances in scholastic texts, such as when discussing treatments for conditions for which rational remedies seemed ineffective. For example, the physician Valesco de Tarenta (fl. 1382–1418) attested to his own successful use of certain religious charms to treat epilepsy, which he says should be recited three times into the patient's ear: "Jesus of Nazareth, crucified king of the Jews" or "Gaspar brings myrrh, Melchior frankincense, Balthazar gold." Furthermore, he claims that the patient should have these phrases written on a clean sheet of paper and suspended from his or her neck to ward off future epileptic fits. In similar fashion, the learned surgeon Teodorico Borgognoni (d. 1298) reported a ritual and incantation for use when extracting arrows from wounds:

> It does not trouble me to write down at the end of this chapter certain empirical experiments, although they have not been tested by me, experiments which I know certain experienced men swear by.
>
> Therefore, for the purpose of drawing out an arrow, let there be said thrice, on bended knee, The Lord's Prayer (that is, the paternoster), and when these have been said, let the arrow be grasped with both hands joined as they are, and let be said, "Nicodemus drew out the nails from our Lord's hands and feet, and let this arrow be drawn out," and it will come out forthwith. (McVaugh 2003, 320)

Teodorico may not have been fully convinced of the efficacy of this ritual, noting that he had not tried it himself, but he still felt the need to include it in his list of treatments for a condition that frequently proved fatal.

4

Women's Health

The single greatest cause of death among women in the premodern world was complications attending childbirth, and premodern societies often recognized that women were prone to different diseases from men and thus required differentiated care. The field of gynecology encompassed not only the treatment of "women's diseases" but almost every aspect of female health care, and it is linked to the field of obstetrics, which focuses on the care of women during pregnancy and childbirth. In premodern societies, the care of women often fell to midwives, especially in the context of managing pregnancies and childbirth, but that was not always the case; male practitioners wrote extensively about how to treat "women's diseases" and also on how to manage complications during birth, and they likely treated female patients in many of these circumstances. In this chapter, we will examine the ways in which women's health care was understood, methods of treating women and managing the birthing process, and the range of practitioners involved in treating female patients.

GYNECOLOGY: WOMEN'S BODIES AND WOMEN'S DISEASES

Mesopotamia and Egypt

It is not clear which practitioners were most involved in providing women's health care in ancient Mesopotamia and Egypt. Midwives, called Sabsutu, assisted in childbirth in Mesopotamia, but evidence indicates that *asu* and *ashipu* were also called in to treat women and attend to complications following childbirth. In ancient Egypt, there are no known words for midwife, gynecologist, or obstetrician, but there is no documentary evidence to indicate that the *swnw* was specifically involved in childbirth, although it is clear they were called on to treat women patients. This raises a question about the extent to which the male practitioners who produced the written medical texts were actually involved in treating women or knew about female anatomy.

Mesopotamian healers did not understand or write extensively about female reproductive anatomy or diseases specific to women. By contrast, several Egyptian medical texts survive that discuss women's health, and the Kahun papyrus is devoted specifically to the subject of gynecology. The Kahun papyrus attributes women's illnesses mainly to the activities of the uterus. This is true not only of what we might consider uterine diseases; for example, a woman whose eyes are aching until she cannot see or one with aching in her molars or ears is diagnosed as having discharges or terrors of the womb. Different medicinal remedies were prescribed for these conditions brought on by the uterus, often including fumigating the uterus with incense or other substances like burning goose fat or dried human excrement. Egyptian texts also offer many remedies for "cooling the uterus" and "driving out heat" or this one: "Instructions for a woman suffering in her vagina, and all her limbs likewise, having been beaten. You shall say concerning her: 'This has loosened her uterus.' You should then prepare for her: oil to be eaten until she is well" (Nunn 1996, 197). These descriptions of women's illnesses and their cures imply that the *swnw* typically viewed all aspects of women's health as being specifically related to the uterus.

Fertility was probably the major concern reflected in Mesopotamian and Egyptian gynecological literature. The Kahun papyrus and other Egyptian medical texts offer a number of tests to determine whether a woman was even fertile like this one: "[To determine] who will [bear children] and who will not [bear children], you should then cause the bulb of an onion to spend the night in her flesh until dawn. If the odor appears in her mouth, she will bear [children]. If [it does not], she will never [bear children]" (Nunn 1996, 192). Likewise, in both medical traditions we find medical prescriptions and magical incantations aimed at helping women conceive or curing sterility. One Mesopotamian prescription for making a barren woman conceive reads, "Total: twenty-one stones to help a barren woman become pregnant; you string them on a linen thread and put them around her neck" (Biggs 2005, 9). The main emphasis of gynecological medicine, therefore, appears to have been to ensure that a woman be able to conceive and bear children.

Greek and Roman Gynecological Literature

The Hippocratic Corpus includes several treatises that consider female physiology and gynecology, including *Diseases of Women*. These texts explain women's health in terms of the regularity or irregularity of menstruation or in terms of the motions of the uterus. Accordingly, retention of the menses, excessive menstruation, and "suffocation" of the womb were considered significant illnesses and therapies (including diet, regimen, and drugs) were provided to alleviate the uterus and restore the proper flow of the menses. Furthermore, according to the Hippocratic *On Generation*, "if [women] have intercourse with men their health is better than if they do not . . . Intercourse by heating the blood and rendering it more fluid gives an easier passage to the menses; whereas if the menses do not flow, women's bodies become prone to sickness" (Lonie 1981, 4). Likewise, in *Diseases of Women I*, the author addresses the importance of intercourse for maintaining women's health and also describes numerous afflictions of the womb:

> If suffocation [of the womb] occurs suddenly, it will happen especially to women who do not have intercourse and to older women rather than to young ones, for their wombs are lighter. It usually occurs because of the following: when a woman is empty and works harder than in her previous experience, her womb, becoming heated from the hard work, turns because it is empty and light. There is, in fact, empty space for it to turn in because the belly is empty. Now when the womb turns, it hits the liver and they go together and strike against the abdomen—for the womb rushes and goes upward toward the moisture, because it has been unduly heated by hard work, and the liver is, after all, moist. When the womb hits the liver, it produces sudden suffocation as it occupies the breathing passages around the belly. . . . When the womb is near the liver and the abdomen and when it is suffocating, the woman turns up the whites of her eyes and becomes chilled; some women become livid. She grinds her teeth and saliva flows out of her mouth. . . . If the womb lingers near the liver and the abdomen, the woman dies of the suffocation. (Hanson 1975, 576)

These diseases of women reflect a societal expectation that women should be engaged in reproduction for the sake of their own health—failure to engage in intercourse and thus maintain regular menstruation and placate the womb could be fatal.

Greek physicians and natural philosophers also considered the physiological differences between male and female bodies, and these discussions often revolved around beliefs about their respective contributions to conception. In his work *Generation of Animals*, Aristotle (384–322 B.C.E.) described female bodies in relation to the humoral and qualitative theories, arguing that female bodies were colder than male bodies. As a result, he maintained, their bodies were unable to produce a fully formed seed and thus they only contributed a lesser, material substance to conception that did not influence the child's physical form. On the other hand, he believed that male bodies, due to their heat, could produce a fully active seed, which impressed itself on the material substance produced by women's bodies to provide the form or blueprint for the future child. Later, Galen of Pergamum (129–ca. 216 C.E.) challenged Aristotle's one-seed theory, claiming that both male and female bodies contributed a seed to conception, and in partial proof of this, he pointed to the fact that offspring often resembled their mothers. These competing theories from the two preeminent medical and biological scholars of antiquity about the differences between male and female bodies would have significant influences on later understandings of sex difference and reproduction in European medicine.

Gynecology in Ayurvedic Medical Literature

As in the Greek world, the *Susruta Samhita* and the *Caraka Samhita* both view menstrual irregularities as the main source of women's diseases. The *Susruta* indicates that menstruation begins at age 12 and ceases at age 50 with the onset of the perceptive deterioration of the body. During those years, the regulation of the menses is deemed crucial because it is the essential factor that makes impregnation possible, along with male semen. Irregular menstruation was usually attributed to derangement of the *doshas* and treated by diet and drugs, when necessary.

Medical and religious texts offer extensive advice to aid with impregnation. Foremost, they recommend a regimen to be followed after the start of the menses: for the first three days, the woman should remain chaste, but after taking a cleansing bath on the fourth day, the following nine days are deemed most suitable for conception. If conception occurs on even days after the onset of the menses (fourth, sixth, eighth, tenth, or twelfth day) she will have a boy, if on odd days (fifth, seventh, ninth, eleventh) she will have a girl. The *Susruta* also indicates that conception under unusual circumstances might present a danger to the future offspring:

> A boneless (i.e., with cartilaginous bones) monstrosity is the outcome of the sexual act in which both the parties are female and their Súkra (sexual secretion) unite somehow or other in the womb of one of them. Fecundation may take place in the womb of a woman, dreaming of sexual intercourse in the night of her menstrual ablution. The local *vata* carries the dislodged ovum into the uterus and exhibits symptoms of pregnancy, which develop month after month till the full period of gestation. The offspring of such a conception is a Kalah (a thin boneless jelly-like mass) on account of the absence of the paternal elements in its development. Such monstrosities as serpents, scorpions, or gourd shaped fetuses delivered from the womb of a woman should be ascribed as the effects of deadly sins. (Bhishagratna 1911, 132)

Sterility and other problems hindering conception are explained as being caused by derangement of the *doshas* that lead to the production of impure sperm or menstrual blood. Therefore, the Ayurvedic texts offer a number of tests to determine the potency of sperm and menstrual blood; for example, incurable impotency can be diagnosed if the sperm or menstrual blood smells like urine or feces. A variety of remedies are otherwise offered to cure impotence, including dietary changes, sweating, and drugs—women are prescribed pastes applied as vaginal suppositories.

Gynecology in Traditional Chinese Medicine

The *Huangdi Neiching* (*The Yellow Emperor's Classic of Internal Medicine*) envisioned male and female bodies in terms of a balance of yin and yang but did not attend extensively to anatomical differences. Indeed, the uterus played virtually no role in early Chinese medical writings—the *zang* and *fu* organs were the main anatomical structures present in both male and female bodies, and the uterus received little attention except in brief discussions of pregnancy. Reproductive powers were associated with the kidneys (a *zang* organ) for both sexes, and they were deemed responsible for fertility and conception. In this learned medical system, male and female bodies were thought to be prone to the same diseases and were treated similarly. In popular practice, however, evidence suggests that women's health care was the domain of a range of female healers (*nü yi*), herbalists, acupuncturists, masseuses, and shamans, suggesting that women did indeed receive differentiated medical treatment.

Sun Simiao (581–682 C.E.) was the first medical author to emphasize the medical importance of sexual difference, arguing that "the disorders of women are ten times more difficult to cure than those of males," and "for women, there are separate prescriptions [from those appropriate for men]" (Furth 1999, 26, 51). Following Sun Simiao's lead, the field of *fuke* (translated as gynecology) arose, examining the range of diseases and therapies of "wives" (a *fu* is a married woman), and it developed into a mature specialization during the Song dynasty (960–1279 C.E.). Gradually, *fuke* became an academic subject and was taught in the state-approved schools of the Imperial Medical Bureau, where learned male physicians sought to establish their own authority to provide for women's health care, especially in the imperial palaces. In 1220, a professor of medicine celebrated the development and spread of *fuke* as a medical specialty:

> For the first time there is specialized knowledge concerning the women's chambers. Surely it should not fail to be written in books? I have made a study of this specialization in medicine. Not daring to be lazy and disregarding my own ignorance, I have gathered many prescriptions and compiled them into a volume called *One Hundred Questions on Medicine for Females*. (Furth 1999, 69)

His book was intended as a kind of bedside manual for family use, not directed specifically at learned physicians, indicating that by his time the field of *fuke* was gaining popular recognition beyond court practice.

With the rise of the specialty of *fuke*, menstruation received greater attention in medical diagnosis as a visible marker of female reproductive functioning, often earning the most extensive coverage in gynecological sections of medical texts. One Song physician, Chen Ziming (ca. 1190–1270 C.E.), maintained, "In treating illness in women, one must first regulate the menses, so I place this first." Furthermore, he advised physicians, "In males one regulates *qi*, in females one regulates Blood [since] . . . in women Blood [function] is the root" (Furth 1999, 75). Following this theory, treatises on *fuke* recognized three broad categories of women's diseases: wind stroke (*zhongfeng*), depletion fatigue (*xusun*, *xulao*), and swellings and accumulations (*jiju*). All of these presumed a deep-rooted pathological disorder of the blood and qi in women that could disrupt the menses or impair sexual and reproductive function. For this reason, *fuke* manuals prescribed drugs for women that were known for their ability to "enliven Blood," "replenish Blood," or "move Blood." One of the most popular, the "Four Ingredients" infusion (*Siwu tang*), contained angelica root and white peony root (both known for their blood-nourishing properties), lovage rhizome (believed to improve the proper movement of blood), and fresh rehmannia root (believed to move qi in the body).

Female Practitioners and Women Patients in the Islamic World

Women healers played an important role in Islamic society, and they did not only treat women patients. Learned physicians often bemoaned the extent to which patients felt free to turn to these women healers:

> How amazing it is [that patients are cured at all], considering that they hand over their lives to senile old women! For most people, at the onset of illness, use as their physicians either their wives, mothers or aunts, or some [other] member of their family or one of their neighbors. He [the patient] acquiesces to whatever extravagant

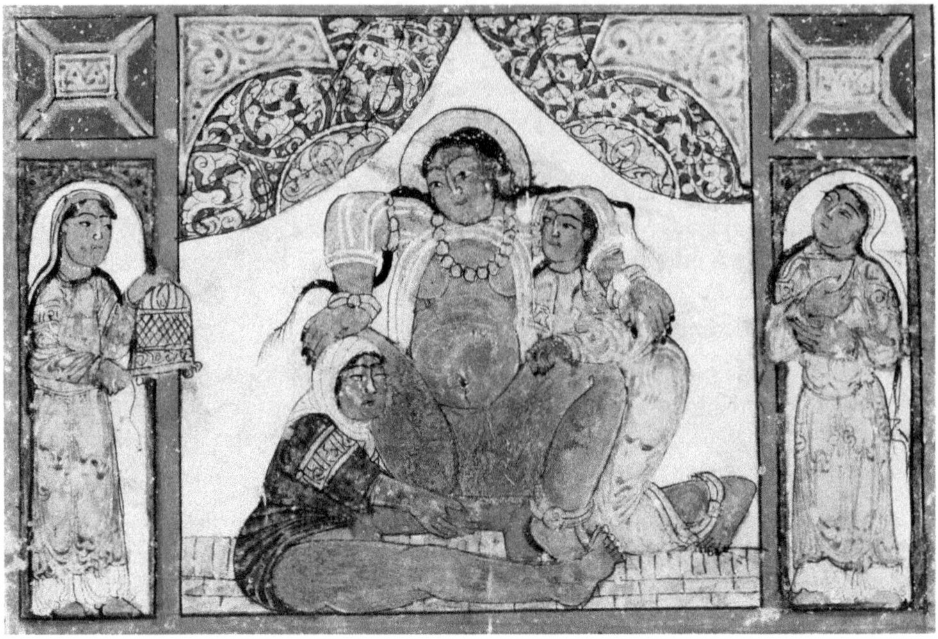

This 13th-century Persian illustration depicts a queen giving birth with the aid of female attendants. Male physicians were not typically present during childbirth. (Bibliothèque Nationale, Paris, France/Archives Charmet/Bridgeman Images)

> measure she might order, consumes whatever she prepares for him, and listens to what she says and obeys her commands more than he obeys the physician. He believes that this woman, despite her lack of intelligence, is more knowledgeable and of sounder opinion than the physician. (Pormann and Savage-Smith 2007, 103)

Learned male physicians, however, were aware that female patients were often unwilling to seek medical care from men, especially for women's conditions. In these cases, it is most likely that women continued to seek the care of female healers.

Male physicians in the Islamic tradition did write extensively on topics relating to gynecology and obstetrics, even if they mostly repeated material found in their Greek sources. Furthermore, it is clear that male physicians were sometimes consulted to treat female patients. Al-Razi (d. ca. 925, known as Rhazes in the Latin West), for example, reports treating a woman with a breast tumor and al-Zahrawi (fl. ca. 1000, known as Albucasis in the Latin West) reports treating a girl with a knife wound in her throat and two other women with growths on their head and neck. Al-Zahrawi even describes the surgical use of forceps to perform a surgical operation on a woman to extract two fetuses that had died in utero. Despite these accounts, however, it appears that the practice of gynecology and obstetrics in the Islamic world remained in the hands of women practitioners.

The "Secrets of Women" and Male Physicians in Medieval Europe

One influential 13th-century text in Europe, the *De secretis mulierum* (*On the Secrets of Women*), erroneously attributed to the Aristotelian natural philosopher

Albertus Magnus, purports to reveal the secret knowledge women have about their bodies that gives them control over human reproduction. Many physicians wrote commentaries on this text, expanding on the ideas it contained, and it was even translated into several vernacular languages, attesting to the popularity of the text among both learned medical men and the literate lay public. The text covers a wide range of sexual, gynecological, and obstetrical topics and elaborates on the power women have to promote or prevent conception, influence the sex of the fetus in utero, procure abortions, and otherwise act against the interests of men seeking male heirs. Furthermore, some passages portray women as sexually avaricious and wicked, warning that, "when men have sexual intercourse with these women it sometimes happens that they suffer a large wound and a serious infection of the penis because of iron that has been placed in the vagina, for some women or harlots are instructed in this and other ill deeds" (Lemay 1992, 88). Menstruating women are described as especially dangerous, and one later commentator expanded upon this point:

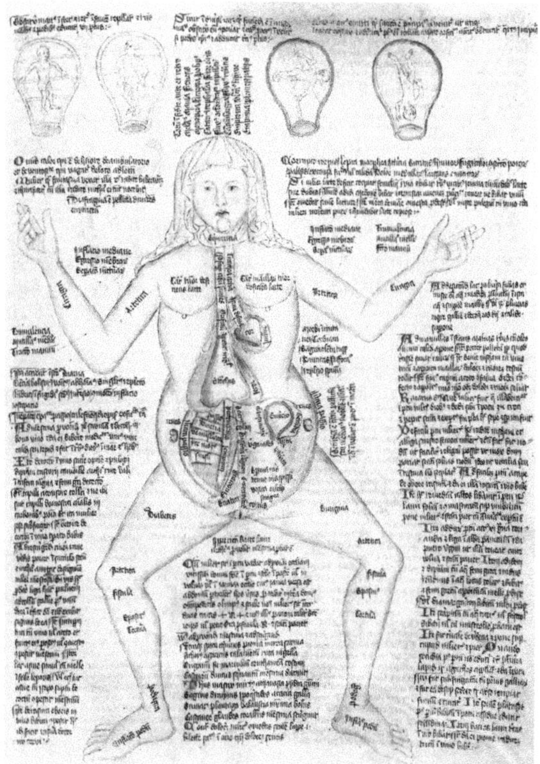

This image of "disease woman" was produced around 1420–1430. The names of various diseases are marked on the parts of the body they affect. Across the top, four images show a fetus in utero, depicting different kinds of fetal presentations one might encounter during birth. (Wellcome Collection)

> When men go near these [menstruating] women they are made hoarse, so that they cannot speak well. This is because the venomous humors from the woman's body infect the air by her breath, and the infected air travels to the man's vocal cords and arteries causing him to become hoarse. It is harmful for men to have sexual intercourse with menstruating women because should conception take place the fetus would be leprous. This also frequently causes cancer in the male member. (Lemay 1992, 130)

Writing in French, Christine de Pizan (1363–ca. 1430), the daughter of a physician at the French royal court, strongly denounced the *De secretis mulierum* for its disparaging portrayal of women. However, in the paternalistic medieval society concerned with producing male heirs, the popularity of this text reflected a general misogynistic fear of the power women had over the reproductive process.

Concurrently with the rising popularity of the *De secretis mulierum* in the 14th and 15th centuries, learned university physicians started to write a number of original texts on gynecology and obstetrics. Many of these texts are written with the stated intention of providing better theoretical gynecological knowledge and training for midwives. However, these books also reflect the male physicians' efforts to establish their own authority to treat all aspects of women's health and to supervise, if not entirely supplant, midwives in these activities. Indeed, their writings suggest that physicians were increasingly active in the treatment of women. One physician, for example, writes about his own experience in applying a rotten hen's egg to cure a woman's prolapsed uterus, boasting, "I marveled at its immediate reduction," and then indicating that he tried it on another woman with similar success (Green 2008, 252). Accounts of male physicians having gained such intimate access to female patients are rare, however; medieval physicians continually lamented the fact that women were reluctant to seek their advice for menstrual disorders until the condition was so advanced that it was difficult to treat.

OBSTETRICS: MANAGING PREGNANCY AND CHILDBIRTH

Childbirth in Ancient Mesopotamia and Egypt

Although medical texts from ancient Mesopotamia offer numerous prescriptions to treat women with difficulties during pregnancy, parturition, and complications after childbirth, care during the delivery of babies mostly rested in the hands of the *sabsutu* ("midwife") who was likely assisted by female relatives and other women. Prior to birth, the *asu* and *ashipu* were concerned with dangers associated with profuse vaginal bleeding, which they feared would lead to miscarriage, and offered a number of medicinal substances (applied as potions, tampons, vaginal fumigations, or salves) used in concert with magical charms to alleviate the bleeding. Mesopotamian healers believed that profuse bleeding leading to miscarriage could be caused by sorcery or evil magic. Therefore, many of the incantations were designed to prevent the evil spells from taking effect:

> If [you want] sorcery not to approach a pregnant woman, [and] for her not to have a miscarriage, you crush magnetite, antimony, dust, subu-stone and dried "fox" grape. You mix [the resulting paste] with the blood of a female shelduck and you take [it] with cypress oil and you rub [it] on her heart, her hypogastric region and her [vulva's] "head" and you tie on a band [made from] a cloth [made] of red-colored wool (or you take a potsherd [found] standing on edge at a crossroads and you bury it in the inner threshold and sorcery will be kept at bay) and you put masculine su-stone on her left hand. (Scurlock 1991, 135–183)

In this case, the use of the red-colored wool likely had magical symbolism associated with blood and the potsherd buried behind the door likely symbolized the intention to ward off intruders from outside. These protective medicines and incantations would have been provided by the *asu* and *ashipu* who knew such rituals and indicates that they did have a role in caring for pregnant women.

It is possible that some women may have wanted to procure an abortion. One Mesopotamian text provides a prescription "to cause a pregnant woman to 'drop' her fetus," listing eight ingredients that should be mixed in wine and given to the woman to drink on an empty stomach and ends with the words, "that woman will 'drop' her fetus" (Biggs 2005, 9). Unlike the evil magic of sorcerers aimed at causing an unwilling miscarriage in women, this drug appears to have been designed for use at the woman's request, but it is not clear how it would have been used. Although this drug could have been used to hasten delivery or to expel a dead fetus, it is also possible that it may have been administered to provoke an abortion. Assyrian law codes specifically demanded the death penalty for women who self-aborted, however, suggesting that the use of such a drug with the specific intention of provoking an abortion would have carried severe risks. The vague way in which the results of the prescription are described may, in fact, reflect this supposition.

The *sabsutu* was expected to perform many rituals in the birthing chamber designed to protect the mother from the dangers of childbirth. For example, for a woman with an overly narrow birth canal, the *sabsutu* could recite this incantation: "The woman in travail is having difficulty giving birth; she is having difficulty giving birth. The infant is stuck fast; the infant is stuck so fast as to end (her) life. The door bolt is secure; the door is made fast against the suckling kid" (Scurlock 1991, 141). She could also apply numerous lubricants in conjunction with massaging the abdomen to help hasten the labor. The lubricants were often composed of substances having magical symbolism such as hailstones, dust from fallen walls, or dust from leaky drainpipes as one text describes: "Like a hailstone (which can never go back to the heavens), may the (fetus) not be able to return to what is behind him. Like one who has fallen from a wall, may he not be able to turn his breast. Like a leaky drainpipe (which cannot hold water), may none of the (mother's) waters remain" (Scurlock 1991, 141). Difficulties during birth could have natural causes, but medical texts also presumed the possibility that evil sorcerers were at work. Such threats would likely have required the use of more powerful incantations that are found in the medical texts, suggesting that the *asu* and *ashipu* probably stood ready to provide assistance as necessary during difficult births.

Although there are no known words for midwife or obstetrician from ancient Egypt, it is likely that women were the ones assisting during childbirth as in other ancient cultures. No documentary evidence indicates the involvement of the *swnw*, but medical texts do offer advice for managing birth. Medical papyri described tests to determine whether a woman was pregnant or determine the sex of the fetus in utero. Mothers wanting a male child would often drink milk from a woman who had recently delivered an infant boy, and mother's milk was sometimes stored in special jars shaped like a mother nursing her baby for such use. Medical texts also included prescriptions that could be used as contraceptives: "Beginning of the prescription prepared for women/wives to allow a woman to cease conceiving for one year, two years or three years: *qaa* part of acacia, carob, dates; grind with one *henu* of honey, lint is moistened with it and placed in her flesh [i.e., in her vagina]" (Nunn 1996, 196). Other recipes for contraceptives recommend the application of crocodile excrement! Finally, there are also several remedies and some incantations for hastening birth and for helping to expel the placenta. Based on these sources, it is clear that the *swnw* was interested in the birthing process, but the descriptions are often vague, suggesting that he would not customarily take part in the delivery.

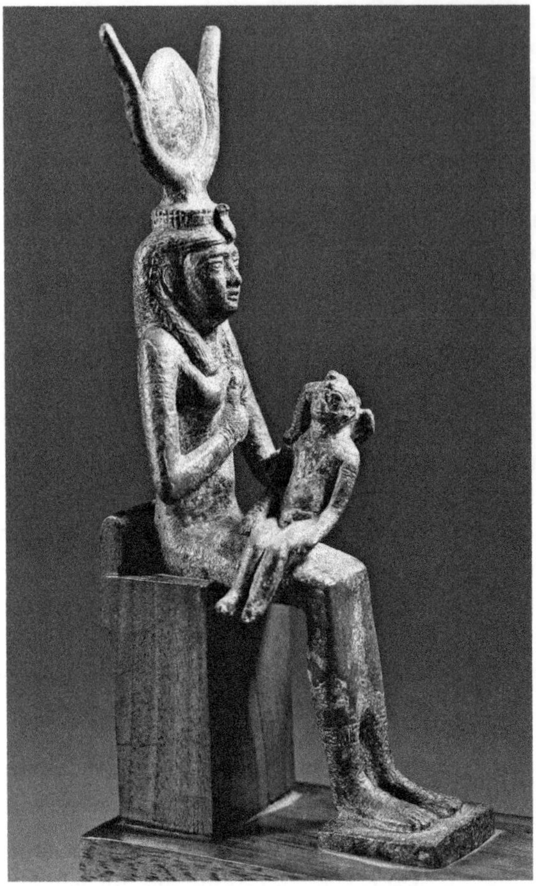

This statue represents the Egyptian goddess Isis nursing her child, Horus. Isis protected Horus from snakes and other predators when he was an infant, and for this reason she was viewed as the ideal mother and was also believed to protect mortal children from harm. Statues like this were kept to provide protection to mothers and children. (G. Dagli Orti/De Agostini/Getty Images)

Childbirth in Ancient Greece and Rome

In ancient Sparta, childbirth was depicted as a glorious act; the Spartans only allowed the names of warriors who died in battle and women who died in childbirth to be inscribed on their tombstones! In other parts of the Greek and Roman world, however, women giving birth were not depicted in such glowing terms. In addition to being dangerous, childbirth was also viewed as being polluting for the mother and child in the ancient Greek and Roman world. Indeed, rules associated with sacred districts stipulated that people could not die and women could not give birth in the precinct for fear of polluting the holy area. As a result, mothers and newborns were regarded as vulnerable immediately after birth and were kept secluded for a period before being reintroduced into the general household after undergoing necessary purification rituals.

Midwives were the ones primarily involved in attending to the needs of pregnant women and assisting in the delivery of babies. Soranus of Ephesus (fl. 100 C.E.) describes the midwife's responsibilities and the birthing process in his work on gynecology and obstetrics. The midwife, he says, was responsible for making certain that the necessary oils, lubricants, sponges, and warm water for cleaning were available, as well as bandages, swaddling, and a pillow for the newborn after birth. She would oversee the woman in labor, providing necessary drugs and comforts to assist until it was time to deliver, at which point the woman would move to a special birthing stool, with a crescent-shaped opening in the bottom and solid crossbars for handles that she could grasp during contractions. The midwife would then be ready to advise the woman on breathing, while directing her assistants and preparing to receive the infant when it appeared. According to Soranus, this was a difficult job, and he listed a number of stringent requirements for any woman who would undertake it: she should be literate (presumably so as to read his book!), physically strong with delicate fingers and short fingernails, able to remain calm under pressure, and be of good moral character. Soranus's text implies that learned doctors would be ready to step in and assist in cases of difficult births, but even then they would have needed to work in concert with the midwife to bring about a safe delivery. He describes in great detail how the midwife would widen the birth canal if necessary and how she should turn the fetus in the womb in cases of difficult presentations. Above all, he advises that she remain calm, "for we see many alive who have thus been born with difficulty" (Temkin 1956, 189). It seems that Soranus clearly intended to imply that he knew more about delivering babies than the midwives!

Soranus expected that midwives would step aside and call in physicians in cases where it was necessary to extract a dead fetus from the uterus, yet another dangerous complication of childbirth, and he describes the tools and procedures for performing this operation. Although popular stories maintain that Julius Caesar was born through a "caesarean" section, giving his name to the procedure, it is unlikely that a true C-section was performed in the Greek or Roman world. As proscribed by Roman law, such procedures were only performed on women who died during childbirth, with the intention of saving the child; this was a measure of last resort, and it was not performed on live women to save the mother's life in cases of difficult births. As Caesar's mother is said to have survived to give birth to other children and to learn of his invasion of Britain, she clearly had not undergone such an operation.

The Greeks and Romans did describe a number of drugs that could be used as contraceptives or to promote abortions. The Hippocratic *Oath* specifically forbids a doctor to provide an abortive suppository to women, but the author of a different Hippocratic text, *On the Nature of the Child*, recommends the "Lacedaemonian leap" in which the woman would leap in the air and kick her heels to her buttocks to expel the seed from her womb, implying that other methods of abortion or contraception were possibly acceptable. Other Hippocratic texts describe recipes for a variety of contraceptive medicines. Soranus, recognizing the discrepancy in these Hippocratic texts sought to distinguish between abortive and contraceptive measures, indicating that the Lacedaemonian leap could be interpreted both ways, and he makes clear the fact that these methods could be controversial in his own day:

> [One] party prescribes abortives, but with discrimination, that is, they do not prescribe them when a person wishes to destroy the embryo because of adultery or out of consideration for youthful beauty; but only to prevent subsequent danger in parturition if the uterus is small and not capable of accommodating the complete development, or if the uterus at its orifice has knobby swellings and fissures, or if some similar difficulty is involved. And they say the same about contraceptives as well, and we too agree with them. And since it is safer to prevent conception from taking place than to destroy the fetus, we shall now first discourse upon such prevention. For it is much more advantageous not to conceive than to destroy the embryo. (Temkin 1956, 63)

Nonetheless, after describing various methods for preventing conception, Soranus also gives detailed advice on how to provoke an abortion—recommending a number of herbal drugs, violent exercise, leaping vigorously, and being shaken around by riding in carriages. Indeed, his apprehension about abortion revolves more around a fear that the drugs could be harmful to the woman than a specific opposition to the goal of provoking a miscarriage. Similarly, many later Greek and Roman texts included recipes for both contraceptives and abortifacient, like this one from the second century C.E.:

> Take 1 drachma iris, 1 drachma Cnidian grain, 1 drachma galbanum, 1 drachma turpentine. Mix in equal parts with lily oil, Cyrian oil (consisting of omphacine oil [Lesbian wine], sweet flag, myrrh, aspalathus, cardamom, and flowers of Cyperus Rose oil). . . . Insert into the vagina before a bath with fenugreek and Artemisia. If this does not produce an abortion, let her repeat the procedure but this time inserting the suppository after the bath with these: wallflower (or stock) seed, soda, and wormwood soaked in wine on wool pad. (Riddle 1992, 95–96, 100)

Other evidence suggests the widespread availability of amulets and charms for the same ends. Thus, although some physicians as well as several legal and literary texts from this period expressed opposition to abortion, it appears that many people made use of such methods.

Childbirth in India

Childbirth was not generally handled by physicians in India but rather by midwives. Nonetheless, Ayurvedic medical texts offer substantial advice on the care and observation of pregnant women. Indeed, the *Susruta* emphasizes that the care of the pregnant woman had dire consequences for fetal development:

> The child of a mother whose wishes are not honored and gratified during pregnancy stands in danger of being born palmless, hunchbacked, lame, dumb or nasal voiced through the deranged condition of the *vata* of its mother's body. The malformation of a child in the womb should be ascribed to the atheism of its parents, or to the effects of their misdeeds in a prior existence, or to the aggravated condition of the *vata*, *pitta*, and *kapha*. (Bhishagratna 1911, 132–133)

Thus, the pregnant woman was supposed to avoid physical labor, sexual activity, sleeping during the day, staying up late at night, and being frightened; rather, she should spend her time in pleasant surroundings, eat good food, and be carried around in a carriage whenever she needed to travel. Advice is also given for recognizing whether a pregnant woman was carrying a male, female, hermaphrodite child, or twins, based on the shape of her belly, development of breasts, facial features, and posture. The sex of the fetus was also thought to dictate the woman's desires (e.g., food preferences) and needs during pregnancy, hence these signs could also be observed to determine the sex of the offspring.

The medical texts also consider cases of difficult labor (*mudhagarbha*) in which the fetus presents in the wrong position leading to an obstructed delivery. Various texts describe a number of abnormal fetal presentations (e.g., the fetus descends with both legs first, with one arm stretched forward, etc.) and indicate that these complications are dangerous and could lead to fetal death. Facing these situations, the midwife's assistants were supposed to recite appropriate mantras while she introduced her hand anointed with ghee (clarified butter) into the vagina and repositioned the fetus. The *Susruta* describes two fetal presentations that should be given up as hopeless since the obstructions cannot be corrected. A fetus in these positions is called *viskambha* ("bolt"), and the text indicates that it will need to be surgically removed. The procedures and tools required for this operation are described in detail. The *Susruta* expects that a male surgeon will perform the operation, although another text indicates that the procedure would be entrusted to a clever midwife. In any case, the mother's survival was probably fairly unlikely, and the texts recognize this, even requiring that the surgeon receive the ruler's permission before starting the operation.

In the event that the mother should die during labor, the *Susruta* provides directions for performing a caesarean section: "A child, moving in the womb of a dead mother, who had just expired (from convulsions, etc.) during parturition at term, like a goat should be removed immediately by the surgeon from the womb as a delay in extracting the child may lead to its death" (Bhishagratna 1911, 58). The indication here is that the surgeon would need to take over in this case, and it implies that the procedure was readily known since it was practiced on animals—possibly why the *Susruta* does not offer any other details of the operation. The earliest recorded case of a caesarean section in India is that of Bindusara (ca. 320–272 B.C.E.), the second Mauryan emperor, whose mother accidentally consumed poison and died when she was about to deliver, necessitating that he be cut from her womb.

Abortion and miscarriage are discussed in the Ayurvedic texts. The medical understanding of embryological development explained that in the first four months, the fetus is in a liquid state so any termination of the pregnancy would be called an abortion; in the fifth and sixth months, the limbs begin to solidify, so after this point it is called a miscarriage. The texts suggest that an abortion could be triggered by many causes, including insufficient food, food that is especially heavy, warm, or pungent (particularly intoxicating beverages), excessive physical exercise, sexual intercourse, suppression of natural excretions, dire emotions (especially anger and fear), and emetic or purgative drugs. Although the medical texts do not explicitly suggest that women might seek to have an abortion, the recognition that certain drugs could provoke an abortion indicates that the possibility of using them in this way existed. Child abandonment was practiced in India, as in other ancient cultures, thus other methods of regulating family size were also available.

Childbirth in China

Chanke (obstetrics) rose to prominence as a medical specialty in China during the Song dynasty, at the same time as the field of *fuke* (gynecology) was developing. Previous works like Zan Yin's (fl. 852–856 C.E.) *Chanbao* (*Treasure of Childbirth*) had indicated increasing medical interest in the subject of childbirth, but it was not until the Song period that it was widely recognized as a distinct medical

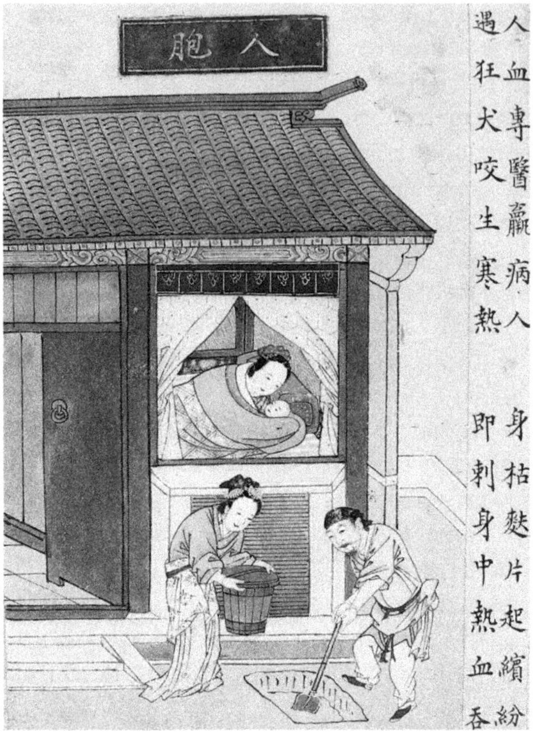

This 16th-century Chinese illustration is titled "Human Placenta." It depicts a mother and her newborn resting in their home, shortly after delivery. Meanwhile, in the foreground a man digs a hole to receive the placenta, which is carried out by another woman in a chamber pot. According to Chinese tradition, the placenta was buried in order to ensure the health of the mother and the newborn. (Wellcome Collection)

subdiscipline within the field of *fuke*, of interest to learned male medical practitioners. Previously, childbirth had been the realm of women healers, the *nü yi*, who did not have access to learned theories on pharmacy or acupuncture. Indeed, popular stories from earlier centuries suggest that physicians were only called in at the last minute to assist with complications arising during childbirth, and their intervention consisted of prescribing drugs and performing acupuncture.

Chen Ziming's *Furen Daquan Liangfang (All-Inclusive Good Prescriptions for Women)* was the best-known text from the Song period on obstetrics. Rejecting what he saw as the spiritualism of Buddhist books and *wu* shamans and the superstitions of old women, Chen Ziming endorsed the natural philosophical model of gestation, envisioning the "ten months of pregnancy" that conformed to the theory of the Five Phases and thus understood the significance of pregnancy within the context of the Chinese zodiac and the greater cosmos. He believed that armed with this knowledge and, by implication the guidance of physicians, pregnant women would be able to know how to ward off the ghostly fetuses and "wandering fetus killers" that threatened the health of the pregnant woman and her fetus. Furthermore, Chen Ziming's advice gave instructions on how to consult the special birth charts (*chan tu*), which would dictate information such as the preparation of the birthing chamber (e.g., the placement of the birthing couch, the curtains, and even the door) and also where the placenta should be buried after delivery to ensure the mother's and child's health. In this way, his work aimed to direct the ritual practices associated with childbirth in accordance with rational natural philosophy and medical theory.

Song physicians also increasingly wrote about intervening in cases of difficult childbirth. Again, Chen Ziming played a leading role, transmitting and augmenting an older text on different kinds of abnormal deliveries in his own medical work. He presents himself as offering advice for the women who would be assisting during delivery, noting, "Few delivery women have subtle and clever hands, and for this reason many [pregnant women] are endangered. Because I grieve for their plight, I must offer assistance" (Furth 1999, 121). While he emphasizes his own authority on the subject of *chanke* (especially in cases of difficult labor and delivery), it is clear that Chen Ziming did not attend to women in childbirth on his own. Rather, he intended his text as an instruction manual for women who would handle the process of childbirth, implying that he would work in concert with them to bring about a successful delivery. Learned male physicians may have been exerting their authority to enter the birthing chamber during this period, but they had not taken it over entirely.

One interesting story from the 12th century C.E. gives some insight into Chinese attitudes toward abortion:

> There was a woman in the capital named Bai; she was beautiful and the city people all called her Peony White. She sold abortifacients for a living. All of a sudden she was afflicted with brain sickness. [Her head] daily swelled larger and none of the famous doctors of the city could cure her. By day it suppurated and stank unbearably, and nightly the neighbors heard her groans. One day she called her household together and said, "You are to burn my entire collection of abortion prescriptions; I warn you, my children and disciples—you cannot carry on this calling." The sons said to their mother, "Our mother has made the family livelihood from this. How can we throw it away?" The mother said, "Every night in my dreams hundreds of infants gnaw at my skull, making me cry out in pain. This is all retribution because I used poisonous drugs to ruin fetuses." Having spoken thus, she died. (Furth 1999, 123)

Bai's final decision suggests that the use of abortifacients could be seen as immoral, leading her to worry that her own illness was brought on by the fetuses aborted by her medicines—indeed, the ghosts of aborted and miscarried fetuses were believed to pose a threat to pregnant women. On the other hand, her family recognized that selling abortifacients was a lucrative business—many people were buying medicines from the lady called "Peony White" (white peony was a known abortifacient). Chen Ziming offered prescriptions to make "nuns, prostitutes, or ailing wives" barren or to "cut off birth" in cases in which the pregnant woman's health was endangered, showing that physicians were also aware of such medicines (Furth 1999, 168). However, physicians were concerned about the dangers of provoking abortions and warned that care should be taken when doing so. Thus, despite laws prohibiting infanticide and abortion in China, the medical stance and story about Bai suggest that abortifacients were commonly available to those who sought them.

Childbirth in Medieval Europe

The birthing chamber continued to be almost exclusively under the control of women during the Middle Ages. Men (male relatives, priests, physicians, surgeons) were only infrequently present in the birth chamber. As a result it seems that this space stirred much fascination, engendering numerous stories from the period about the escapades of men who dressed up as women in order to infiltrate this feminine world and discover its secrets (although court records indicate that these men were often sneaking into birth chambers in order to find eligible women companions). Male physicians also tried to assert their authority to enter this feminine realm. Over the course of the 14th and 15th centuries C.E., physicians increasingly wrote about the need to instruct and supervise midwives. For example, in addition to his Latin texts on the subject, Michele Savonarola (1385–1468) wrote a manual in Italian, the *Regimen for the Women of Ferrara*, with the explicit aim of instructing midwives and other women in the city of Ferrara on matters of obstetrics. Although male physicians and surgeons probably did not wish to displace midwives in most cases of obstetrical care, their texts imply that they were skilled in handling a variety of obstetrical difficulties, especially those that might require surgical intervention.

The management of difficult labors and obstetrical surgery received extensive coverage in Latin medical texts. The performance of caesarean sections to extract a living fetus from a woman's womb after she had died received particular attention. Theologians and priests emphasized the benefits of this operation since it would allow the child to be baptized, ensuring its eternal survival, even if there was little expectation that the child would survive long after the baptism. Furthermore, medical authors described a number of different methods for performing this operation, suggesting that male medical practitioners (physicians and surgeons) were increasingly performing or at least supervising such procedures. The texts also describe methods for dismembering a dead fetus so that it could be extracted surgically to save the life of the woman, thereby emphasizing their expertise in surgical care during obstetrical emergencies.

Contraception and abortion were controversial subjects, especially as far as priests and theologians were concerned in the Middle Ages. General consensus, however, seems to have been that women knew how to prevent conception or procure abortions whenever they chose. Regarding abortion, the popular *De secretis mulierum* (*On the Secrets of Women*), which existed in numerous vernacular translations, reported that excessive physical exertion on the part of pregnant women could provoke the menses and cause a miscarriage. The author follows this observation in typical misogynistic fashion, impugning the morality of women:

> For this reason harlots, and women learned in the art of midwifery, engage in a good deal of activity when they are pregnant. They move from place to place, from town to town: they lead dances and take part in many other evil deeds. Even more frequently they have a great deal of sex, and they wrestle with men. They do all these things so that they might be freed from their pregnancy by the excessive motion. The reason for their great desire for coitus is that the pleasure that they experience will help them blot out the grief that they feel from the destruction of the fetus. (Lemay 1992, 102)

However, many medical authors were less worried about the morality of sexual activities. While acknowledging the religious and moral mandates against sexual intercourse and various practices that might encourage nonreproductive sexual activities, many physicians still felt free to describe recipes for contraceptive medicines and different drugs and methods that could be used to "provoke the menses," which in many cases may have been intended to produce an abortion in pregnant women. Nonetheless, even if physicians chose not to pass on their knowledge about contraceptives and abortifacients, evidence suggests that they were indeed available and well known in the Middle Ages.

5

Infant and Children's Health

AGING AND THE LIFE CYCLE IN PREMODERN MEDICAL THEORIES

Infant and child mortality rates were high in premodern societies; some estimates suggest that 30–40 percent of children died before the age of five, most of those before age one. If a person survived childhood, he could achieve an old age, but average life expectancy was still low. As might be expected, given the high infant and child mortality rates and lower life expectancies, far greater attention is given in the medical texts to considering the health care needs of infants and children, but physicians did also consider some conditions of old age and the treatment of the elderly. In many cases, children and the elderly were viewed as similarly weakened and thus in need of similar medical accommodations, for example, in terms of the dosage of drugs provided.

The Ayurvedic tradition recognizes a correlation between the *doshas* and age, noting that *vata* (wind) predominates in old age, *pitta* (bile) in middle age, and *kapha* (phlegm) in childhood. Childhood lasts to age 16 and is characterized by rapid growth; in adulthood, vitality achieves its high point, lasting to age fifty-five after which old age ensues with a period of mental and physical deterioration. The *Susruta Samhita* advises physicians to tailor all drugs according to the age of the patient so that "the use of strong or drastic purgatives, and cauterization are alike prohibited in cases of children and old men. They should be used only in weakened or modified forms if found indispensably necessary" (Bhishagratna 1907, 323). This recommendation reflects the general concern that the young and the old face different medical concerns and require different forms of treatment.

In traditional Chinese medicine, the aging process is attributed to the waning of yin in the body, so that by age 40, the yin is reduced to half its natural capacity and vitality starts to degenerate. According to the *Huangdi Neiching*, "At the age of fifty the body grows heavy and the ears no longer hear well nor is the vision of the eyes clear any longer. At the age of sixty the life-producing force of *yin* declines and impotence sets in." Furthermore, reflecting its Taoist influences and the importance of following "the Way" to achieve a healthy harmony in life, it maintains that those who achieve the appropriate balance in their lives can prevent the depletion of yin and thus "will retain good hearing and clear vision, their bodies will remain light and strong, and although they grow old in years they will remain able-bodied and flourishing" (Veith 1972, 121).

The Western medical tradition, guided by the theory of the relationship among the four humors and four qualities in the body, reflects similar notions about the life cycle and aging to those seen in Ayurvedic and Chinese medicine. Aristotle (384–322 B.C.E.) had observed that the innate heat of a body gradually diminishes the body's moisture over its life span, and Galen of Pergamum (129–ca. 216) later expanded upon this idea to identify the innate heat as the primary quality necessary for life. In the 13th century in Europe, a number of scholastic physicians took up this notion and further developed it to consider how an individual's complexion or personal humoral balance would change throughout life and lead to a natural death. In brief, these theories maintained that nutrition was necessary not only for growth but also to repair parts of the body consumed by the innate heat. The *humidum radicale*, otherwise known as the "radical" or "seminal" moisture, was deemed the other fuel necessary for maintaining the body's innate heat. Although the exact nature and abundance of this substance was the subject of much theoretical debate, in general, the radical moisture was thought to be the most fundamental fluid, which derived from the seminal seed involved in reproduction and as such carried the formative virtue of the soul. Thus, once the body was unable to assimilate nutrition properly and/or had been drained of the vital *humidum radicale*, the body's innate heat would run out of "fuel" and be extinguished, resulting in a natural death. Defined in this way, aging is viewed as a process of drying out characterized by the youthful age of intense heat and activity, followed by a gradual decline in middle age, and then the drying out (and shriveling up) associated with old age. At each stage of life, therefore, people's complexions would change, making them susceptible to different diseases as well as necessitating different forms of therapeutic intervention.

PEDIATRIC MEDICINE

Mesopotamian Cures for Children

The Mesopotamians feared that children, newborns in particular, were in danger of assault by demons that would result in disease. Many different medical practitioners had roles in protecting infants and children from such dangers. From the beginning, midwives were expected to perform protective rituals on newborns soon after delivery. A midwife would cut the umbilical cord with a special knife or sliver of reed, wash the infant, and apply oils to its chest while reciting special incantations. After these protective rituals had been performed, the infant would be presented with objects appropriate for its sex: weapons for a boy, a spindle or other domestic items for a girl. After the initial protective rituals performed by the midwife, the *asu* (physician) might be asked to treat sick children with his incantations and herbal medicines, but in most cases, the care of infant illnesses seems to largely fall to the *ashipu* (exorcist), who specialized in performing the necessary rituals to expel invading demons.

One ancient Mesopotamian tablet was devoted entirely to the medical problems of infants, and others also had specific cures for treating the diseases of children. A number of specific demons were believed to threaten the lives of infants and were associated with particular conditions; the most widely recognized being the Kubu-demon, lilu-demons (and their female counterparts, lilitu-demons), and the most fearsome demoness, Lamastu. Kubu-demons were ghoulish beings that especially directed their malevolence against newborns. References to Kubu-demons as ones who were "not buried in a grave" or as "little ones who do not know their own names (and) who never saw the sun" suggest that they were conceived of as demonic manifestations of stillborn children. They were commonly believed to cause harm to newborns: "If it [the infant] cries during the evening without interruption and does not want to drink milk, it is the hand of Kubu. If (the infant) wheezes before it is put to bed, it is the hand of Kubu. If it continually cries and wheezes, it is the hand of Kubu" (Scurlock 1991, 135–185). In order to dispel these demons, parents would provide personal names for stillborn children in an attempt to make them feel welcome in the family and thus less inclined to inflict harm on their live sibling. Furthermore, it appears that midwives worked a protective ritual on the afterbirth, symbolic of a stillborn twin to the newborn, to turn its attention away from the baby, which had been separated from it when the umbilical cord was cut.

Lilu-demons and lilitu-demons were the ghosts of young men and women who had died before they had the opportunity to marry or have children themselves. They were supposed to sneak into people's homes seeking other children to become the husbands or wives they never had. The *ashipu* could perform a ritual to unite lilu-demons and lilitu-demons in marriage and send them to a properly provisioned home in the underworld, thus placating them and turning their attention away from snatching living children.

The most frightening threat to infants and children was the demoness Lamastu, a minor divinity and daughter of the sky-god Anu. Lamastu is often described as a hideous woman seeking to steal children to nurse as her own. No wonder that the symptoms she causes are sometimes associated with nursing: "If the infant is continually frightened at its mother's breast (and) cries continually, or if it is continually disturbed (and) he jumps from the lap of his mother and cries a lot, the daughter of Anu has chosen him" (Scurlock 1991, 155). Furthermore, she was associated with fevers, abdominal distension, cramps, diarrhea, dizziness, and convulsions in children. The *ashipu* would make offerings to Lamastu in order to induce her to turn her attentions away from the sick child or to fulfill her need to be a mother. One elaborate cure directed at Lamastu requires the *ashipu* to speak an incantation and perform a ritual:

> [Speak the incantation] "I have married you to a black dog, your slave; I have poured out well water for you, (so) let up, go away, withdraw and distance yourself from this little one, child of his god." . . . [The ritual to go with the incantation]: (On the first day in the morning), you make a Lamastu represented as imprisoned. You arrange offerings; you put twelve breads made from unsifted flour before her.

> You pour out well water for her. You marry her to a black dog. For three days you have her sit at the head of the patient. You put the heart of a piglet in her mouth. You pour out hot broth for her. You put out dried bread for her. You give (her) a wooden *sikkatu*-vessel full of oil. You provide her with (provisions). You recite the spell (every day) in the morning, noon, and evening. On the third day in the late afternoon you take her out and bury (her) in the corner of a wall. (Scurlock 1991, 157)

Many dedicatory plaques made for Lamastu show her riding in a boat filled with her various presents and accompanied by a dog and a piglet, which she is suckling. Interpreted in relation to the plaques, the ritual appears as a kind of bribe and an effort to get her to turn her maternal attentions toward the piglet.

The selection of wet nurses posed another significant consideration for parents seeking to maintain their infant's health. Indeed, the use of wet nurses was prevalent enough in Mesopotamian society to merit attention in the Code of Hammurabi (ca. 1750 B.C.E.): "When a seignior gave his son to a wet-nurse and that son has died in the care of the wet-nurse, if the wet-nurse has then made a contract for another son without the knowledge of his father and mother, they shall prove it against her and they shall cut off her breast because she made a contract for another son without the knowledge of his father and mother" (Meek 1969, 175). Given the health dangers associated with nursing, parents would want to be certain that the nurse did not take on other children, possibly reducing the care and feeding their own child would receive.

Egyptian Cures for Children

Like the Mesopotamians, the ancient Egyptians employed a variety of religious and magical cures to protect infants and children. One example:

> Mayest thou flow away, she who comes in the darkness and enters in furtively, with her nose behind her, and her face turned backwards, failing in that for which she came!
>
> Hast thou come to kiss this child? I will not let thee kiss him! Hast thou come to silence (him)? I will not let thee set silence over him! Hast thou come to injure him? I will not let thee injure him! Hast thou come to take him away? I will not let thee take him away from me!
>
> I have made his magical protection against thee out of clover (that is what sets an obstacle), out of onions (what injures thee), out of honey (sweet for men, but bitter for those who are yonder), out of the roe of the *abdju*-fish, out of the jawbone of the *meret*-fish, and out of the backbone of the perch. (Wilson 1969, 328)

The Egyptian medical papyri also reflect the importance of religious and magical rituals designed for the care of infants and children. In the Ebers papyrus, we find a number of tests to assess the viability of the infant immediately after birth: if the baby cries *ny* (yes), it will live, but if it cries *mebi* (no), it will die; or, if when turned head downward it groans, it will die. The Ebers papyrus does not specify what to do in response to these tests, but in the Ramesseum IV papyrus, which is devoted to problems of childbirth and neonatal care, a different test is proposed: the *swnw* is advised to give a piece of the placenta rubbed in milk to the newborn, and if it is vomited, the child will not survive. This test is followed by

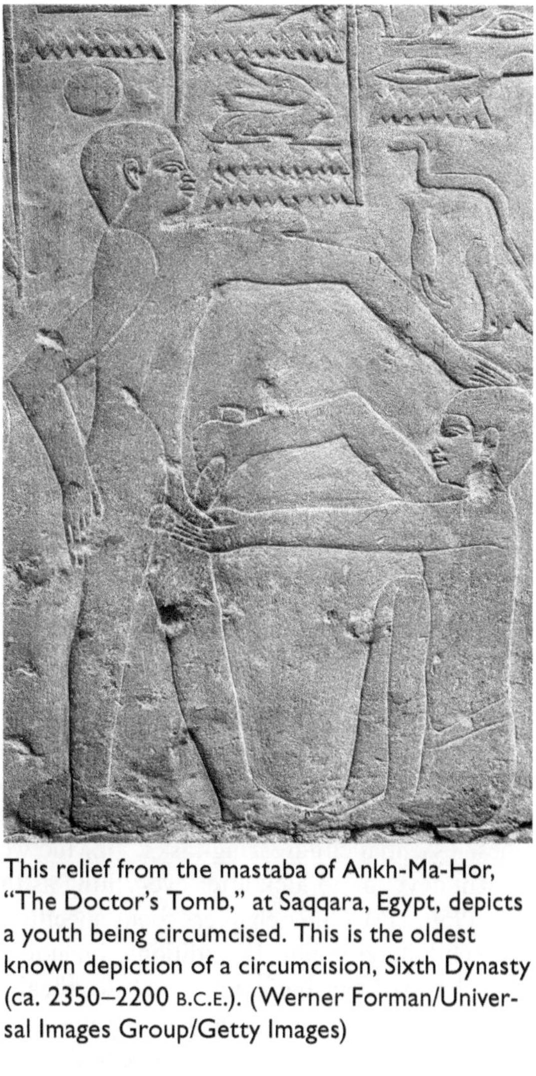

This relief from the mastaba of Ankh-Ma-Hor, "The Doctor's Tomb," at Saqqara, Egypt, depicts a youth being circumcised. This is the oldest known depiction of a circumcision, Sixth Dynasty (ca. 2350–2200 B.C.E.). (Werner Forman/Universal Images Group/Getty Images)

recommendations for protective incantations and rituals that should be performed for the child on the day it is born. Magico-religious cures are not uncommon in the medical papyri, but the high proportion of them among cures for infants suggests just how tenuous early life was.

Medical papyri also offer more naturalistic cures and treatments for children. They explain common procedures like the ligation of the umbilical cord in some detail and discuss alternative methods for giving drugs to newborns, who cannot swallow pills—the medicine could be rubbed with fresh milk on the mother's nipples prior to nursing or the mother could take it directly, suggesting the belief that its curative powers would be passed on to the child through her milk. Certain drugs are prescribed for infants to induce them to accept the breast, another remedy prescribes a medicine including poppy to stop children from crying, and sucking on a fried mouse was recommended for children with teething pains. Different remedies (combining drugs and incantations) are offered for the medical conditions of older children, such as retention of the urine, cough, the *baa* disease (characterized by fatigue of the heart, green lips, and weak knees), as well as to stop bed-wetting.

The ancient Egyptians also performed circumcisions on some young male children. The Greek author Herodotus reports that the Egyptians were the first people to practice circumcision, and the operation is depicted in a relief from around 2345 B.C.E. on the doorway to the tomb in the city of Memphis of Ankh-Ma-Hor, vizier of King Teti, the only surgical operation depicted in Egyptian art. This operation was likely performed as a ritual initiation into manhood or as an initiation ceremony for the *hem-ka* priests, rather than for medical reasons. It is not clear why Ankh-ma-hor might have wanted this scene in his tomb, or if it is supposed to depict his own circumcision. In either case, evidence from mummies indicates that the operation was normally performed in late puberty, and it was not done to all male members of the social classes who were mummified. The practice was probably introduced to the Hebrews during their bondage in Egypt, for whom it signified the covenant between the Hebrew people and the Lord (as explained in Gen. 17:10–14). Another scene in the Bible describes Moses's wife, Zipporah, cutting off the foreskin of their son with a sharp flint stone while journeying from Midian to Egypt (Exod. 4:25–26).

Children and Medicine in Ancient Greece and Rome

Greek and Roman medical texts also expressed concern for the differentiated treatment of children and especially the care of newborns. Some, like the Roman Pliny the Elder (23–79 C.E.), provided advice that mixed naturalistic medicinal remedies with amulets and magical cures. For example, Pliny explained, "The tooth of a wolf tied on as an amulet keeps away childish terrors and ailments due to teething, as does also a piece of wolf's skin. . . . The brain of a she-goat, passed through a golden ring, is given drop by drop by the Magic to babies, before they are fed with milk, to guard them from epilepsy and other diseases of babies" (Jones 1963, 173–175). By contrast, the physician Soranus of Ephesus (fl. 100 C.E.) focused more on offering naturalistic medical advice. He wrote a treatise on gynecology in Greek in which he dedicated several chapters to the appropriate treatment of newborns. He describes how to sever the umbilical cord, how to breastfeed and wean the infant, how one should swaddle a baby, and how to teach it to walk so as to promote the proper development and shape of the limbs. Betraying his own biases, Soranus notes that in Rome people were more likely to mishandle these essential childrearing tasks, "for the women in this city do not possess sufficient devotion to look after everything as the purely Grecian women do" (Temkin 1956, 116). Other chapters focus specifically on the treatment of certain infant and childhood medical conditions, including teething, thrush, inflamed tonsils, and illnesses causing coughs and diarrhea. Furthermore, Soranus explains how one should select an appropriate wet nurse, taking into account not only the state of her breasts and supply of milk, but also her character,

> Since by nature the nursling becomes similar to the nurse and accordingly grows sullen if the nurse is ill-tempered, but of mild disposition if she is even-tempered. . . . For the same reason the wet nurse should not be superstitious and prone to ecstatic states so that she may not expose the infant to danger when led astray by fallacious reasoning, sometimes even trembling like mad. (Temkin 1956, 93)

Soranus also draws attention to the practice of exposure or child abandonment in the ancient Greek and Roman worlds. He writes,

> The majority of barbarians, as the Germans and Scythians, and even some of the Hellenes [i.e., Greeks], put the newborn into cold water in order to make it firm and to let die, as not worth rearing, one that cannot bear the chilling but becomes livid or convulsed. . . . We, however, reject all of these. For cold, on account of its strong and sudden condensing action the like of which the child has not experienced, harms all; and though the harm resulting from the cold escapes notice in those more resistant it is, on the other hand, demonstrated by those susceptible to disease when they are seized by convulsions and apoplexies. Certainly, the fact that the child did

> not withstand the injury does not prove that it was impossible for it to live if unharmed; more resistant children will also thrive better if not harmed in any way. (Temkin 1956, 82)

Despite his misgivings about this harsh treatment, Soranus begins his account of the care of newborns by explaining how to recognize "whether it is worth rearing or not" based on whether it was deemed strong enough to survive. The Greek author Polybius (ca. 203–120 B.C.E.) had previously noted that some Greek families tried to limit themselves to having only one or two children and Aristotle (384–322 B.C.E.) implied that employing contraceptives or abortifacients to control family size was acceptable so long as they were used prior to the formation of the fetus (which he believed occurred in the middle of the second trimester). Soranus's advice reveals that exposure, abandoning weak or sickly infants in the wilderness, was also a common method for preventing family growth in the ancient world. Plutarch (ca. 46–ca. 120 C.E.), a Greek historian, makes it clear that this custom was regularly practiced by the Spartans, who wished to raise only those who would become strong warriors, but it was likely common throughout the Greek and Roman world.

The ultimate decision in both the Greek and Roman worlds as to whether to raise the child rested with the father. In both cultures, ceremonies were held some days after the birth in which the baby was revealed to the community, symbolically marking its acceptance into the family. In Athens, a ritual called the *amphidromia* was held on the seventh day after birth, which entailed performing sacrifices to the gods followed by a ceremony in which the father carried the infant through the doorway to the house, which would often be decorated with wool for a girl and with an olive garland for a boy, and placed it before the household hearth. Similarly, in Rome on the eighth day after birth for a girl and the ninth day after birth for a boy, the ritual of the *dies lustricus* (purification day) was held in which the mother and child were both purified and the child was given a name, marking its acceptance into the family.

Pediatric Care in the Ayurvedic Tradition

Ayurvedic medical texts contain extensive information devoted to the care of infants and children. According to the *Susruta Samhita* and the *Caraka Samhita*, immediately after birth, the newborn should be cleansed, and its mouth should be washed with a mixture of rock salt and clarified butter, after which the umbilical cords should be cut. The postnatal ceremony of *jatakarman* would also be performed in which the infant is given an electuary of honey, butter, some plant juices, and powdered gold with the recitation of specific mantras, to provide intelligence, long life, and strength to the baby. In the following days, a series of further rituals would be performed to protect the infant and mother from demons; the room in which they slept would be strewn with various aromatic substances (crushed sesame seed, mustard, and linseed), a purifying fire would be maintained to fumigate the chamber, and a Brahman would perform atonement prayers for 10 days, during which time friends and relatives were expected to keep watch, sing songs, and do their best to create a cheerful environment. Furthermore, a bundle of twigs and plants called *raksoghna* (demon-killing) was to be tied above the door to the room and also placed on the child's body to ward off evil spirits. On the 10th day after birth, the woman was allowed to rise from bed, and the naming ceremony (*namakarana*) would take place in which the child would receive its popular name and another name, derived from the constellation at the time of its birth. In the months after birth, further ceremonies were performed: in the fourth month the "first going out" rite (*niskramana*) occurred, when the child was dressed in fine clothes and taken out of the room to worship the gods, then in the sixth to eighth month a physician would make a hole in its earlobes (in the right ear first for boys, the left ear first for girls) from which golden rings would be hung.

The *Caraka* has further advice on how the child's room should be constructed and furnished. The author emphasizes that it should be well ventilated, filled with sunlight, fumigated with aromatic substances and kept clean and free of insects. In addition to attending to the child's physical environment, the *Caraka* also expresses concern for attending to the child's emotional well-being. Appropriate toys are described, with emphasis on making them safe and entertaining: they should be colorful, produce fun noises, be easy to handle, and not be too heavy, sharp, or otherwise dangerous or frightening. Furthermore, the author urges parents to take precautions against frightening the child by wakening it suddenly or handling it violently and not to threaten it with demons even when it is disobedient or become angry when it cries or does not eat, lest this disturb the balance of the *doshas* in the body, making it vulnerable to demonic possession.

Possession by demons was believed to be one of the greatest threats to the health of infants and children. Symptoms of demonic possession included fever, crying, biting the nurse, vomiting, inability to sleep soundly, diarrhea, hoarseness, and loss of appetite. The *Susruta* describes nine different *grahas*, demons that caused disease in children, especially those children who lived in an unclean environment, with dirty wet nurses, or those who are angry, frightened, or in a bad mood. Thus, the precautions described in the *Caraka* for the careful maintenance of the room and toys for children can be seen as a means of warding off the threat of *grahas* and other evil spirits. In addition to managing the child's living space, certain medicines, baths, sacrifices, and invocations are called for to drive out demons from those children who are possessed.

Ayurvedic medical texts also attribute children's diseases to the influence of the mother's or nurse's milk. Thus, the *Susruta* explains,

> A child nursed at the breast of any and every woman for want of a nurse of the commendable type, may fall an easy prey to disease owing to the fact of the promiscuous nature of the milk proving uncongenial to its physical temperament. The milk of a nurse not being pressed out and spelled off at the outset may produce cough, difficulty of breathing, or vomiting of the child, owing to the sudden rush of the accumulated milk into its throat choking up the channels. Hence a child should not be allowed to suck in such milk. (Bhishagratna 1911, 227)

The wet nurse was supposed to be chaste, to come from a good family of the same caste as the infant's family, and to have a living male child of her own. The nurse was also expected to attend to her hygiene and diet to ensure that her milk would not become unhealthy. Bad milk could induce the derangement of the *doshas* in the child leading to various diseases, such as *ksiralasaka* (milk-tympany), a disease recognized by watery, frothy and bad-smelling diarrhea, white-yellow and sticky urine, fever, vomiting, and flatulence.

Pediatrics in Traditional Chinese Medicine

The earliest medical texts in traditional Chinese medicine, like the *Huangdi Neiching*, do not give much attention to the diseases or treatment of children as distinct from general medicine. The development, however, of a meritocratic system of advancement for civil and military officials during the Han dynasty (206 B.C.E.–220 C.E.), which highlighted the need to educate young boys in preparation for future government service, drew increased attention to children and childhood. Han leaders called for the establishment of a public school system and numerous books were written to advise mothers on the best methods of child-rearing and early childhood education. One of these texts even declared "learning begins in the womb" and offered advice on appropriate activities for pregnant women to prepare their fetus while it was still in the uterus. The education of girls received far less attention since they would not have been able to assume public duties in the military or in the civil service.

The *Book of Rites*, compiled originally by Confucius (551–479 B.C.E.) and re-edited during the Han dynasty, describes a number of rules or rituals for conduct, including passages concerning the incorporation of newborn children into the family, and rituals to mark the growing development of the child and its relation to the family. According to the text, the mother and newborn were to be confined to a separate room until the third day after birth when a divinatory ceremony, including necessary sacrifices and rituals, would be held to identify a good man (not the father), who would receive the child and carry him out of the birth chamber to his bedroom. After three months, another ritual was held in which the child's hair would be shaved off (leaving certain portions, depending on whether it was a boy or girl) and then it would be taken from the bedchamber and presented to the father, who would only then give the child a name. These rituals recognize the gradual introduction of the child into the family and public life. Other celebratory rituals, like the hair-pinning and capping of teenage boys and girls and marriage rituals, marked the child's further progress into later life stages (adolescence and adulthood).

These developments regarding views of children during the Han period likely stimulated growing medical interest in the treatment of children. Under the Sui dynasty (581–618 C.E.) and more so under the Tang dynasty (618–907 C.E.), the specialized field of pediatric medicine (*erke*) developed rapidly. The physician Sun Simiao (581–682 C.E.) devoted a chapter in his *Qianjin Yaofang (Prescriptions of the Thousand Ounces of Gold)* to maternal and infantile disorders. Declaring that nothing was more important than raising children well, Sun Simiao described appropriate methods for bathing infants, selecting wet nurses, and regulating feeding. Reflecting the growing interest in diseases of children, the Imperial Medical Academy during the Tang dynasty created a new department of pediatrics for training specialized pediatricians. Pediatric medicine took greater steps during the Song dynasty (960–1279 C.E.) and Yuan dynasty (1271–1368 C.E.). The physician Qian Yi (1035–1117 C.E.) devoted 40 years of his life to the treatment of children, and his student Yan Xiaozhong recorded his observations in the *Xiao'er Yaozheng Zhijue* (*The Appropriate Way of Recognizing and Treating Infant Maladies*), which focused on the physiological, pathological, and therapeutic aspects of pediatric medicine. Among other things, Qian Yi distinguished between the symptoms and treatment of measles, chickenpox, and smallpox. He viewed smallpox as a disease of children (reflecting the fact that it was an endemic disease in China by this time) and described it in particular as being produced by a fetal toxin, passed from parents to children. He also developed specialized medical formulas for use in treating children, emphasizing that they required different treatment than adults. His book was followed by a number of other texts focused on pediatric medicine, reflecting the fact that this field was well established during the Song dynasty.

The philosopher Han Fei Tzu (ca. 280–233 B.C.E.) observed that it was common in his day for couples to expose infant girls rather than raise them. Laws from the Qin dynasty against infanticide confirm this practice. In a legal text from 217 B.C.E., we learn that parents had the right to kill newborns that were deformed, but the law did not condone infanticide when "the child's body is whole and without deformity [and the child is killed] merely because [the parents] have too many children and do not wish it to live" (McLeod and Yates 1981, 151). Later texts also denounce infanticide. In the mid-seventh century C.E., the *Nan Shi (History of the Southern Dynasties)* reports that the governor of Ren Fang passed a law declaring that parents who refused to bring up their child should be judged as if they had committed murder. These condemnations likely reflect a desire to maintain a strong population to protect imperial power. Nonetheless, other sources suggest that child abandonment and infanticide were prevalent in ancient China. Indeed, the *Yili* (*Book of Etiquette and Ceremonial*), a Confucian compilation on social rituals composed during the Han dynasty, discusses mourning rituals for children, recognizing different procedures depending upon the age of the child when it died. For those that died between the ages of three months and seven years, it indicates that the parents should wear no mourning garments; it implies through silence that those who die when younger than three months of age (prior to being received and named by the father) would not be mourned at all. Given these accounts, it appears likely that child abandonment and infanticide were common in China, as in other parts of the ancient world.

Childcare and Pediatric Medicine in Medieval Europe

Medieval Europe witnessed a dramatic increase in the number of texts concerned with childcare and childhood from the 12th to the 15th centuries. Medical texts also gave greater attention to the specific medical needs of children and the treatment of childhood diseases. The proliferation of these writings reflects the importance given to providing for the physical, psychological, and spiritual well-being of children during this period, both among church leaders and the wider community in general. In fact, the vast attention given to children in this period

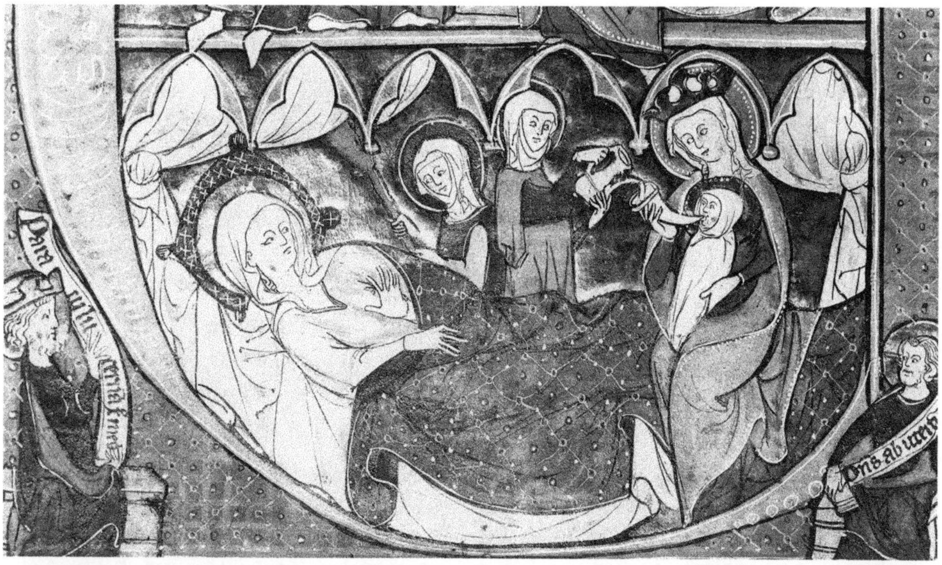

In this 13th-century French manuscript illustration, a mother is shown in bed attended by another woman. On the right, two women use a cow's horn to feed her infant. (Wellcome Collection)

challenges some earlier historical scholarship suggesting that people did not value children or the concept of childhood during the Middle Ages.

Physicians wrote extensively on infant and child health care, not only within their more general medical manuals but also in treatises dedicated specifically to child and infant care, such as the *Practica puerorum in cunabulis* (*Practical Manual on Children in Cradles*) and the *De passionibus puerorum* (*On the Diseases of Children*). The physician Michele Savonarola (1385–1468) recognized that the treatment of infants and children presented a distinct challenge because the patients were often unable to articulate their complaints, making the task of diagnosis more difficult, and, furthermore, he felt that the normal diagnostic measures of taking the pulse and studying the urine were not as useful in children since they were smaller and their bodies behaved differently. Savonarola and other authors recognized a wide range of diseases specific to children such as *marasmus* (what we might recognize as a severe form of malnutrition), which was believed to be caused by the untimely consumption of the body's radical moisture (*humidum radicale*). Other conditions like "*parvitas corporis*" (achondroplasia, or dwarfism), smallpox, and measles were also described as children's diseases, along with a wide range of conditions causing vomiting, wheezing, coughing, and fevers. Cures were always supposed to be gentle, and bloodletting and cautery were deemed inappropriate, especially for infants. There were also many remedies to stop infants from crying, like the magical-astrological cure of putting an image of Capricorn on the infant's navel; the best remedy, however, was nursing—hence why Savonarola called the nurse's nipple the "baby-pacifier."

The authors of medical texts did not limit themselves to offering medical advice about disease; they also discussed different aspects of child-rearing and some even addressed the appropriate moral education of children. Physicians, following their Greek sources, offered advice on the selection of wet nurses but advocated that mothers should nurse their own children; Bernard de Gordon (active in the late 13th and early 14th centuries) complained that "women nowadays are too delicate or too haughty, or they do not like the inconvenience" of nursing their own children (Demaitre 1977, 474). They also offered advice on how and when children should be weaned. Savonarola, for example, argued that boys should be weaned at around age three, six months to a year later than girls, because, he said, males live longer than females. Other physicians suggested that in order to encourage weaning, the mother or wet nurse should apply unpleasant substances like mustard to their nipples, although many indicated that this could be dangerous and warned that one should not wean a child too suddenly. Finally, medical texts that considered children's health also frequently discussed methods for teaching them how to walk, speak, and learn good manners.

Numerous accounts of divine intervention or miraculous cures for children survive, providing insight into the kinds of dangers they faced. According to these accounts, children received miraculous cures for a wide range of illnesses or disabilities, indicating the extent to which they were susceptible to disease and confirming modern impressions of the high infant mortality for this period. In many cases, children, especially those under the age of six, received miracle cures after having been injured in the course of normal childhood activities rather than for diseases (e.g., drowning, burns, choking or suffocation, fractures, lacerations). Older children faced dangers not only from play but also from working with adults alongside large farm animals in fields or in the course of performing other chores, such as collecting firewood or water.

Records of miracle cures may suggest that young boys and girls were often poorly supervised, but they also make clear the extent to which parents loved their children. Parents would go to great lengths to achieve a miracle cure for their children, often taking the child on an extended pilgrimage in order to pray at a saint's shrine. Many saints were known for curing children, but the story of Saint Guinefort is especially surprising. According to legend, a greyhound that had been defending his child from attackers was unjustly killed by its master, who thought the dog had been trying to harm the child. Peasants in the nearby region learned of this event and began to venerate the dog as a saint, Saint Guinefort, and brought their ailing children from miles around to pray at his "shrine," and they reported many successful cures. The cult of Saint Guinefort continued to thrive in the 13th century, despite efforts by the church to denounce the veneration of the dog as sacrilegious superstition.

In the 13th and 14th centuries, it became common practice to have infants baptized soon after birth, replacing previous practice of performing baptisms only twice per year. The religious ceremony of baptism performed by a priest marked the formal, public recognition of the child and its entry into the Christian community. The religious belief that anyone who died without being baptized would not be accepted into heaven placed particular importance on performing this ritual soon after birth. Indeed, recognizing the dangers facing unbaptized children, Church authorities even allowed midwives to perform emergency baptisms (even in utero) when it appeared that the child would not survive the birth process. As the child grew, other sacraments marked different life stages, such as confirmation when the child reached adolescence and then the sacrament of marriage marking entry into adulthood.

Although infanticide and child abandonment were practiced in medieval Europe, parents still often expressed a concern for the survival of the child's soul. One story from the 15th century recounts the desperate case of a young woman named Denisette Bieart, who gave birth in a courtyard outside an inn and after delivering a daughter,

> went into the inn, where she took a basin and water . . . and having done this she climbed up to the privies, and there she took the said child by one of its arms and threw the water on its head, saying, "My child, I baptize you in the name of the Father, the Son, and the Holy Spirit" . . . and then threw her child in the privies of the inn. (Park 2010, 25–26)

This account of infanticide reminds us of the importance of baptism in medieval society; indeed, a mother could face harsher penalties for killing an unbaptized child. More typical accounts tell of children abandoned on church steps or outside monasteries. In many of these cases, the child was left with a little bag of salt, which served as an indication that the child had not yet been baptized and as payment for its baptism. These stories reflect the general hope that the child would survive and be raised elsewhere, even if the parents could not afford to raise it themselves.

6

Diseases

STUDYING DISEASE IN HISTORY

Studying the patterns of infectious diseases in the premodern world is fraught with difficulties. Paleopathologists offer some insight into the prevalence of diseases in early societies by observing signs of pathological lesions in human skeletal remains, yet only chronic, degenerative diseases (e.g., tuberculosis, leprosy, and syphilis) leave visible evidence of infection in hard tissues that can be studied today; individuals who die from an infectious disease typically do so long before the condition could cause deformation in teeth or bones. These efforts are further complicated by the fact that it is not always easy to know with certainty which disease may have caused a particular pathological lesion. Advances in techniques to extract DNA samples from human remains (e.g., from surviving dental pulp tissue or mummified remains) have made it possible to look for signs of other infectious organisms that do not otherwise cause damage to hard tissues (e.g., finding the DNA for the agents causing diseases such as bubonic and pneumonic plague or smallpox). Nonetheless, these techniques still only allow a fragmentary picture of the patterns of disease in early societies.

Another means of learning about the incidence of infectious diseases in premodern societies is to examine the written evidence. Interpreting premodern accounts of disease presents its own challenges, however. These accounts do not always list enough specific symptoms to allow modern physicians to make a clear diagnosis of what the disease may have been. A case in point is the disease *di'u*, described in ancient Mesopotamia as being a summer affliction characterized by fevers, sweating, and headaches. Based on the general symptoms, we might associate *di'u* with a range of different infectious diseases, parasitic diseases such as malaria, or with heat stroke. Thus, Mesopotamians seem to have recognized a range of conditions under the heading of a single disease entity, *di'u*, whereas modern physicians would wish to distinguish among them. When looking at diseases in history, differential diagnosis, the systematic practice of discerning the specific cause of a disease from a number of related possibilities, is further complicated by difficulties in translation or understanding what is meant by specific words, like the reference to "Khonsu's tumor" (*aat net Khonsu*) discussed in the Egyptian Ebers papyrus; different scholars have translated this phrase variously to describe bubonic plague buboes, the growths associated with tubercular leprosy, or possibly cancer. Thus, accurately determining disease patterns in the premodern world based on the written evidence is not always possible.

For historians of medicine, the task of identifying the actual disease described in the written records is often less important than trying to learn how a disease was understood in a given society and how that might shape an individual's experience of illness. With these goals in mind, it is worth considering the comparative theories of disease in different cultures and the social responses to some specific diseases within those cultures. Epidemic diseases posed a constant threat, and a variety of plagues spread regularly through premodern societies. Smallpox and bubonic plague rank among the most deadly epidemic diseases in world history, and they elicited a variety of responses in different cultures. Although it did not claim as many lives as smallpox or bubonic plague, leprosy was prevalent throughout premodern societies and created its own set of challenges. In this chapter, we will consider the medical and social responses to these diseases in world history.

EPIDEMICS AND THEORIES OF DISEASE CAUSATION

Premodern societies had a number of ways for explaining the cause and process of disease in a single person. A range of explanations might be offered to account for the onset of disease in an individual, including the role of personal sin, invading demons or evil spirits, or inadequate diet and regimen. These theories, however, could not easily explain why hundreds and thousands of people could all suddenly fall ill and die at around the same time, while exhibiting the same symptoms. The sudden appearance and rapid spread of epidemic disease within a large population requires a different explanation for how disease spreads that not only accounts for the nature of an individual body but also makes clear why multiple people would be infected by the same ailment.

Today we are accustomed to thinking of the multiple vectors by which diseases can be transmitted. In the face of fears of a possible deadly influenza pandemic, the spread of viruses like HIV and SARS (severe acute respiratory syndrome), and the rise of drug-resistant strains of bacteria causing infectious diseases like tuberculosis, we are continually reminded of the dangers of contagion, the human-to-human transmission of disease. Despite the fact that people in premodern societies no doubt recognized that certain diseases could be transmitted from a sick person to a healthy one, in general, theories of contagion played only a minor role in early explanations for the spread of disease. Even in cases in which premodern people employed terminology to express a concept of contagion, they did not necessarily conceive of the mechanisms of transmission in the way that we do today, that is, by touch or other contact with an infected person that could pass along a "germ." In the Greek world, Galen of Pergamum (129–ca. 216 C.E.) was well aware of the fact that some diseases could be caught from other sufferers and considered the possibility of "seeds" of disease that could be transmitted between people, but he did not give much weight to it in his considerations on the spread of disease, and the concept was not developed in later Roman, Islamic, or medieval European medical writings that built upon the Greek philosophical tradition. Likewise, Chinese and Indian medical texts reflect an awareness of diseases that can be transmitted by human-to-human contact, but place far greater emphasis on other explanations for the spread of disease.

Healers in premodern societies generally did not believe that contagion was sufficient to explain how so many people could acquire the same illness so swiftly. Most often, doctors emphasized the role of environmental factors when discussing the cause and rapid spread of epidemic disease. The Greek Hippocratic text, *Airs, Waters, Places*, examined the different diseases that might be caused by seasonal changes, different winds (depending on the direction of the winds and whether they are hot or cold), proximity to bodies of water (e.g., spring waters vs. marshlands and swamps), or by other astronomical and meteorological factors. The author claims that attending to these factors will allow the physician "to tell what epidemic diseases will attack the city either in summer or in winter. . . . For knowing the changes of the seasons, and the risings and settings of the stars, with the circumstances of each of these phenomena, he will know beforehand the nature of the year that is coming" (Jones 1984, 73). Building upon these ideas, Greek physicians developed the theory of miasmas, fetid or corrupted airs, which could arise in a region and cause many people to contract the same disease in a short period of time by adversely affecting everybody's humoral balance. Traditional Chinese medicine and Ayurvedic medicine also attributed the spread of epidemic diseases to the negative effects environmental factors might have on people's bodily systems. The *Huangdi Neiching* (*The Yellow Emperor's Classic of Internal Medicine*), for example, offered the following advice:

> Huang Di asked, "As extremes and disharmonies occur during the interplay of the natural elements, plagues and disease arise to cause suffering in people. What are the ways that can help to prevent the effects of imbalance from the macrocosm upon human beings?"
>
> Qi Bo replied, "You have asked a question that deserves an answer in depth. Generally, a physician needs to be versed in the laws of the universe and its interactive dynamics, and to have a firm grasp of the knowledge of acupuncture, in order to know when to fortify a deficient and when to reduce an excessive state and how to maintain constancy of energy flow in patients." (Ni 1995, 273)

Therefore, doctors needed to known how to counteract the adverse effects of the environmental factors by fortifying the body through changes in diet and regimen or through other means such as the use of prophylactic acupuncture or bloodletting.

Epidemic diseases were also regularly attributed to divine or supernatural causes in premodern sources. In the Ayurvedic tradition, the *Susruta Samhita* categorizes diseases according to their various causes and details a range of causes for epidemic diseases:

> Sometimes a town or a city is depopulated by a curse, anger, sin, or by a monster or a demoness conjured up by a spell or incantation. Sometimes the pollens of

> poisonous flowers or grasses, etc., wafted by the winds, invade a town or a village, and produce a sort of epidemic cough, asthma, catarrh, or fever, irrespective of all constitutional peculiarities or deranged bodily humors agitated thereby. Towns and villages are known to have been depopulated through malignant astral influences, or through houses, wives, beds, seats, carriages, riding animals, gems and precious stones assuming inauspicious features. (Bhishagratna 1907, 52)

This full range of both environmental and supernatural explanations for epidemic disease is followed by a similarly wide range of therapeutic advice, including the use of drugs, but with special emphasis on performing rituals of purification and penance, praying and making sacrificial offerings to the gods, showing self-control, kindness and obedience to elders, and following other such rules of conduct which "may prove beneficial to the affected community" (Bhishagratna 1907, 52). Clearly, epidemic diseases could be explained in many ways and responses to them varied.

SMALLPOX

The earliest evidence for the origins of smallpox come from ancient Egypt and the Indus Valley; significantly, three mummies from the Eighteenth and Twentieth dynasties in Egypt (1570–1085 B.C.E.), including the pharaoh Ramses V (d. 1157 B.C.E.), show marked signs of pustular eruptions indicative of smallpox. Smallpox, caused by the *variola major* virus, had a mortality rate of 25–30 percent, and it was, therefore, especially feared. Those who survived acquired a natural immunity to the disease and so would not be subject to repeat infection. Consequently, the natural history of smallpox suggests that it probably did not exist until the rise of civilizations with sufficient populations to sustain it. After an initial incubation period of roughly 12 days, people infected by the disease would develop a high fever, headaches, and body pains, followed by the eruption of a distinctive rash developing first on the face before spreading over the arms, chest, back, and legs. The rash itself would give rise to raised pimples, then blisters, and then pustules, which dried up and turned into scabs. Those who died from the disease typically did so within three to five days, but others could succumb to complications attributed to the disease 18 days or more after the first symptoms appeared. Survivors were often left with pockmarked faces and sometimes were blinded in one or both eyes. The high mortality coupled with the danger of permanent disfiguration for survivors made this a particularly fearsome disease in the premodern world.

Hindu mythology suggests that smallpox was likely present in India at roughly the same time as in Egypt. Religious texts make numerous allusions to the worship of Shitala, the goddess of smallpox, who was supposed to possess the body of individuals, thereby causing the disease. The *Atharvaveda* also describes a series of services and prayers that Brahmin priests would offer for the worship of Shitala, which included a ritual of inoculation in which people would breathe in dried scabs from smallpox lesions to induce a mild case of the disease. These unsystematic rituals likely led to the death of many and were probably not effective enough to have thwarted large-scale outbreaks of the disease, but they offer the earliest account of inoculation measures in the world. The practice of inoculating against smallpox was later introduced into China from India during the Sung dynasty (960–1279 C.E.), where the procedure was known as "planting the flowers" since the Chinese often called smallpox pustules the "Heavenly Flowers." The earliest medical description of *masurika*, or smallpox, in the Ayurvedic tradition is found in the *Susruta Samhita*, which describes the disease as being caused by a derangement of the *doshas*. Later medical texts continued to develop diagnostic accounts of the disease, offering a range of diet, drugs, and other forms of therapy designed to correct the imbalances of the *doshas*. Both the naturalistic and divine explanations of the disease coexisted in the Indian tradition and both methods of treatment were followed.

Smallpox likely first entered China in the north with the invading of the Huns around 250 B.C.E., shortly before the Chinese had completed the protective barrier of the Great Wall. The second major outbreak entered from the south in 48 or 49 C.E. when the emperor's army went to suppress an uprising in the modern-day Hunan Province where an epidemic was in progress. More than half of the Chinese army died from the disease and the survivors brought the disease back with their prisoners. These epidemics were variously called the "Hun pox," "captive's pox," or "barbarian pox," reflecting the belief that they represented diseases brought to China from the outside world. The Taoist adept Ge Hong (ca. 281–341 C.E.) provides the earliest detailed clinical description of the disease in his *Zhouhou Beijifang* (*Emergency Prescriptions*), noting that, "this [disease] is due to poisonous air. The people say that it was introduced in the reign of Chien Wu when that king was fighting with the Huns at Nang Yang. The name of 'Hun pox' has been given to it" (Hopkins 1983, 104). In 610, Chao Yuanfang compiled a medical text, the *Zhu bing yuan hou fun* (*Compilation on the Origins of Disorders*), in which he explained that the disease was caused by an excessive accumulation of heat toxin in the body, caused by cold damage during the winter or by unseasonal noxious qi.

By the Song and Yuan periods (907–1368 C.E.), smallpox was increasingly recognized as a pediatric disorder in China, indicating that it had become endemic so that most adults had already survived exposure to it and were thus immune. Chinese physicians began to attribute the disease to the *tai du* (fetal toxin), a heat toxin introduced into the fetus by way of the mother, father, or both parents—in other words, a hereditary disease. A number of factors were proposed to account for this; for example, the mother's diet, the father's drinking, or the parents continued sexual activity during pregnancy all might elevate the amount of heat toxin in their bodies that could then be passed to the fetus. The *tai du* would remain dormant in the child's body until activated by disorderly climactic conditions, at which point it would spread through the channels of the body and cause smallpox. Recognizing that the disease used not to exist in China, physicians explained that the ancient Chinese forebears had led a purer lifestyle, which had prevented the elevation of heat toxins in their bodies so that they did not contract the disease. By implication, the decadent present-day lifestyle was responsible for the continued spread of smallpox in China and the cure required greater discipline and morality in terms of diet and other behaviors.

Smallpox entered Japan in the sixth century C.E., probably brought by Buddhist missionaries from Korea, who came with statues of the Buddha and several sacred Buddhist books sent as gifts from Korean rulers. Favoring the new religion, Japanese rulers encouraged their subjects to worship the Buddha over their indigenous Shinto gods. The fact that the missions from Korea roughly coincided with the outbreak of smallpox epidemics in Japan led many people to believe that the disease was a punishment for turning away from the Shinto gods. In response, they destroyed the Buddhist statues, burned Buddhist temples, and flogged Buddhist monks and nuns. When the epidemics did not abate, however, others feared that the pestilence was sent as punishment for destroying the images of the Buddha, so later emperors, who converted to Buddhism, erected monasteries and statues of the Buddha to help ward off the disease. In 981 C.E., a Japanese medical book, the *I Shinho*, discussed treatments for those suffering from the disease, advocating isolation in hospitals and wrapping patients in red cloths or hanging red cloths from the walls of the sickroom as a means of curing the affliction by magical influence.

Although there were likely outbreaks of smallpox in Europe, introduced from Egypt, during the early Greek and Roman periods, the earliest substantive evidence of a smallpox epidemic occurred during the reign of the Roman emperor Marcus Aurelius Antonius in the early third century C.E. Smallpox epidemics are reported in later centuries in Europe, but the population was likely not great enough to support regularly recurring epidemics of the disease until the 13th century. Prior to this, the Arabic physician Abu Bakr Muhammad ibn Zakariya al-Razi (d. ca. 925, known as Rhazes in the Latin West) wrote a medical treatise, *On Smallpox and Measles*, in which he distinguished between smallpox and measles for the first time in the Greek medical tradition. By the 13th century, several European physicians also described the causes and cures of smallpox in their medical texts, some of whom, like Gilbertus Anglicus in his *Compendium Medicinae* (ca. 1240), advocated treating patients by wrapping them in red blankets in a fashion similar to the practice in Japan. By the 15th century, smallpox was increasingly known for afflicting children, suggesting that it had become endemic in Europe by this time, just before European conquerors were to introduce the disease into the Americas.

BUBONIC PLAGUE, OR THE BLACK DEATH

The Origin and Spread of the Bubonic Plague

In the mid-14th century C.E., a pandemic spread throughout the Near East, Europe, and North Africa. The disease, known as the Black Death in Europe, is generally assumed to have been bubonic plague caused by the *Yersinia pestis* bacterium. The symptoms could be horrifying, as described by Gabriele de' Mussis (d. 1356) in his *Historia de Morbo*:

> Those of both sexes who were in health, and in no fear of death, were struck by four savage blows to the flesh. First, out of the blue, a kind of chilly stiffness troubled their bodies. They felt a tingling sensation, as if they were being pricked by the points of

arrows. The next stage was a fearsome attack which took the form of an extremely hard, solid boil [i.e., plague bubo]. In some people this developed under the armpit and in others in the groin between the scrotum and the body. As it grew more solid, its burning heat caused the patients to fall into an acute and putrid fever, with severe headaches. As it intensified its extreme bitterness could have various effects. In some cases it gave rise to an intolerable stench. In others it brought vomiting of blood, or swellings near the place from which the corrupt humor arose: on the back, across the chest, near the thigh. Some people lay as if in a drunken stupor and could not be roused. Behold the swellings, the warning signs sent by the Lord. All these people were in danger of dying. Some died on the very day the illness took possession of them, others on the next day, others—the majority—between the third and fifth day. There was no known remedy for the vomiting of blood. Those who fell into a coma, or suffered a swelling or the stink of corruption very rarely escaped. But from the fever it was sometimes possible to make a recovery (Horrox 1994, 24).

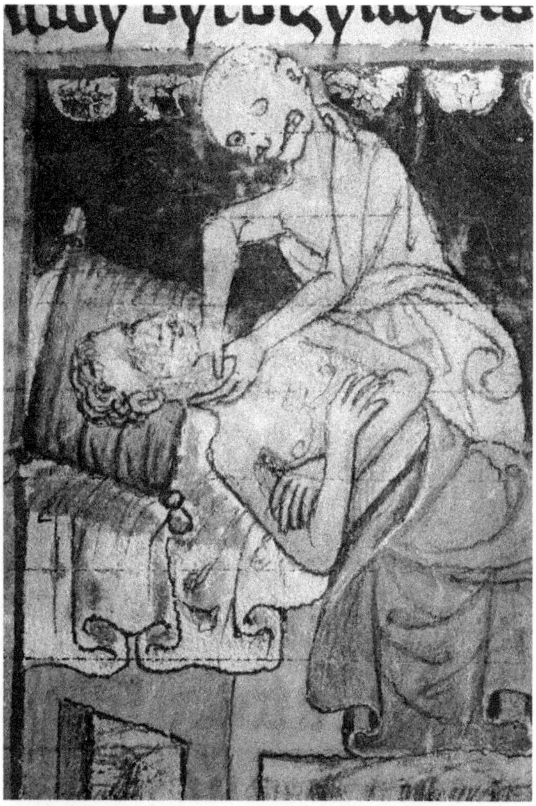

In this manuscript illustration from 1376, Death, depicted as a rotting corpse, strangles his victim. In the years following the first wave of the Black Death, the figure of Death was often portrayed spreading the plague by shooting plague arrows or dragging away those who died from the disease. (Werner Forman/Universal Images Group/Getty Images)

The Justinian plague that struck Europe in the mid-sixth century C.E. and described by the Byzantine author Procopius in his *History of the Wars* was likely an outbreak of bubonic plague. Thereafter, large bubonic plague epidemics were rare in the West until the Black Death in the 14th century, after which the plague was endemic in Europe with near yearly occurrences until the late 17th century. Unfortunately, it is difficult to distinguish outbreaks of bubonic plague from other epidemic diseases in Chinese sources, but it seems that the earliest description of bubonic plague in China was by Cha'o Yuan-fang in 610 C.E. and that the disease was endemic in the region between China and India from at least that point forward.

The 14th-century pandemic likely originated sometime during the 1330s in the Eurasian steppe, where it had been harbored in populations of burrowing rodents, from where it was carried by Mongol horsemen to other parts of the world.

Chinese records suggest that an epidemic swept through the province of Hopei in 1331, killing nine-tenths of the population, and then another epidemic swept more widely through eight different parts of China in 1353–1354 killing up to two-thirds of the population. It seems likely that these epidemics can be tied to the early spread of bubonic plague out of the Eurasian steppe. Otherwise, records reveal little about the spread of the disease in China or into the Indian subcontinent. However, it appeared in the eastern parts of the Muslim world in the mid-1340s, arriving in the Mediterranean by 1347, in Italy, Spain, and southern France by 1348, and in Germany and England by 1349. Estimates suggest that one-quarter to one-third of the population died during this initial wave of the Black Death, and thereafter recurrences continued in more localized regions roughly every 10 years killing around 10–20 percent of the inhabitants with each outbreak.

Medical Responses to the Black Death in Europe and the Islamic World

Physicians in the Islamic world and in Europe both sought to explain the rapid spread of the plague as a humoral disturbance induced by miasmas, or bad airs; for example, according to one Arabic physician,

> The pestilence resulted from a corruption occurring in the substance of the air due to heavenly and terrestrial causes. In the earth the causes are brackish water and the many cadavers found in places of battle when the dead are not buried, and land which is water-logged and stagnant from rottenness, vermin, and frogs. As regards the heavenly air, the causes are the many shooting stars and meteorites at the end of the summer and in the autumn, the strong south and east winds in December and January, and the signs of rain increase in the winter but it does not rain. (Dols 1977, 88–89)

In Europe, the faculty of medicine at the medical school in Paris explained that an unusual planetary alignment had caused the corruption of airs on earth and induced earthquakes that had released foul vapors from underground. In this way, they tried to account for the sudden onset of this particularly deadly disease in terms of their rational, scientific theories that explained the relationship between the microcosm and the macrocosm. Other physicians also employed the astrological theories to account for the seemingly random way in which the disease spread, affecting some towns and not others, and even seeming to affect people living in one street more than others. One medical astrologer suggested that "each city, town and home has fixed stars and planets ruling it . . . therefore wherever the rules of these places agree in power and effect with the planets and stars bringing the general mortality, those subject to them will have been made ready to receive that celestial influence upon their bodies" (Horrox 1994, 170).

Although, as we have seen, contagion played a minor role in explaining the spread of epidemic disease in the Greek tradition, physicians could not help but recognize that this disease seemed to spread through contact with infected persons. Muslim religious scholars wrote many plague tracts following the initial outbreak of the epidemic, considering the possibility of contagion. Referring to the Prophetic tradition, some scholars maintained that Muhammad had proclaimed that there was no possibility of contagion since this would imply that disease might spread independent of the will of God. However, this issue was complex, and numerous Muslim authors supported the possibility of contagion revealing that there was no single Islamic position on this issue. Ibn al-Khatib (14th century), for example, specifically argued that experience revealed that plague was spread by contagion, and outbreaks often coincided with the arrival of people traveling from regions where the plague was raging. He supported his empirical observations by citing hadith (prophetic sayings) that he felt endorsed the possibility of contagion. The debate over the possibility of contagion continued far beyond the period of the Black Death, but those physicians who supported a contagion theory found it necessary to reconcile it with the miasmatic theory, by arguing, for example, that the sick contaminated the air around them, as well as their clothing, bedding, and utensils. European physicians also sought to reconcile contagion theory with the belief in miasmas. One physician at Montpellier offered a miasmatic explanation of contagion through eye contact with a sick individual:

> But sometimes the brain expels the windy and poisonous matter via the optic nerves at the eyes. This is agony, and the sick man stares fixedly ahead, as if he cannot move his eyes. Amazingly, as it stands in the eyes, the primary windiness assumes the characteristics of a poisonous vapor, and seeks a new home in some other body, which it can enter and be at rest. And if a healthy person sees this visible vapor, he is stamped with the pestilential illness. The man is poisoned faster than air can leave the sick man, for the thin poison moves faster than the heavy air. (Horrox 1994, 183)

The medical response, therefore, focused on mitigating the harmful influences of the miasmas. Most physicians advocated that patients preserve health by regulating their diet and physical activity in order to fortify their bodies against the detrimental effects of the noxious vapors. Another prophylactic measure endorsed by physicians was the use of aromatic substances in a nose pomander or to fumigate rooms in order to cleanse the air. Indeed, the emphasis on miasmas led to efforts to clear cities of the sources of foul smelling air, such as the waste produced by overflowing latrines and butcher shops. Those who fell ill received more direct treatment through bloodletting, cupping, and the administration of drugs, including the much-praised compound medicine, theriac.

Religious Responses to the Black Death

The dramatic appearance, terrifying symptoms, and high mortality of the plague no doubt gave additional support to arguments for the divine cause of the Black Death. Many Christians viewed the plague in apocalyptic terms, as signifying the end of the world and the coming of Judgment Day when the faithful would be taken into heaven. Similarly, some Islamic theologians described the plague as a mercy and martyrdom for faithful Muslims and a punishment for infidels, relating it to the ideology of the *jihad*, or holy war. However, far greater emphasis was given to the belief that the plague was sent as a divine punishment for individual and communal sin. Several possibilities were offered to explain divine displeasure. In Europe, for example, priests preached from the pulpit about humanity's general sinfulness, but they also identified some specific examples of activities that would merit God's wrath, such as people wearing indecent clothing, women dressing in men's clothes, and disobedient children. Some people responded by pointing to the sins of the clergy as the real reason for divine displeasure.

Belief in the divine origin of the plague led to a number of efforts to restore moral behavior and atone for sin. Religious leaders in many cities in Europe led intercessory processions through the streets or sang special Masses as a means of expressing communal pleas for mercy and atonement for sin. Individuals offered their own prayers, often directed toward the saints specifically recognized for healing those afflicted with plague, Saint Sebastian and Saint Roche. Saint Sebastian was an early Christian who was martyred by Roman soldiers for his faith. According to legend, the soldiers first attempted to execute Sebastian by shooting him with arrows, but he survived this attack, and they needed to resort to different means to complete the execution. The arrows themselves were viewed as symbolic of the spread of plague, and by extension, Sebastian was known for having survived the assault of the plague, hence why he was considered an appropriate plague saint. Saint Roche, who lived in the 14th century, was known for surviving his own infection with the Black Death after which he dedicated his life to caring for other plague victims. Saint Roche is often depicted in artwork raising his robes to reveal the plague bubo in his groin, with the dog that was said to have brought him food while he endured the disease alone in the wilderness.

Another manifestation of religious responses to the plague in Europe was the appearance of groups of laymen and women known as the flagellants, who traveled in processions from town to town, denouncing sinners. During the processions, the flagellants would publicly scourge themselves with whips (*flagella*) to atone for the sins of humanity and beg for God's mercy. One witness attests to the ghastly scenes enacted by a troop of flagellants:

> Each whip consisted of a stick with three knotted thongs hanging from the end. Two pieces of needle-sharp metal were run through the center of the knots from both sides, forming a cross, the ends of which extended beyond the knots for the length of a grain of wheat or less. Using these whips they beat and whipped their bare skin until their bodies were bruised and swollen and blood rained down, spattering the walls nearby. I have seen, when they whipped themselves, how sometimes those bits of metal penetrated the flesh so deeply that it took more than two attempts to pull them out. (Horrox 1994, 150)

Although some people were impressed by the flagellants' fervent displays of piety, many members of the clergy were concerned that these actions only revealed the pride and excess of the participants and saw them as a threat to the authority of the church. Ultimately, Pope Clement VI forbade the practice in 1349, and authorities sought, often unsuccessfully, to suppress the flagellant movement in Europe.

Popular and Civic Responses to the Black Death

In his *Decameron*, Giovanni Boccaccio (1313–1375) describes a common response to the appearance of the plague in a city—flight. Citizens refused to help their neighbors and sometimes even deserted members of their own families and, as Boccaccio notes with horror, "even worse, and almost incredible, was the fact that fathers and mothers refused to nurse and assist their own children, as though they did not belong to them" (McWilliam 1995, 8–9). His description vividly portrays the fear evoked by the appearance of the plague.

Driven by fear, local inhabitants sometimes identified scapegoats, including foreigners, the poor, and Jews, whom they could blame for the disease. One general accusation was that people were poisoning local wells, thus causing the plague. In cities throughout Europe, many Jews were tortured into confessing to well-poisoning and were burned or otherwise executed for the crime. In response to the merciless massacre of Jews, Pope Clement VI issued a papal bull in 1348 condemning Christians who had falsely accused and impiously slain Jews for spreading the plague and extending papal protection over Jewish communities in Christendom.

Civic and lay authorities also tried to limit the spread of plague. In many towns, lay leaders enacted legislation aimed at cleaning up the source of foul airs in cities, reflecting the prevalence of the belief in miasmatic theory. For example, some cities passed ordinances that banned butchers from dumping the entrails and blood left over from their trade into the streets, since this waste was viewed as a source of corrupt air, and in other cases, tanners' shops were relocated outside city walls—tanners used large, foul-smelling vats of urine in the tanning process. New regulations were also passed requiring that "the bodies of the dead shall not be removed from the place of death until they have been enclosed in a wooden box, and the lid of planks nailed down so that no stench can escape," and that "to avoid the foul stench which comes from dead bodies each grave shall be dug two and a half armslengths deep" (McWilliam 1995, 196). Acknowledging the possibility that the plague was contagious, many cities attempted to establish quarantines, preventing foreigners and linen products from infected regions from entering.

LEPROSY

Leprosy, or Hansen's disease, is a bacterial infection, which results in skin and nerve damage that can lead to severe disfigurement to the face and deformity of the extremities. The pathogen responsible for Hansen's disease, *Mycobacterium leprae*, may have evolved in East Africa or India before spreading eastward to China and, at a slightly later date, northwest into Europe. Although ancient Mesopotamian and Egyptian medical texts do not provide enough descriptive detail of disease symptoms to positively prove the incidence of leprosy, paleopathologists have discovered skeletons in Egypt that exhibit characteristic symptoms of the disease dating to the second century B.C.E. Indeed, it is often difficult to rely upon premodern diagnoses of "leprosy" since in many cases, they are just as likely describing otherwise harmless skin disease like psoriasis as actual cases of Hansen's disease. Greek and Roman authors use a number of terms to identify conditions that might have been leprosy, including the words "lepra" (which means in Greek "a scaly disease") and "elephantiasis" (referring to a disease causing the thickening of the skin and changes to the bones). Likewise, the biblical word *sara'at*, which appears thirty-five times in various forms in the Hebrew Old Testament, generally refers to certain skin conditions inflicted on humans for sin (although the term is also applied to house walls and clothing) and has regularly been translated as "leprosy" in the English Bible, although the descriptions do not necessarily support this diagnosis.

Leprosy in India

In 2009, a team of paleopathologists reported finding evidence of leprosy in the skeletal remains of a middle-aged adult male who lived in India around 2000 B.C.E.—the oldest documented skeletal evidence for leprosy in the world (Robbins et al. 2009). Given that it is not common to find adult burials in this region after 2000 B.C.E., the paleopathologists suggest the burial may imply that it was not considered appropriate to cremate the diseased body as a sacrifice to the Hindu gods. The earliest documentary evidence for this disease in India would seem to confirm this possibility. The condition *kustha*, a dangerous skin condition that has often been thought to be leprosy, is first described in the *Atharvaveda*:

> Born by night art though, O plant, dark, black, sable. Do thou, that art rich in color, stain this leprosy [*kustha*], and the grey spots! . . . The leprosy which has originated in the bones, and that which has originated in the body and upon the skin, the white mark begotten of corruption, I have destroyed with my charm. (Bloomfield 2004, 19)

References to the condition *kustha* are also found in later Hindu religious scriptures, which declare that the disease is a punishment for sinners in their future birth.

Ayurvedic medical texts confirm the religious beliefs about *kustha* found in the *Atharvaveda*, but they also offer a naturalistic explanation that it is caused by a derangement of the *doshas*. The *Susruta Samhita* also suggests that *kustha* is contagious (although the risk of contagion of actual Hansen's disease is slight), transmitted by touch, breath, sexual intercourse, or by sharing utensils, or that it is a hereditary disease passed from parents to offspring. Perhaps unsurprisingly, the remedy reflects a blend of natural and religious measures:

> Wise men hold that, for killing a Brahman, or a woman, or one of his own relations, for theft, as well as for doing acts of impiety, a man is sometimes cursed with this foul disease by way of divine retribution. The disease re-attacks a man even in his next rebirth in the event of his dying with it. Uncured *Kushtham* (leprosy) is the most painful, and most troublesome of all diseases.
>
> A Kushthi (leper), getting rid of this foul malady by observing the proper regimen of diet and conduct and by practicing expiatory penances and by resorting to proper medicinal measures, gets an elevated status after death. (Bhishagratna 1911, 42)

Leprosy in China

Leprosy was known in China from at least the sixth century B.C.E. in the Zhou dynasty. A bamboo strip containing a number of legal records discovered in a tomb from the third century B.C.E. describes a court case where a doctor was called to confirm whether a person had *li* (leprosy), responding with this diagnosis: "[The villager] has no eyebrows; the bridge of the nose is destroyed; his nasal cavity is collapsed; if you prick his nose, he does not sneeze; . . . the soles of both feet are defective and are suppurating in one place; his hands have no hair; I ordered him to shout and the *ch'i* of his voice was hoarse. It is *li* [leprosy]" (McLeod and Yates 1981, 153). Chinese criminal law from this period indicates that criminals afflicted with *li* could expect a more severe punishment than others convicted of similar offences, including being drowned or buried alive. The different penalties suggest a deeper religious significance attached to those suffering from *li*. Indeed, in this period, *li* was associated with possession by a ghastly spirit that personified moral vileness and manifested the external symptoms of the disease on the patient. Thus, burying alive or drowning a criminal afflicted with *li* was a ritual performance to suppress the ghastly spirit. *Li* patients convicted of lesser, noncapital crimes, would still be transferred to special prisons for lepers. Furthermore, those with *li* were deprived of their right to marriage and were often expelled from their communities.

From the 4th through 13th centuries C.E., numerous accounts of people suffering from *li* reflect the religious responses to the disease in the Buddhist and Taoist traditions. Stories from the Buddhist tradition emphasize that the disease was a punishment for moral transgressions committed in this life, a former life, or by one's forebears. Buddhist monasteries established special quarters to house *li* sufferers in the sixth and seventh centuries C.E., and many Buddhist monks dedicated their lives to caring from them. For example, around 581, the monk Daoxun was said to travel among those with *li*, selflessly caring for their needs: "Whenever he saw pus flowing out of corrupted sores, he did not have any second thought and cleaned them with his mouth. He washed their clothes, and purified the sins of their hearts" (Leung 2008, 70). In addition to their physical care, Buddhist healers also provided the necessary purification rituals to cleanse the afflicted of their sins. The Taoist tradition, by contrast, places greater emphasis on the role of the sick individual in self-healing by means of practicing bodily and spiritual discipline. The Taoist physician Sun Simiao (581–682) spoke of the healing process for *li* in these terms: "There is an auspicious and an inauspicious meaning to this illness. If the sufferer of the disease cultivates good, he will have an auspicious end. If he maintains the same habits as other worldly beings, he will certainly have an inauspicious end" (Leung 2008, 74). Similarly, Taoist stories tell of *li* sufferers who achieved cures by traveling into the mountains and learning to follow a simple spiritual life.

Leprosy in Medieval Europe

Leprosy entered Western Europe sometime around the fourth century C.E. and spread along expanding mercantile routes and in the developing urban centers. In the 12th and 13th centuries, social and medical responses to leprosy suggest a massive increase in awareness or incidences of the disease. The late 14th and 15th centuries, by contrast, witness a steep decline in social and medical reports of the disease. This brief upsurge in reports of leprosy in Europe, peaking in the 13th

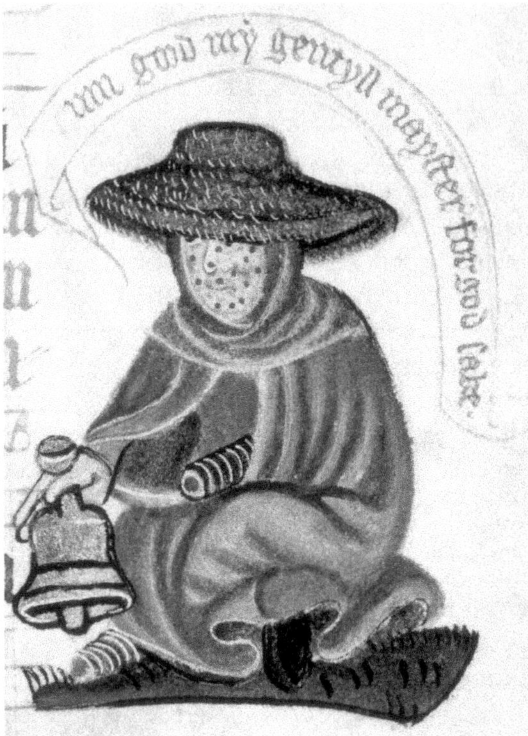

This 14th-century illustration depicts a leper with facial disfigurement and amputated limbs. The leper carries a bell to warn others of her approach. (The British Library)

century, is difficult to explain. Some scholars have argued that the seeming explosion of leprosy cases represents increased social fear of the disease rather than a real rise in the disease's prevalence. Other explanations suggest that more accurate methods of diagnosis led to fewer people being diagnosed with leprosy in later centuries or that a greater number of people afflicted by the disease had died as a result of the Black Death due to their weakened immunity, reducing the number of infected individuals. In any event, by the 16th century, the writings of physicians in Western Europe reflected less concern with leprosy and turned increasingly toward consideration of other diseases such as syphilis.

During the height of leprosy's prevalence in Europe, however, the afflicted often suffered severe social stigmas, as happened in other cultures. Fear that the disease was extremely contagious and biblical references that supported the expulsion of lepers from society meant that those diagnosed with leprosy could face social exile. Furthermore, whereas bubonic plague was sometimes interpreted as a sign of communal sin, leprosy in medieval Europe was often interpreted as an indication of individual sin, justifying a leper's isolation. In conformity with these beliefs, the Third Lateran Council (1179) explicitly declared that lepers should be cut off from society and have their own churches and burial places. On the other hand, many authors described leprosy as a gift from God, a trial to test the faith of the afflicted and the charity and compassion of other Christians. As a result, far from being vilified and persecuted, lepers received compassionate support from Church authorities, and those who cared for lepers were often viewed as having an aura of sanctity. Indeed, it is significant that archaeologists have found remains with signs of leprosy buried alongside other bodies in local graveyards, suggesting that lepers were not always completely cut off from the community. One highly visible expression of Christian piety toward lepers was the establishment of numerous *leprosaria* throughout Europe for housing lepers. These charitable institutions were frequently located within the precincts of a town or city and provided a place where lepers could receive spiritual and physical care, while minimizing contact and the possibility of spreading the disease to others.

Despite the charitable attitudes, a diagnosis of leprosy could still have profound consequences for individuals in the Middle Ages—social exile. Initially, the determination as to whether a person was leprous, and hence whether the person should face expulsion from the community, fell to local priests or boards of lay officials, leading several physicians to express a concern that cases of leprosy were judged very poorly in their day. The famous Montpellier physician and surgeon, Guy de Chauliac (1298–1368), summarized these views, writing, "Great attention should be paid to the examination and judgment of leprosy, for it is extremely unjust to sequester those who should not be sequestered and to send the infected among the people" (Demaitre 2007, 40). In line with these views, during the 13th and 14th centuries, physicians wrote extensively on how to make an accurate diagnosis of leprosy and distinguish it from other skin disorders, asserting their authority to judge cases of leprosy. Furthermore, although they viewed it as contagious and incurable, physicians still offered extensive advice on treatments to prolong the patient's life and to avoid becoming infected in the first place. Through these efforts, medical men intervened in the process of identifying and treating lepers with the intention of minimizing the social consequences of what was viewed as a frightening disease.

7

Environmental and Occupational Hazards

Environmental and occupational hazards also posed a different range of threats to health in daily life. Authors of the ancient Greek, Ayurvedic, and traditional Chinese medical traditions all asserted the important role played by environmental conditions on individual health. Hippocratic authors warned of the dangers of living in close proximity to swamps, which might be a source of unhealthy miasmatic airs, and the differing influences of the four winds. The author of *Airs, Waters, Places* even indicates that environmental factors accounted for the cultural and physical differences between Greeks and people of other races, like the Scythians. Therefore, the author advises that cities seeking to send out colonies ensure that the new city be built in a salubrious location. Similarly, the *Huangdi Neijing* (*The Yellow Emperor's Classic of Internal Medicine*) considers dietary and health effects on people living in different regions:

> The people of the regions of the East eat fish and crave salt; their living is tranquil and their food delicious. Fish causes people to thirst, and the eating of salt injures the blood. Therefore the people of these regions are all of dark complexion and careless and lax in their principles. Their diseases are ulcers, which are most properly treated with acupuncture by means of a needle of flint. . . .
>
> The North is the region of storing and laying by. The country is hilly and mountainous, there are biting cold winds, frost and ice. The people of these regions find pleasure in living in this wilderness, and they live on milk products. The extreme cold causes many diseases. These diseases are most fittingly treated with cauterization by burning the dried tinder of the artemisia (moxa). (Veith 1972, 147–148)

In the premodern world, most people lived in rural settings and were usually involved in some form of agricultural labor, facing environmental and occupational hazards particular to these conditions. By contrast, life in cities offered a vastly different experience. Urban dwellers had a greater diversity of occupational opportunities (although requiring a higher degree of specialization), and for this reason, villagers from the countryside were often drawn to these centers. However, the confined spaces of cities and the masses of people in them generated new environmental hazards peculiar to urban life.

LIVING AND WORKING CONDITIONS IN RURAL COMMUNITIES

The vast majority of the population in the premodern world was engaged in agricultural labor. Depending upon the climate and soils, different staple crops were produced: for example, wheat, barley, and millet were grown in northern regions, while rice production was common in the wet regions of Southeast Asia. In some cases, peasant farmers owned and worked their own land (a field large enough to provide for a family or possibly larger) as freeholders. However, in other cases slaves or serfs (an individual obligated to work the land but who could not be bought or sold like a slave) worked in the fields held by a wealthy landowner. Serfs were allowed to keep a portion of the produce from the lands they worked for themselves, while delivering the lion's share to their lord, and even freeholders owed taxes or other obligations.

Peasant farmers necessarily made do with minimal possessions. Dwellings were typically small, consisting of no more than one or two rooms. In parts of the world where timber was scarce, people made dwellings out of clay or mud bricks, and in northwest China, some people lived in artificial caves, digging chambers into the sides of hills. Elsewhere, dwellings were made of wood or bamboo and were likely built to last only one generation before they would disintegrate and be replaced. Such temporary structures often posed threats to inhabitants, and many peasants had their homes collapse on them during strong windstorms. In India, evidence suggests that astrologers were often consulted when determining where a house should be built and what layout it should follow (e.g., the door should not face west since that region belonged to the dead). In other parts of the world, such as medieval England, peasant villages followed a haphazard design, and houses were not necessarily placed so as to align with village streets, to be near to water sources, or to minimize or maximize contact with other dwellings. One part of the house would serve as a byre for farm animals and to store farm equipment, meaning that animals and humans lived in very close proximity. Wealthier peasants might be able to afford to build a separate outbuilding to shelter animals, but this was not often the norm. Indeed, the Chinese symbol for "home" is a pictograph of a roof with a pig under it. Hearths for cooking and heat were common and were made of clay or stone where possible, but ventilation was not always adequate, and they were also a significant cause of house fires and other injuries. One coroner's report from medieval England relates that a baby died when pigs in the home knocked over its crib and it rolled into the family hearth. In general, a peasant home did not necessarily provide for the safest or most hygienic living conditions.

Rural life and the activities of peasants were typically structured by the agricultural calendar. During the spring months, men would be involved mostly in plowing fields and planting crops; during the late summer months, they turned to harvesting, carting, and storing their crops, and then in the fall, they would be involved in preparing fields for winter crops, butchering animals, and salting or smoking meats. The winter months of December and January, by contrast, were a lull time in terms of agricultural production, but this time was often used to construct and repair fences, homes, and outbuildings. All of these activities presented different hazards.[1] The most dangerous time of the year was around the harvest, when men worked long and exhausting hours and might be prone to making careless mistakes. Many men were injured or killed by accidental cuts from the scythes and reaping hooks used to gather the crops, while others were crushed by the heavily laden carts used to carry the harvested crops from the fields, which easily overturned while being drawn across the uneven furrows. The task of storing the loads was also tricky; for example, straw and hay often needed to be stacked in storage barns, and it was not uncommon for men to fall from ladders while putting crops into storage lofts at this time of year. In addition to the dangers present at harvest time, farmers were often injured by the large animals they raised for food or employed in the fields to pull plows or carts.

Women frequently assisted men in the fields, especially during harvest time, and were thus exposed to the same kinds of occupational hazards. For the most part, however, women were injured while engaging in daily activities closer to home, suggesting that this was their chief sphere of work. Although it may seem strange today, one of the most dangerous tasks was drawing water from wells and ponds for drinking, cooking, and washing; the earth around these water sources was often slippery and many women slipped and drowned in them. Women were also commonly injured while preparing the family meals; cooking, baking, and brewing required women to work around large open hearths and carry large vats of boiling liquids. Milking cows, doing laundry, and gathering firewood presented further dangers to women engaged in routine household work. In sum, although women's work was not always as dangerous as men's, we must recognize that they engaged in far more dangerous activities than simply spinning and weaving.

In general, agricultural production existed at little more than a subsistence level for most peasants. They would typically supplement the meager amount of food grown in their fields by raising livestock (chickens, geese, pigs, sheep, etc.) growing vegetables or fruit in home gardens, hunting and fishing, or gathering nuts, herbs, and wild fruits. However, even in the best of times, the margin between survival and starvation was thin, and in these conditions, natural disasters could easily lead to ruin. Farmers along the Nile River in Egypt relied on the predictable flood season to renew the soils and irrigate the crops in their lands, allowing for abundant harvests, hence Egypt's reputation as the breadbasket of the ancient Mediterranean world. The reliable and life-giving floods of the Nile aside, swarms of locusts or other pests, hail, excessive rains and flooding, or droughts could destroy an entire harvest and lead to widespread famine. Years of farming the same fields could also lead to soil depletion, when necessary nutrients were gradually leeched from the ground so that once fertile lands were no longer as productive as they once had been. Furthermore, marauding armies would often burn fields or steal the little food peasants had stored to feed the soldiers as they passed through an area, not to mention the fact that invading armies would burn villages and slay any peasants they found in an effort to wreak destruction on their enemy's territories. These unpredictable conditions meant that peasants often lived in a chronic state of instability; the lack of food reserves and the inadequate means for transporting supplies to stricken regions meant that famine was an almost endemic scourge in the premodern world. In France between 970 and 1100 C.E., there were no less than 60 years of famine, England reported terrible famines from 1086 to 1125 C.E., and poor harvests lead to famine and privation throughout Europe for much of the 14th century C.E., coinciding with frequent plague epidemics. Likewise, China witnessed a series of poor harvests in the seventh century C.E. (brought on by floods and plagues of locusts), and the 14th century was also troubled by a series of widespread famines that coincided with the spread of epidemic disease.

Chinese emperors in the Tang dynasty (618–907 C.E.) regularly assumed responsibility for natural disasters, and the government created a series of granaries in strategic locations throughout the empire from which food could be distributed in the event of natural disasters. Not all governments were as prepared to assist starving peasants in times of disaster, and in most cases people were left to fend for themselves. Under such difficult circumstances, villagers might turn to eating their seed supplies, set aside for the next season's planting, which would only compound the problem by diminishing future harvests. Stories relate that peasants facing starvation turned to eating grass roots and tree leaves, while some may even have resorted to cannibalism. In other cases, peasants might abandon their villages and move into towns in search of employment and the hope for a better life.

Mining was another of the important rural occupations in the premodern world. People mined for metal ores (gold, silver, copper, iron, red lead, mercury, etc.) as well as precious and semiprecious stones (diamonds, rubies, topazes, sapphires, emeralds, and a variety of crystals). Mines were often operated as a government monopoly, where the state (or an administering official) would claim the proceeds of the mine. Labor in the mines was dangerous. In addition to accidents, miners faced a variety of health hazards including lung diseases from breathing in too much dusty air, exposure to toxic levels of lead (from working in lead and silver mines), or arsenic poisoning (from working with copper ores or arsenic). Lucretius (ca. 99–ca. 55 B.C.E.), a Roman poet and philosopher, commented on working conditions and the noxious airs produced by mines:

> And where there is mining for veins of gold and silver
> Which men will dig for deep down in the earth
> What stenches arise, as the Scaptensula [a mining town in Thrace]!
> How deadly are the exhalations of gold mines!
> You can see the ill effects in the miners' complexions.
> Have you not heard and seen how short is the life
> Of a miner compelled to remain at this terrible task?
> All these exhalations come from the earth and are breathed forth into the open light of day. (Nriagu 1983, 110)

Labor in mines was so hazardous that it was often consigned to slaves and criminals, especially in the Greek and Roman worlds. In other parts of the world miners were paid laborers, but not necessarily paid well, and mutinies among miners were not uncommon. As new technologies were invented, such as devices to pump water out of deep mine shafts, mines progressed from being open pit to underground operations, which only compounded the dangers faced by miners, who could be trapped by tunnel cave-ins.

LIVING AND WORKING CONDITIONS IN URBAN CENTERS

Cities and towns in the premodern world were not large by modern standards. The largest capital cities of the ancient world may have had populations exceeding a half-million inhabitants. Estimates suggest that by the end of the first century B.C.E., Rome and the city of Alexandria in Egypt each had populations of about 1 million people; the Chinese capital city of Hangchow had a population in excess of 1 million when Marco Polo visited it toward the end of the 13th century C.E. By contrast, Paris, the largest city of medieval Europe had a population of perhaps 90,000 or 100,000 in the 14th century. A city with a population of 10,000 or more inhabitants would have been considered large, and most towns had a population of no more than around 2,000 or 3,000 people. Throughout the premodern period, the population of towns and cities was not self-sustaining. Deaths brought on by incidences of epidemic disease and general living conditions served continually to whittle down a town's inhabitants. In these circumstances, urban centers required a regular influx of new inhabitants from the countryside to maintain or expand their populations.

Waste and Sewage Removal

One of the most pressing problems faced by any city is the removal of sewage and other waste. The Romans built a complex network of sewers in their cities to help with waste removal, and they were flushed by the water that overflowed from public fountains fed by a system of aqueducts. Although these sewers were remarkable by comparison to other premodern cities, they were not without their own dangers. Indeed, when the Tiber River flooded, it would often back up into sewers and thence into peoples' homes, and it was not unheard of for a buildup of sewer gases to cause explosions. Latrines connected to sewers also served as an entry point for criminals into the home. Not all homes had latrines served by sewers, however, and most people were likely to use chamber pots, which they would empty into the open streets, despite laws against this practice in many towns. Indeed, the satirist Juvenal (d. early second century C.E.) commented that simply going out to dinner in Rome was dangerous because one risked as many deaths as there were windows to pass under! Much of the waste thrown into streets was washed away by the overflow from public fountains, but more likely the water and sewage were churned together into the ground by the passage of humans, animals, and carts so that the streets were filled with mud and excrement—indeed, several Roman authors commented upon the muddy and filthy condition of Roman streets. Furthermore, the bodies of dead animals and the offal produced by butchers' shops could not easily be removed through the sewers and might be left to decompose in the streets. Although families were expected to pay for the burial or cremation of deceased family members, it was not uncommon to find dead bodies rotting in the streets, if comments by some Roman authors are to be trusted. Authorities might hire workers to clean out cesspits that were not serviced by the network of sewers and to remove dead bodies (human and animal) and other waste (at least from major roadways) to open pits outside the city, but this was not typical.

In the Chinese city of Hangchow in the 13th century C.E., public authorities hired street cleaners and paid to have garbage carried by boats that traversed the network of canals to a designated wasteland outside the city. In Hangchow, the wealthy had private cesspits near their homes and would pay to have them emptied when necessary. Most people, however, made do with "horse buckets," which would be left outside their homes and collected by scavengers or night soil collectors, commonly called "the pourers," who would sell the contents as manure for gardens around the city. As in other towns, however, it is probable that much of the waste found its way into streets and canals.

Not all cities developed the efficient means of waste removal found in Rome and Hangchow. Indeed, most medieval European cities had an open ditch through the center of main streets that people could empty night soil and other waste into, but these channels would often become clogged and municipal authorities did not always pay for workers to keep them clear. Cesspits with privies located in yards or cellars were also typical, and individuals would need to pay to have them cleaned out and the waste carted away every couple of years—in many cases, excrement collected from cesspits was simply dumped into the river (e.g., the Thames River served as the main dumping ground for London sewage and other waste for centuries). Latrines could often be dangerous places, and numerous reports indicate that children and even adults fell into cesspits and drowned. Tenants in upper stories of buildings might not wish to go to the trouble of descending stairs in the middle of the night to use a latrine, such as one servant in the city of London who "rose naked from his bed and stood at a window of the solar 30 ft. high to relieve himself towards the High Street," and fell to his death (Hanawalt 1993, 29). Although urban leaders passed laws to regulate the placement of latrines, these laws were irregularly enforced and authorities likely only became involved in questions of sewage removal in extreme cases. For example, at an Assize of Nuisances in London in 1347, two men were brought to trial for piping their waste into a neighbor's cellar—the neighbor had not become aware of this until his cellar was overflowing! The city itself must have smelled awful for this homeowner to have failed to notice the smell coming from his own cellar.

In addition to sewage, other waste could quickly accumulate in city streets. Butchers would throw offal from their shops into the streets—one estimate suggests that some 250,000 head of livestock were slaughtered per year in Paris during the 13th century—that might collect along with the bodies of dead animals and overflowing sewage channels to putrefy in the sun. The tanning industry, which used urine, tannic acids, lime, and other chemicals in the tanning process, also produced extensive pollution that was washed into streets and nearby streams. The brewers and ale makers, among others, regularly complained about the corruption of fresh-water sources (from which water was used for drinking and to make ale). Many towns passed regulations mandating where the butchers and tanners dumped their wastes or confining them to the outskirts of town, but they were not always enforced. It is little wonder that one 16th-century traveler remarked that he could smell the city of Paris two days before he could see it on the horizon!

Fresh Water and the Risk of Lead Poisoning

Providing fresh water to urban inhabitants presented another range of difficulties. Natural springs and dug wells might provide fresh water for a number of inhabitants, but the quickly growing populations of cities required that additional water be brought in from elsewhere. Once again, Roman engineers excelled in this realm, building vast aqueducts to bring fresh water into cities from great distances. Other cities maintained nearby reservoirs or lakes from which they could draw fresh water. Hangchow, for example, created a nearby artificial lake known as the "Six Wells" and jealously guarded its purity. During the years 1265–1274, the court brought charges against two high officials who had built houses on stilts over the lake where they washed their hair and did their laundry, charging that "in this way the wines offered up in libation to Heaven and Earth and to the Imperial Ancestors cannot have the required purity. Moreover, the townspeople, who drink no other water but this, run the risk of epidemics" (Wright 1962, 45). Not all towns were as careful about where they drew their water supply, however; for example, many inhabitants of London received water drawn from the Thames River downstream from where the city dumped sewage until the mid-19th century.

In addition to the risk of piping in contaminated water, the pipes themselves may have posed a danger to the drinking water. The pipes were made of different materials, including earthenware (as in Hangchow), wood (as in Basel in 1266), or even lead. Vitruvius Pollio (ca. 50–26 B.C.E.), a Roman architect and military engineer, composed a treatise, *De Architectura,* in which he described the way in which water was delivered to Rome. Concerning the materials used to make pipes, he noted, "Water is much more wholesome when delivered in earthenware pipes than it is when lead pipes are used, for it seems to be made injurious by lead, because white lead is produced by it and this is said to be harmful to the human body" (Cruse 2004, 81). Despite his advice, lead was easier to work with and relatively cheap, so it was widely used in the Roman world for water pipes, as well as for kitchenware and vessels for storing wine and other liquids. The widespread use of lead pipes may have caused increased cases of lead poisoning among inhabitants who drank water supplied by them.

Lead pipes were not the only possible source for lead poisoning. In fact, Romans regularly imbibed a syrup called *sapa,* which was produced by simmering unfermented grape juice in lead vessels and contained a high concentration of lead. *Sapa* was known for being an effective preservative as well as for adding an appealing color, fragrance and sweet taste to wines, and it was also added to many foods to sweeten them. Debate continues among scholars concerning the extent to which lead poisoning among the Roman aristocracy contributed to the fall of the Roman Empire. Nonetheless, even if rates of lead poisoning were not high enough to reduce the fertility of the Roman aristocracy as dangerously as some have suggested, it seems clear that many in the Roman world were exposed to far higher levels of lead than would have been healthy. Furthermore, in addition to the risk of lead poisoning from contaminated food and drink, workers who used lead in industries such as painting, plumbing, roofing, sculpture, pewter ware, shipbuilding, enameling, and glazing pottery would have regularly risked occupational exposure.

The Risk of Fire

Fire was an ever-present danger for the residents of premodern cities. The homes of wealthier urban residents may have been larger, with walls around them and slightly wider streets to allow some space and privacy from neighbors, but the majority of buildings in premodern cities were made of wood (or other flammable materials such as bamboo), multistoried, and crowded around a twisting network of narrow streets and alleyways. To gain extra room in upper stories, some buildings had projections that hung out over the street, further narrowing the distance between them and giving an even more claustrophobic feel at the street level (although some cities, like London, passed ordinances stating that projections had to start high enough up from street level to allow a man riding on a horse to pass under them). In a world where everyone had to cook over open flames and used candles or oil lamps to provide light, it is not surprising that fires were extremely frequent, and once started they could quickly spread, causing enormous destruction. In addition to cooking fires, blacksmith shops were often cited as the source of blazes, as were scholars who stayed up late at night, reading by candlelight.

The great fire of 64 C.E. in the city of Rome raged for six days, and by the time it was extinguished, 10 of Rome's 14 districts had been severely damaged, three of which were completely leveled. Tacitus (56–117 C.E.), a contemporary historian who witnessed the fire, reports that following the fire the emperor Nero (r. 54–68 C.E.) mandated that homes be more spaced out and built of brick to help prevent the spread of future fires. During the years of the Roman Republic, Rome had no fire brigade, but Marcus Crassus (ca. 115–53 B.C.E.), who would later be a member of the First Triumvirate with Julius Caesar and Pompey Magnus, notoriously made a large part of his vast fortune by creating a for-hire fire-fighting force. When he learned that a house was on fire, he would rush to the location and offer to purchase the home and surrounding buildings for an outrageously low price; if the owners agreed to the sale, he would have his men extinguish the fire, but if not he would leave it to burn—a true fire sale! Later, the emperor Augustus (r. 27 B.C.E.–14 C.E.) established a force of about 7,000 watchmen (called *vigiles*), who were given buckets, ladders, axes, and other fire-fighting equipment and required to patrol the city at night looking for fires.

The city of Hangchow in China saw numerous fires in the 12th and 13th centuries, sometimes with several large fires noted for the same year. After two major fires (one in 1132 and another in 1137), which destroyed 13,000 and 10,000 houses respectively, the court erected a series of watchtowers in the most overcrowded districts and manned them with a brigade equipped with fire-fighting tools. This brigade would watch for smoke and signs of fire and then use a series of flags and lanterns to indicate the location of the fire so that fire fighters from other towers could join them to help extinguish it. Furthermore, they would patrol the city at night and exact fines on anyone who had fires burning in their homes after lawful hours. Although these measures undoubtedly helped, they could not eliminate the risk of fire, and in 1208, another great fire spread through the city, this one destroying 58,097 homes along a three-mile corridor. Wary of these dangers, merchants in Hangchow opted to construct warehouses for their goods in districts that were surrounded on all sides by canals that could work as natural fire breaks, or provide a handy source of water to extinguish any fires.

Although some cities like Rome and Hangchow did develop official fire-fighting forces, most cities continued to rely on citizens to watch for fire and organize unofficial bucket brigades. One monk described the spread of a fire in Canterbury in 1174, noting that it started in one house, and while the citizens gathered to fight it, a violent wind quickly spread sparks and cinders to neighboring houses setting them alight too. Some of the sparks and cinders landed on the church roof and got between the joints of the lead tiles (lead was sometimes used in roofing in part since it was fire resistant, as opposed to thatch or wooden roofs) until it caught the underlying wooden frame on fire. The account continues:

> Then the people and the monks assemble in haste, they draw water, they brandish their hatchets, they run up the stairs, full of eagerness to save the church, already, alas, beyond help. When they reach the roof and perceive the black smoke and scorching flames that pervade it throughout, they abandon the attempt in despair, and thinking only of their own safety, make all haste to descend. . . .
>
> And now the people ran to the ornaments of the church, and began to tear down the *pallia* and curtains, some that they might save, some to steal them. The reliquary chests were thrown down from the high beam and thus broken, and their contents scattered; but the monks collected them and carefully preserved them against the fire. . . .
>
> Not only was the choir consumed in the fire, but also the infirmary, with the chapel of Saint Mary, and several other offices in the court. (Gies and Gies 2002, 166–167)

In addition to highlighting the bravery of the citizen fire fighters, this author also makes clear the fact that fires were also invitations for looting for some citizens. Indeed, merchants might have had cause to fear the volunteer firefighters as much as the fire!

Violence and Crime

Premodern cities never had a police force in the modern sense, dedicated to preventing crimes or investigating crimes that had been committed. Many cities did employ night watchmen, however, who were charged with patrolling the streets at night to enforce the curfew. For example, the Gold Bird Guards patrolled in the capital cities during the Tang dynasty in China and maintained a watch post with guards at every intersection. These watchmen would provide a show of force to deter riots and mob violence, and they would be involved in apprehending criminals perceived as a threat to the state, but they were not otherwise charged with investigating crimes or apprehending criminals. Rather, private citizens needed to see to their own protection and capture any thief, murderer, or other criminal and take him before a magistrate themselves.

In Rome, homeowners were allowed to kill any thief that broke into their home at night, but if the thief broke in during the day, they were expected to raise an alarm and apprehend him with the assistance of neighbors. Similar rules existed in most cities and suggest that neighbors worked together to patrol and protect their own streets. In some cases the townsfolk could act as a mob, and captured criminals might be torn apart before they could be delivered to any magistrate. At other times, however, neighborhood watches were not especially effective. One story from India relates that a tradesman awoke at night to find a thief fleeing his shop and dashed into the streets crying, "Stop thief!" The neighbors rushed out with torches to help pursue him. The thief, however, ran through the street's sewage canal, something no upper class Hindu would have dreamt of doing, and then he fled through a graveyard, considered a haunted spot that no one ever dared visit at night. His pursuers, deciding not to risk defiling themselves, allowed him to escape. For this reason, wealthy citizens often hired personal guards to provide for their own personal protection and the protection of their shops.

In addition to individual crimes, many cities witnessed a high level of gang violence. In the Byzantine Empire's capital city of Constantinople, for example, youths divided into *demes*, or associations, which were linked to the different factional chariot-racing teams, denoted by the color of their uniforms: Blues, Reds, Greens, and Whites. Political factions in the city often tried to manipulate these gangs to their own ends so that they were not only social but also political associations. As a result, these gangs were often involved in hooliganism and causing riots in the city. The most famous riot occurred in 532, when people gathered at the Hippodrome to watch the races and the Blues and Greens joined forces crying out "*Nika*" (meaning "conquer") and started to assault the palace with the intention of overthrowing the emperor, Justinian I (r. 527–565), with the support of various senators. After five days of rioting, Justinian sent word (along with bags of gold) to the Blues, reminding them that he had always supported their faction and pointing out that the new emperor they hoped to install was a Green. After this, the Blues broke off their alliance with the Greens and ceased to riot, and Justinian sent his armies in to kill and dispel the remaining rebels—about 30,000 rioters were reported killed.

In other cities, guilds provided the primary social unit by which people identified themselves. In medieval Europe, it was common for rivalries to develop between youth gangs from different guilds. Apprentices from one guild would sometimes band together and make forays into neighborhoods of rival guilds to start fights, and many of these apprentice gangs engaged in prearranged mock battles that often ended in severe injuries or even deaths. Gangs of male youths were also known to attack and rape vulnerable women. Students were perhaps the most notorious of all youths, widely condemned for the violence and mayhem they caused in cities. In many European universities, students were expected to enter clerical orders, signified by the tonsure or the shaving of the crown of the head. Clerical status conveyed important privileges in medieval society, including protecting the individual as sacrosanct—any violence perpetrated against someone with clerical status was punished with immediate excommunication. Furthermore, clerics were not subject to civil law but rather to the canon law of ecclesiastical courts, which often gave lighter punishments for crimes than civil courts (the most extreme punishment was to be stripped of one's clerical status, whereas the death penalty was common for a variety of offenses under civil law). Together these privileges allowed students a great margin for causing trouble without the expectation of serious retribution. In Paris at the beginning of the 13th century, for example, students were known for provoking brawls in taverns with guild apprentices, relying upon their clerical status to protect them from any response and with the knowledge that they would face a lighter punishment than the lay youths for their actions. No wonder that King Philip Augustus (r. 1180–1223) marveled at the bravery of students who waded into fights carrying swords but not wearing any armor or helmets—their shaved heads advertising their clerical status were armor enough!

NOTE

1. Barbara A. Hanawalt, *The Ties That Bound: Peasant Families in Medieval England* (Oxford: Oxford University Press, 1986) offers extensive insight into the hazards faced by agricultural laborers. She examines records produced after coroners' inquests into cases of accidental deaths in medieval England to learn about the daily lives of peasants. Although she focuses on medieval England, her findings about the occupational hazards faced by agricultural laborers are likely similar to conditions in other premodern agrarian communities.

8

Surgery and Medical Procedures

Humans have been performing a variety of surgical operations and physical manipulations on the body for a very long time. Archaeologists have discovered evidence that Neolithic humans were performing trephinations, carving holes into the cranium, as early as 10,000 B.C.E., and the indication of new bone growth along the cut edges of the skull indicate that the individuals who underwent such operations had a high survival rate. Indeed, many skulls have been trepanned more than once. Today, trephination is used to relieve pressure on the brain caused by internal bleeding from head wounds, for example. While it is not clear why these operations were performed among prehistoric peoples, they may have been performed for religious as well as medical reasons, perhaps to release malign spirits from the head or as a form of ritual mutilation, similar to cutting off joints from fingers as is done in some primitive societies (e.g., to placate ghosts or honor the recently dead). In any event, the practice indicates the extent to which prehistoric peoples developed and employed surgical techniques.

As remarkable as the practice of trephination might seem, it was likely an elective procedure, and prehistoric peoples probably needed to treat injuries such as fractures and dislocations far more often. Archaeologists have discovered bones from the Neolithic period with healed fractures, indicating that prehistoric peoples could also treat broken bones. Indeed, they may have used some kind of splint, as is done among many primitive tribes today, using tree branches or even soft clay that hardens into a protective cast around the injury. It is not inconceivable that prehistoric tribes also employed various means for reducing dislocations; indeed, primitive societies today often treat dislocations through massage or employ more active manipulations to alleviate these conditions.

Although we have no evidence for how prehistoric man dealt with lacerations and other kinds of open wounds, it is likely that they employed techniques similar to those seen used in primitive tribes today. Anthropologists have found that some primitive peoples employ a variety of means for stanching the flow of blood, for example, using herbs or roots, often with astringent or antibacterial qualities, that they apply to the wound in the form of powders or poultices. In other cases, they also apply heat, in the form of hot stones or needles, or even the direct application of fire, to stanch blood flow. Suturing wounds with stitches was likely rare among prehistoric peoples, and they were probably left open during treatment. Premodern tribes in different parts of the world today, however, display several other methods for closing wounds, which may have been employed in some early societies. For example, some tribes in South America and in parts of India have used large ants to close wounds; the edges of the wound would be brought together and grasped in the ant's mandibles, after which the ant's body would be removed, and the jaws, stiffening in death, would remain to hold the wound closed. Another means of suturing is employed among the Masai in Africa, who use a long acacia thorn, which is struck through both open edges and then the ends are united and twined together, drawing the wound closed. In the absence of suturing, however, a variety of substances might have been used as wound dressings (including animal substances, such as milk, fat, and even excrement) to keep the wound covered and aid in healing. It is therefore likely that through the empirical process of trial-and-error, our prehistoric forebears developed a number of methods of wound treatment.

In the early civilizations we examine, surgeons were predominantly concerned with treating fractures and wounds. However, as surgeons became more adept at healing injuries, they also expanded their skills to treat other physical conditions through surgery, including bladder stones, cataracts, and hernias. In some cases, surgeons even developed techniques for cosmetic surgery. As the theories and activities of healers became increasingly complex and specialized, those who focused on curing diseases and internal disorders (physicians or doctors) were distinguished from those who treated external conditions or provided physical treatments (surgeons). In this chapter, we will examine the activities and status of the surgeon in different cultures.

SURGERY IN ANCIENT MESOPOTAMIA

There are very few references in medical texts from ancient Mesopotamia to surgical activities or treatments suggesting that this knowledge was learned through apprenticeship and practice rather than through reading texts. The Code of Hammurabi, however, does offer some insight into surgical practice. It consists of 282 laws, which enumerate a range of regulations and prescribe punishments for various crimes, inscribed in the cuneiform script on a roughly seven-foot-tall, black diorite stone dating to about 1750 B.C.E. While it says nothing about the use of drugs or other treatments for internal diseases, it does include several regulations stipulating the *asu*'s fee for various procedures and thus giving a sense of the range of surgical operations he might be called upon to perform.

> 215: If a physician performed a major operation on a seignior with a bronze lancet and has saved the seignior's life, or he opened up the eye-socket of a seignior with a bronze lancet and has saved the seignior's eye, he shall receive ten shekels of silver.
>
> 216: If it was a member of the commonalty, he shall receive five shekels.
>
> 217: If it was a seignior's slave, the owner of the slave shall give two shekels of silver to the physician.

221: If a physician has a set a seignior's broken bone, or has healed a sprained tendon, the patient shall give five shekels of silver to the physician.

222: If it was a member of the commonalty, he shall give three shekels of silver.

223: If it was a seignior's slave, the owner of the slave shall give two shekels of silver to the physician.

Furthermore, punishments for unsuccessful cures or medical malpractice are also recorded.

218: If a physician performed a major operation on a seignior with a bronze lancet and has caused the seignior's death, or he opened up the eye-socket of a seignior and has destroyed the seignior's eye, they shall cut off his hand.

219: If a physician performed a major operation on a commoner's slave with a bronze lancet and has caused (his) death, he shall make good slave for slave.

220: If he opened up his eye-socket with a bronze lancet and has destroyed his eye he shall pay one-half his value in silver. (Meek 1969, 175–176)

Clearly, the risks were great for the *asu*, but so were the rewards—it would take a carpenter 450 working days to earn ten shekels!

In specifically medical texts, we find a few more detailed references to treating wounds with the bronze knife. In most cases, they refer to using the knife to make incisions to release pus from abscesses or boils. For example, one text, *Prescriptions for Diseases of the Head*, describes a typical procedure:

If the ailment mentioned above is painless, and the very surface of the flesh is intact; if, when you open, pus squirts out and keeps flowing: the name of this disease is "little she-fly." If the wind has blown onto the patient, it is a case of Pabil-sag [the god]: you can operate [on] it. To remove it, attack this disease with the point of the knife. After cutting it open grind boiled plaster, salt of ammonia and powder of [unknown mineral]. Apply all this onto the diseased surface and make a dressing of it. If the disease has reached into the bone, cut all around, scrape and remove. (Majno 1975, 52)

As this passage makes clear, the Mesopotamian *asu* learned how to make wound dressings to wrap and protect injuries. Surviving texts describe a few examples of the ointments or salves that could be made to wash and cover the wound, along with recommendations for how often to change bandages, but there is no specific mention of suturing wounds in the medical texts.

Other surgical procedures might have been performed by different kinds of practitioners. The code refers to the *asu alpim u lu imerim* ("physician of an ox or an ass," a veterinary surgeon), specifying the fee he could receive for performing a major operation on an animal to save its life and also the fine the veterinary surgeon would pay if his operation caused its death. It is likely that castration was one of the tasks the *asu alpim u lu imerim* might perform on animals, and other documents indicate that humans were also castrated, either as a form of punishment or because many court employees were expected to be eunuchs. The code also recognizes the *gallabu* (barber), who would perform minor manual operations. In the law codes, the *gallabu* is associated with branding or cutting the mark of the owner onto slaves, but some scholars have suggested that he might also perform other kinds of minor surgery such as extracting teeth, a function carried out by barbers in other early civilizations. Whether or not the *gallabu* was responsible for doing dental operations, we know that this was one of the kinds of surgical procedures regularly performed in ancient Mesopotamia. Dental problems were often associated with larger medical concerns, and tooth extraction was regarded as the necessary treatment, as can be seen in this letter from an *asu* to the king:

> Replying to what the king my lord wrote me, "send me your true diagnosis." I have given my diagnosis to the king my lord in one word: "Inflammation!" He whose head, hands, and feet are inflamed, owes his state to his teeth: his teeth should be extracted. On this account his insides are inflamed. The pain will presently subside; the condition will be mostly satisfactory. (Sigerist 1951, 435)

This interesting passage suggests that the *asu* might try to cure some internal disorders through physical operations, but it is unclear whether he would perform the extractions himself or leave this to another specialist.

SURGERY IN ANCIENT EGYPT

The medical papyri reveal a good deal about the surgical abilities of the *swnw* and the kinds of instruments they might employ. In most cases, the surgical operations described in the papyri are for treating traumas or lancing abscesses, but otherwise surgery was fairly limited in scope. No uniquely surgical instruments have been found from the period of the pharaohs, reinforcing the impression that the ancient Egyptians did not conduct difficult surgeries that might require specialized equipment. Most of our information about Egyptian surgery comes from the 48 surgical cases described in the Edwin Smith papyrus, which appears to have been aimed at teaching.

Dislocations and fractures are among the most prevalent conditions described in the Edwin Smith papyrus. The *swnw* is advised on how to reduce dislocations of the shoulder and the jaw and on how to reduce fractures so that broken bones could be set. Case 35 provides an elaborately detailed description of how to reduce a fractured clavicle:

> If you should examine a man having a break in his collar-bone, and you should find his collar-bone short and separated from its fellow. You should say concerning him: "One having a break in his collar-bone, an ailment which I will treat." You should place him prostrate on his back, with something folded between his two shoulder-blades; you should spread out with his two shoulders in order to stretch apart his collarbone until that break falls into its place. You should make for him two splints of linen, and you should apply one of them both on the inside of his upper arm and the other on the under side of his upper arm. You should bind it with *ymrw*, and treat it afterward with honey every day, until he recovers. (Breasted 1930, 350–352)

An analysis of 6,000 bodies buried in cemeteries in Aswan from 4000 B.C.E. to 500 C.E., found 200 with united fractures. Although some revealed perfect alignment of the bones, most instances were less successful, and several display excessive shortening of the limb and misalignment of the bones, revealing how difficult it was to sustain the traction necessary to maintain alignment (Jones 1908,

455–458). The accounts of treating fractures suggest the use of bandages and also of some form of splint as described for the clavicle fracture, to hold the bones in place while they healed.

Bites and stings from a variety of creatures, including snakes, scorpions, lions, crocodiles, and humans, defined the other major category of traumas sustained by ancient Egyptians. The first concern for snake and scorpion bites was whether the person might expect to survive the venom, depending upon what kind of snake bit him. Treatment included using a combination of magical incantations and surgical remedies. One papyrus offers this advice, "What is to be done for the bite of the male snake? Incise his wound/bite with the knife treatment many times. Then you should apply a bandage to it (with) red natron . . . salt, etc." Or, "Another [remedy] to drive out the swelling. Incise his wound/bite with the *des*-knife many times on the first day. Apply salt 1/8 or natron. Bandage the wound with it" (Nunn 1996, 188). The emphasis on swift treatment (numerous applications on the first day) and the need to cut around the swelling at the wound would serve to reduce the swelling and possibly to minimize the absorption of the venom. For bites where there was no concern for venom, treatment mainly consisted of bandaging various drugs over the injury, as was done with other forms of wounds, and there is no mention of cutting around the site. For example, the doctor is told, "If you examine the bite of a crocodile and you find it [with] his flesh piled up and its two sides being separated, then you should bandage it with fresh meat on the first day, likewise all wounds of a man" (Nunn 1996, 190).

The treatment for a crocodile bite is indicative of the approach to curing all kinds of gaping wounds: bandage with fresh meat on the first day. Following the initial treatment with fresh meat, the *asu* might bind other substances (such as honey, grease, and lint) over the wound. These procedures were likely effective since fresh meat has been shown to contain coagulants that could help stanch bleeding and the antibacterial quality of honey would likely serve to reduce the chance of infections and thus accelerate healing.

SURGERY IN ANCIENT GREECE AND ROME

Hippocratic Surgeons

The Hippocratic texts reveal that the *iatros* was prepared to perform a wide variety of surgical procedures to treat injuries and wounds. For example, two entire texts, *On Fractures* and *On Joints*, were dedicated to explaining methods for realigning broken bones and reducing dislocations. While two strong men would serve to carry out the procedure in most cases, the texts also discuss the construction of an innovative apparatus that could mechanically draw the limb back into alignment. For example, in order to repair a spinal distortion, the *iatros* is advised to give the patient a warm bath, presumably to help relax the muscles, and then strap him down to a plank, with straps under the armpits and around the hips so that they could be drawn apart, while the *iatros* massaged the spine back into alignment. If necessary, the author says that a wheel and axle could be attached to either end of the board and to the straps so that they could be turned to stretch the spine; furthermore, he notes, "This reduction apparatus is easy to regulate as regards greater or less force, and has such power that, if one wanted to use such forcible maneuvers for harm and not for healing, it is able to act strongly in this way also" (Withington 1944a, 301). Clearly, the author recognized another potential use for this device and was not thinking of the directive in the Hippocratic *Oath* that the physician should do no harm.

Hippocratic surgery was not limited to the treatment of wounds and injuries, however; indeed, the authors also discussed a number of elective operations. In addition to lancing boils, the knife was used for the surgical removal of nasal polyps, for removing swollen tonsils, and for cutting ulcerated varicose veins. Cautery was also used to treat certain surgical conditions such as hemorrhoids: "Force the anus out as far as possible with your fingers; heat the irons red-hot, and burn until you so dry the hemorrhoids out that you do not need to anoint: burn them off completely, leaving nothing uncauterized" (Potter 1995, 381–383). The *iatros* might also undertake more daring procedures, such as that described in *On Diseases II* for draining pus from the pleural cavity:

> Cut as low as possible so that the pus may flow out more easily. Cut between the ribs, the skin first, using a knife with a rounded blade. Then take a pointed knife, wrap its blade in a cloth so that only the point will protrude as much as the length of a thumb's nail, and cut through [to the pleural cavity]. Let out as much pus as you think best, then put in a tent of raw linen attached to a thread. Let out the pus once a day. On the tenth day, having removed all the pus, put in a tent of fine linen; then inject warm wine and oil through a small tube, so that the lung, accustomed to be moistened by the pus, may not remain suddenly dry. Remove in the evening the oil and wine injected in the morning; that injected in the evening, remove it on the following morning. When the pus becomes as thin as water, slippery to the finger, and scanty, put into the wound a hollow tin drain. When the pleural cavity becomes dry cut the drain shorter little by little, and allow the incision to heal as you retrieve the drain. Signs that the patient will escape death: if the pus is white and pure and contains streaks of blood, there are good chances of healing. But if pus . . . on the next day flows thick, greenish and fetid the patients die after the pus has run out. (Majno 1975, 157)

Aside from this extreme case, however, most Greek surgery was fairly conservative and fairly limited in scope.

The Greeks also applied surgery for treating internal disorders. The humoral theory, which explained disease as caused by an imbalance in the body's humors, dictated that treatment should aim at restoring the balance through dietary changes or by purging the excess harmful humor. One means of removing excess humors was through the application of bloodletting (also referred to as phlebotomy or venesection), and several Hippocratic treatises recommend the use of the knife to let blood from veins. Although some texts merely recommend phlebotomy without specifying a location, others advise that veins be opened in different parts of the body, depending on the condition. For example, *On the Nature of Man* recommends that for pain in the loins and testicles blood should be let from behind the knee or the inner side of the ankle, but in other conditions, it is recommended that blood be let from the inner arm at the elbow. It appears that the application of the knife to let blood for the purposes of treating internal disorders was likely one of

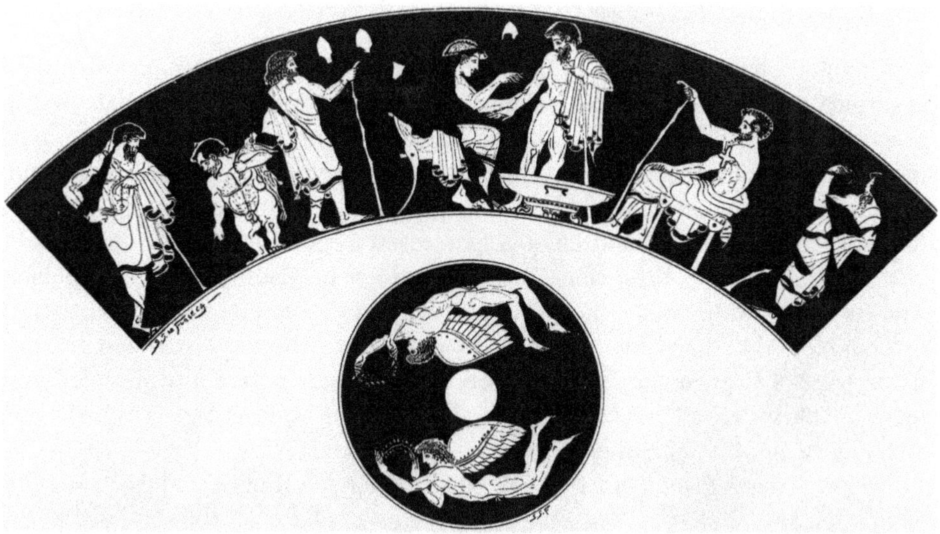

This is a flattened view of the images on a Greek vase from ca. 480–460 B.C.E. It depicts a doctor letting blood from a patient in the center, while other patients, including a dwarf and an amputee, wait for assistance. Some patients use crutches or walking sticks and wear bandages on their arms or legs. The small white shapes in the space above the doctor are the vessels used for cupping. (Wellcome Collection)

the most common surgical procedures performed by the Hippocratic doctors. In a later period, Galen (129–ca. 216 C.E.) wrote no fewer than three treatises dedicated to bloodletting: *On Venesection*, *On Venesection against Erasistratus*, and *On Venesection against the Erasistrateans*. He elaborated upon the Hippocratic theories, making phlebotomy not only the preferred treatment for a wide range of internal disorders, but also the main tool for preventative health. Galen advocated letting blood from different veins in the body, depending upon the location and nature of the internal disorder, and argued that other factors, such as the season and the age of the patient, should also be taken into consideration when determining when and how much blood to let. Following Galen, bloodletting became a fundamental method of treatment throughout the Greco-Roman world and continued to be practiced in the Islamic world and during the European Middle Ages.

Cupping was another manual practice in the Greek world that, like phlebotomy, required physical application on the body to treat internal disorders. Cupping entailed putting a piece of burning material into a little metal cup so that when applied to the skin, the flame would be extinguished and create a vacuum, holding the cup to the skin. These could be applied to the skin to help draw humors to the site, to help rectify localized humoral imbalances in the body. The practice of "wet" cupping (as opposed to "dry" cupping) entailed scarifying the skin to cause bleeding before applying the cup so that excess humors could be drawn out of the body. This treatment was so closely associated with doctors that the cupping vessel became one of the main symbols of a doctor, very much as the stethoscope might be a symbol of the doctor today.

Roman Surgeons

Although often suspicious of Greek theoretical medicine, Romans were adept at surgical practice. Archaeological discoveries have revealed that Roman medical practitioners possessed surgical kits with a number of specialized surgical tools, including scalpels, probes, hooks, forceps, bone levers, cautery needles, cupping vessels, trephining saws, and rectal or vaginal specula. Indeed, a surgeon in the town of Rimini from around 257 C.E. possessed a kit with over 150 instruments with many versions of the same instrument each displaying subtle differences. The variations in the instruments suggest that they were adapted for specialized procedures (or perhaps for operating on people of different sizes) and attest to wide range of Roman surgical expertise. Archaeologists have also revealed false teeth (made with both real and artificial teeth) and a variety of artificial limbs attesting to the Roman ability to make prosthetic devices.

Although he was not a practicing doctor himself, the Roman author, Aulus Cornelius Celsus (ca. 25 B.C.E.–ca. 50 C.E.) offers an excellent account of the extent of Roman surgical practice in the seventh book of his *De Medicina*, where he considers "the third part of the Art of Medicine . . . that which cures by the hand." Celsus holds surgical skill in high regard, declaring that it is more reflective of the doctor's expertise than other forms of treatment since people often recover from diseases as much from luck as from any medicines, whereas it is obvious when the surgeon's actions are the reason for success (Spencer 1961, 295). He reveals that Roman surgeons were more adventurous than their Hippocratic forebears and were willing to attempt many more difficult procedures. These included the surgical removal of cancerous tumors (although he lamented that using corrosive substances to burn them out only made them grow faster and that cutting them out was often ineffective because they only grew back after scar tissue had formed), hernia repair, removal of bladder stones, and amputation. Celsus also describes in great detail the operation for couching cataracts (moving aside or extracting a lens that has become so cloudy that it blocks light from reaching the retina), which he claims is the most delicate of procedures. The patient should be seated and have his healthy eye covered so he will not see what is about to happen next:

> Thereupon a needle is to be taken pointed enough to penetrate, yet not too fine; and this is to be inserted straight through the two outer tunics [layers of the eye] at a spot intermediate between the pupil of the eye and the angle adjacent to the temple, away from the middle of the cataract, in such a way that no vein is wounded. The needle should not be, however, entered timidly, for it passes into the empty space and when this is reached even a man of moderate experience cannot be mistaken, for there is then no resistance to pressure. When the spot is reached, the needle is to be sloped against the suffusion itself and should gently rotate there and little by little guide it below the region of the pupil; when the cataract has passed below the pupil it is pressed upon more firmly in order that it may settle below. If it sticks there the cure is accomplished; if it returns to some extent it is to be cut up with the same needle and separated into several pieces, which can be the more easily stowed away singly, and form smaller obstacles to vision. After this the needle is drawn straight out; and soft wool soaked in white of egg is to be put on, and above this something to check inflammation; and then bandages. (Spencer 1961, 345–353)

The range of complex surgical procedures described by Celsus reveals the extent to which surgical expertise had advanced in the Greco-Roman world by his time. Not to diminish the Roman surgeon's skills, we should remember that these operations were carried out without the benefit of anesthetics. Therefore, it should not come as a surprise that when Celsus describes the qualities of an ideal surgeon, he recommends that while the surgeons should feel pity for the patient, he should not be "moved by [the patient's] cries, to go too fast, or cut less than is necessary; but he does everything just as if the cries of pain cause him no emotion" (Spencer 1961, 297). Patients must have been suffering indeed to decide to undergo any form of elective surgery!

SURGERY IN INDIA

Surgical Training and Procedures

Early Ayurvedic medical texts, the *Susruta Samhita* in particular, contains several chapters on a variety of surgical procedures. The author of the *Susruta* praises surgery as the oldest and most important of all the branches of the Ayurveda, since "it contains all that can be found in the other branches of the science of medicine as well, with the superior advantages of producing instantaneous effects by means of surgical instruments and appliances" (Bhishagratna 1907, 8). Furthermore, the author maintains that the surgeon, "skilled in the art of using surgical instruments, is always successful in his professional practice, and hence the practice of surgery should be commenced at the very outset of medical studies" (Bhishagratna 1907, 70).

Becoming a successful surgeon, however, was not an easy task. First, the surgeon needed to become familiar with the use of a wide range of instruments, including knives, probes, and implements for cautery; the *Susruta* recommends that young surgeons learn how to use their instruments by practicing on dead animals, gourds, cucumbers, watermelons, or filled water skins. Furthermore, while acknowledging that religious prohibitions against contact with dead bodies posed a difficulty, the author of the *Susruta* maintained that the surgeon should familiarize himself with anatomy by examining a dead body in the following manner:

> The excrementa should be first removed from the entrails and the body should be left to decompose in the water of a solitary and still pool, and securely placed in a cage (so that it may not be eaten away by fish nor drift away), after having covered it entirely with the outer sheaths of *Munja* grass, *Kusa* grass, hemp or with rope etc. After seven days the body would be thoroughly decomposed, when the observer should slowly scrape off the decomposed skin etc. with a whisk made of grass-roots, hair, *Kusa* blade or with a strip of split bamboo and carefully observe with his own eyes all the various different organs, external and internal, beginning with the skin as described before. (Bhishagratna 1911, 172)

Despite this advice, it is likely that most surgeons did not acquire much anatomical knowledge beyond what they could learn by treating wounds, however. As a result, the surgeon's basic knowledge of anatomy most likely revolved around learning the locations of the 107 *marmas*, vital parts or seats of life in the body.

Injury to any of these sites was supposed to lead to rapid death without judicious treatment, and the surgeon needed to carefully avoid damaging these areas when performing operations.

Bloodletting and cautery are perhaps the two most common surgical procedures described in the *Susruta*. Phlebotomy could be accomplished with the knife or with leeches—indeed, in one chapter, the author explains the classification, selection and appropriate care of leeches, as well as their application for bloodletting. Cautery could also be accomplished by different means, either with caustic substances or hot-irons. Both of these forms of what we might consider minor surgery might be used to treat an internal disorder (e.g., an imbalance of *doshas* leading to disease), to stanch bleeding or to treat an external ulcer. Indeed, so far as the author of the *Susruta* was concerned, surgery and internal medicine were closely related, and therefore, the surgeon needed to be familiar with the written tradition of theoretical medicine.

Early Methods of Reconstructive Surgery

The *Susruta* describes a number of difficult elective surgical procedures, including operations for removing anal fistulas, reducing inguinal hernias, and couching cataracts. Perhaps the most remarkable procedures covered in Indian medical texts are those for plastic surgery. Piercing the earlobes for wearing jewelry as ornamentation and to ward off malign influences was a common practice in ancient India. The piercing procedure and post-operative treatment are portrayed in the text along with advice on how to cope with complications caused by profuse bleeding or infection (including the risk of tetanus). Once pierced, the earlobes were gradually stretched over time by carrying heavy ornaments and in some cases, whether by the weight or in the course of an argument, the earring would tear through the lobe. This condition appears to have occurred regularly enough to merit extensive coverage in the *Susruta*. Indeed, the author classifies no fewer than 15 varieties of tears and 10 different diseases that affect torn earlobes!

In response to these conditions, Indian surgeons developed methods of reconstructive surgery to repair the torn lobes. Taking the type of tear (e.g., whether the ends of the bifurcated lobes were of equal size, thick or shriveled, short or extended, etc.) into consideration, the surgeon would scarify the two parts of the torn lobe and wash the bleeding ends with different substances, depending upon which of the *doshas* was deemed to be disordered. Then the surgeon would adhere the two ends, anoint them with honey and clarified butter, wrap them in cotton, tie them together with string, and leave them to heal (with continued application of medicines and appropriate attention to diet and regimen). If all went well, the two ends of the lobe would grow together over time, but the *Susruta* offers advice on what to do should further complications arise. Thus, we find a pioneering account of plastic or reconstructive surgery from the ancient world.

The *Susruta* also describes an even more difficult technique for rhinoplasty, replacing noses cut off in battle or, more often, as a common form of punishment for adultery. A flap of skin would be cut from the patient's forehead, leaving a strip attached at the bridge of the nose. The flap would then be twisted down and sewn over the scarified skin around the hole on the face, with two tubes inserted to help mold the nostrils. The strip of skin at the top of the nose would provide nourishment through blood vessels, until the scarified tissue of the flap and around the hole grew together and produced new blood vessels. The ability to carry out this procedure successfully would be very valuable, as the author notes, since "the physician, who is well conversant with these matters, can be alone entrusted with the medical treatment of a king" (Bhishagratna 1907, 154). Essentially the same procedure is still used today.

Surgery and the *Vaidya*

The *Susruta* is certainly remarkable for its detailed description of several elaborate surgical procedures and for the effort to unite the practice of surgery with the theoretical concepts of Ayurvedic medicine. It is, however, unlikely that the surgical activities described continued to be practiced by the *vaidyas* ("doctors") much beyond the time when the *Susruta* was composed. Later Ayurvedic medical texts do not reflect any further development of surgical techniques, and those that do cover surgery are mainly based on sections copied from the *Susruta*. Historians believe that as the caste system developed during the first millennium C.E., taboos against cutting into the body may have led *vaidyas*, trained in the Sanskrit literary tradition and coming from the upper social castes, to avoid the practice of surgery. The result was that surgery gradually ceased to be represented in the written tradition of Ayurvedic medicine as *vaidyas* focused their attention on internal medicine.

There is evidence, however, that the surgical practices discussed in the *Susruta* were continued by members of lower social castes, who functioned as barber-surgeons. These barber-surgeons would not have been trained in the learned, written tradition of Ayurveda; rather, they would have learned and passed on their surgical skills via apprenticeship. The argument in favor of the continuation of surgery outside the literary tradition is supported by the example of the famous rhinoplasty operation witnessed by British army surgeons in India in 1793. A Maratha named Cowasjee, who had been a bullock-driver with the British army, had been captured by the forces of the Tipu Sultan and had his nose and hand cut off. In the following year, he and his associates who had suffered the same fate sought the aid of a man from the brick-maker's caste near Poona, who performed the reconstructive surgery. The British surgeons, thoroughly impressed by this operation, wrote up a description of it, along with diagrams and an engraved illustration, for publication in Europe. The fact that the procedure was performed by a member of the brick-maker's caste, who probably knew no Sanskrit, strongly suggests that the techniques first recorded in the *Susruta* persisted outside the written medical tradition.

CHINESE SURGERY

The Low Status of Surgery and Surgeons

Little written evidence exists concerning the practice of surgery in ancient China. Within traditional Chinese medicine, even skin disorders and wounds were treated according to the theory of systematic correspondence, and as a result, the medical literature contains few references to any kind of surgical procedures. It may be too simplistic to blame the Confucian dogma against opening the body for the apparent lack of attention to surgery, but in any event, it does appear that surgical skill was not highly regarded and the surgeon was considered inferior to the physician. As a result, surgery existed outside the learned tradition of Chinese medicine and therefore was typically practiced by illiterates, who learned their technical skills through apprenticeship and were unfamiliar with the theoretical, written medical tradition.

The written tradition of Chinese medicine does celebrate the possibly legendary activities of one learned surgeon, Hua Tuo (110–207 C.E.). He is said to have traveled widely in China, learning from popular medical traditions wherever he went and to have served as physician to kings. Among other things, Hua Tuo is recognized for his advocacy of acupuncture and physical exercise as remedies, but he was most famous for his surgical skills. One famous story attributes to him the discovery of an anesthetic known as *mafeisan*, a powder dissolved in a fermented beverage, which he used on a patient on whom he performed some form of abdominal surgery. Another legend relates that Cao Cao, ruler of the Cao Wei kingdom in northern China, requested Hua Tuo's presence at court, but the physician refused to attend him. Infuriated, Cao Cao had Hua Tuo imprisoned and sentenced for execution. While in prison prior to his execution, Hua Tuo wrote down his medical learning, but when he could not smuggle it out of prison, he had it burned. Another legend relates that a few pages were snatched from the flames, containing his explanation for the procedure of castration, but otherwise all of his medical learning, including the recipe for *mafeisan*, was lost!

Moxibustion and Acupuncture

Although the practice of surgery was not highly regarded in ancient China, the application of acupuncture, which was a physical operation, became a highly valued therapeutic practice favored by physicians. The origin of acupuncture is not clear, but it seems to have developed out of early surgical activities. The earliest Chinese medical texts discovered in the Mawangdui gravesites, which date to about 168 B.C.E., do not mention acupuncture, but they offer insight into the development of theories that would later support the practice. These texts describe a series of 11 *mai* (vessels) running through the body and emphasize that disease arises from disturbances in the flow of qi (vapor) through them. The therapeutic practice advocated for treating disorders is cauterization by means of applying burning materials on the body along the path of the affected *mai* in order to influence the movement of qi. This form of cauterization soon developed into the practice of moxibustion, the specific use of mugwort tinder (moxa) to cause the burn. The practice of bloodletting may also have provided a precursor to the use of acupuncture. The Mawangdui texts do not mention bloodletting (although it is discussed in the *Huangdi Neijing*), but they do discuss the use of lancing stones to open abscesses. Furthermore, those texts indicate that the *mai* contain both qi and blood and the congruence between blood vessels and *mai* is suggestive. The *Huangdi Neijing* recommends bloodletting to release bad blood and to stimulate the flow of qi. In this regard, the practice of bloodletting may also have contributed to the development of acupuncture therapy.

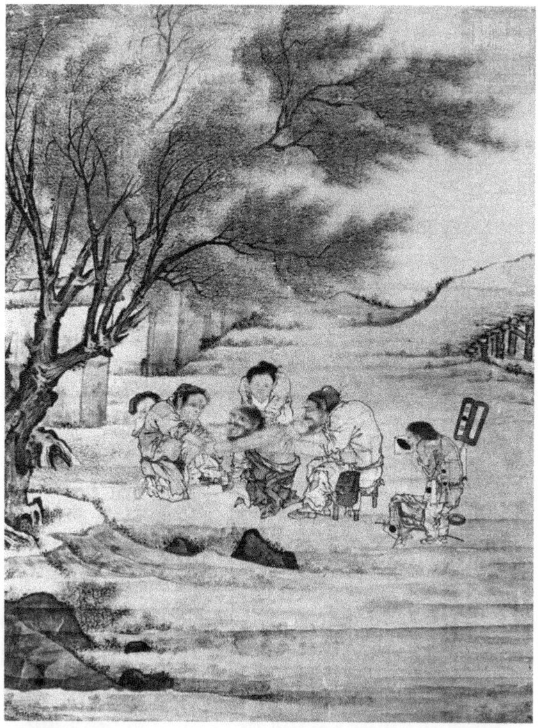

In this painting by Li Tang (1049–1130), a Chinese village doctor is shown applying moxibustion to a patient, who is shouting with pain while being held still by another man. (Takeyoshi Tanuma/Time Life Pictures/Getty Images)

It is clear, however, that by the first century B.C.E. acupuncture was adopted as a supplement to moxibustion as the primary means of correcting the flow of qi in the body. The *Huangdi Neijing* provides an elaborate explanation of the procedure, although it does not always clearly distinguish between the use of moxibustion or acupuncture. This text identifies twelve channels or meridians in the body through which qi flows and identifies 365 specific points on the body along these channels for applying moxibustion or acupuncture. According to the theoretical system, the body was in a constant flux between a state of *shi* (fullness) and *xu* (emptiness), and acupuncture could be used to either deplete or drain off fullness or stimulate the flow of qi to combat emptiness. Unlike bloodletting, therefore, acupuncture was used either to remove excesses and sedate the body or to correct deficiencies and to tonify the body. Indeed, as it developed, acupuncture became a bloodless form of surgery—any bleeding from the needlepoint would represent a lapse in technique. The acupuncturist needed to consider a number of factors when applying the needles, as one passage in the *Huangdi Neijing* makes clear:

> The nine needles are of different size, shape, and use. When acupuncturing excess, one must sedate. Insert the needles and await the arrival of *yin qi*. When one feels a cooling sensation under the needle, remove the needles. In deficiency, one must tonify. After needle insertion, await the arrival of *yang qi*. When there is a warming sensation, remove the needles. Once you grasp the *qi* with the needle, be very attentive and listen so as not to lose the opportunity to manipulate the effects. Treat disease according to where it is located; determine whether to insert deeply or shallowly. When the disease is located deep, insert deeply. When the disease is superficial, needle shallowly. Although there is a difference in depth of penetration, the principle of awaiting the *qi* is the same. (Ni 1995, 192–193)

Later texts, including the *Nanjing* and Huangfu Mi's (215–282 C.E.) *Zhenjiu Jiayijing* (*The ABC of Acupuncture and Moxibustion*), provide more detailed descriptions of the use of needles applied to specific points to restore health and more fully relate the use of acupuncture to the paradigm of systematic correspondence that forms the theoretical basis of traditional Chinese medicine. Over time, the number of points identified for acupuncture rose. Finally, during the Song dynasty (960–1279 C.E.), Wang Weiyi (ca. 987–1067) produced two bronze statues of a man into which 657 holes were drilled representing acupuncture points, which could be used for teaching. These models were filled with water and then covered with wax and students would be expected to practice their acupuncture skills, knowing that if they hit water, they had found the proper acupuncture point. Wang Weiyi also compiled the *Tongren Shuxue Zhen Jiu Tujing* (*Illustrated Manual of the Bronze Man Showing Acupuncture and Moxibustion Points*), as a guide to teaching for those who did not have access to the bronze models.

SURGERY IN THE ISLAMIC WORLD

Arabic medical literature from the 10th and 11th centuries provides extensive coverage of surgery. These texts draw extensively upon the Greek and Roman written tradition, and as a result, Islamic books on surgery cover many of the same procedures without additions or emendations. Despite the lively medical literature, some question remains concerning the extent to which the written works on surgery reflected actual surgical practice in the Islamic world. In several surgical writings, physicians described a surgical procedure but then commented that they did not know anyone who actually performed the operation or indicated that they themselves chose not to do it. Indeed, it is suggestive that although the famous physician, Abu Bakr Muhammad ibn Zakariya al-Razi (d. ca. 925, known as Rhazes in the Latin West), described 900 case histories from his own practice in his formal medical texts, he did not discuss performing any surgical procedures aside from bloodletting and cauterization.

One explanation for the lack of innovation or indication of personal experience in surgical writings may be attributed to the fact that Arabic literature recognized distinct medical specialties and a division of labor, whereby physicians did not undertake surgery themselves. One physician noted,

> As for the handling of these matters with surgery, that is a function of some of the assistants to the physician. The same is true for bloodletting, cautery, and phlebotomy . . . All these are functions of the physician's attendants. As for the physician, he should be concerned with treating the patient by means of diet and medicaments and he should not include manual techniques [that is, surgery]. (Pormann and Savage-Smith 2007, 122)

Indeed, by the 14th century, Arabic authors recognized a number of specialized medical practitioners apart from physicians, who focused on particular manual operations, including oculists, circumcisers, phlebotomists, cuppers, bonesetters, cauterizers, and those who administered enemas. These practitioners would have a lower status than the physicians, trained in the written medical tradition, and they likely developed their own skills through apprenticeship and practice.

Abu al-Qasim al-Zahrawi

Not all physicians eschewed surgical practice, however. Abu al-Qasim al-Zahrawi (fl. ca. 1000, known as Albucasis in the Latin West) was one of the physicians who earned a reputation for his surgical skills in Islamic Spain. Although he often expresses caution about undertaking surgical procedures and does not suggest many innovative surgical techniques in his encyclopedic work, *The Arrangement of Medical Knowledge for One Who Is Not Able to Compile a Book for Himself*, al-Zahrawi does describe 18 surgical case histories from his own practice. Eleven of the cases were for the treatment of wounds (from arrows, spears, and knives), four involved the removal of tumors or growths, two were cases where he chose not to operate (including a man who amputated his own foot and hand), and for the final case, he provides no details about treatment. His texts make it clear that despite his status as a physician, al-Zahrawi did not hesitate to perform surgical treatments himself. For example,

> My own experience was this: a slave-girl seized a knife and buried it in her throat and cut part of the trachea; and I was called to attend her. I found her bellowing like a sacrifice that has had its throat cut. So I laid the wound bare and found that only a little hemorrhage had come from it; and I assured myself that neither the jugular vein nor an artery had been cut, but air passed out through the wound. So I hurriedly sutured the wound and dressed it until healed. And no ill befell the maid except for a hoarseness in the voice, but nothing more; and after some days she was restored to the best of health. Hence, we may say that tracheotomy is not dangerous. (Spink and Lewis 1973, 338)

Al-Zahrawi's encyclopedia is remarkable for its inclusion of a number of illustrations of surgical instruments. His surgical chapters describe the use of a number of sophisticated instruments for use in typical surgical procedures. Modifying a procedure for the removal of stones in the duct carrying urine from the bladder, al-Zahrawi describes the use of a fine drill that would be inserted through the urinary passage to break up the stone, as an alternative to the procedure described in Greek sources that required making an incision to remove the obstruction. In another case, he describes using a scissorlike instrument with transverse blades for removing tonsils: the surgeon would hold the tongue with a tongue depressor, grasp the swollen tonsil with a hook, and then cut through the gland with this ingenious instrument. Al-Zahrawi also invented a knife for lancing abscesses, which was designed so as not to alarm the patient. The instrument, which he called the "deceiver," was made by concealing the blade between two curved plates attached to a handle so that it could be extended for use only as needed. The development of such specialized instruments for use in these more common operations makes clear that some Islamic surgeons did continue to advance their craft in this period.

SURGERY IN THE MEDIEVAL WEST

Surgeons and Physicians

During the European Middle Ages, surgery flourished as a craft tradition, and surgeons were trained through apprenticeship. Following the rise of universities in the 12th century, many physicians made a categorical distinction between the *physicus* ("physician") trained in the written tradition of learned medicine at the university, and the *chirurgicus* ("surgeon"), who learned his skills in practice, with little if any exposure to the medical works of the Greek, Roman, and Arabic authors.

The physician claimed expertise in the practice of internal medicine, prescribing drugs to cure the humoral imbalances that caused disease, while the surgeon was expected to limit his practice to the application of manual procedures to treat wounds and external conditions, including skin disorders. Although physicians claimed the prerogative to regulate the practice of phlebotomy, since it was undertaken to treat internal disorders and therefore depended upon the physician's extensive theoretical knowledge, surgeons were the ones who would typically apply the knives and often did so without a physician's supervision. Thus, patients might also turn to surgeons when looking for cures to a variety of internal diseases through bloodletting.

In addition to the professional *chirurgicus*, a number of other individuals in medieval society might offer surgical cures. Barber-surgeons would not only offer a shave and a haircut but would also be ready to let blood or pull teeth as part of their regular services—indeed, the barber's bowl could serve both to hold warm water for shaving and to catch blood drained through phlebotomy. Furthermore, a wide range of empirics, who specialized in the treatment of a particular condition, including fractures, bladder stones, cataracts, and hernias, also flourished. Faced with competition from these other practitioners, surgeons often sought to protect their own craft knowledge. For example, after relating his cure for hemorrhoids in his book, the English surgeon, John of Arderne (1307–1380 or 1392), advised, "The doctor should be careful in case any of the bystanders see how it is done as the excrescences are opened up. Since once the barbers grasped the method they would usurp this cure for themselves to the considerable shame and harm of the master surgeons" (Jones 1994, 304).

The Rise of Rational Surgery

From the 12th to 15th centuries, there was an explosion of new treatises on the practice of surgery, written in both Latin and vernacular languages by physicians. This explosion was in part fueled by the rapid influx of translations of Arabic and Greek surgical texts into Latin (the writings of al-Zahrawi, known as Albucasis in the West, were especially influential) that provided a theoretical foundation for the practice of surgery. One of the first to write a surgical text was Roger Frugard (before 1140–ca. 1195), a physician and surgeon at Parma, who produced his *Chirurgia* (*Surgery*) around 1170. The *Chirurgia*, which covered the treatment of injuries in a head-to-toe arrangement, became a standard text for Latin instruction in surgery in the universities in Italy and at Montpellier until the late 13th century when it was supplanted by newer Latin books on surgery and the direct study of Greek and Arabic texts, especially that of Albucasis.

Frugard's *Chirurgia* helped to spawn a new genre in medical writing in Western Europe, the Latin general surgery. Many of the authors of these new Latin surgical texts self-consciously sought to elevate the study and practice of surgery to the status of a learned science, founded upon abstract rational principles (McVaugh 2006). Two physicians working in Bologna sought to describe surgical practice with reference to the Greco-Arabic surgical texts, the procedures used by their contemporaries and their own practice: Teodorico Borgognoni (ca. 1205–1298), who started writing handbooks on surgery in the 1240s, and Bruno Longoburgo, who produced his *Cyrurgia magna* (*Great Surgery*) in 1252. Both authors expanded the study of surgery beyond the treatment of wounds to include the treatment of cancers and conditions such as arthritis and gout. Furthermore, their goal was to situate the study of surgery within the learned tradition of medicine and to consider significant earlier surgical scholarship from authors including Galen, Albucasis, Avicenna, Rhazes, Haly Abbas, and Roger Frugard. Thus, both authors argued that surgery was a subject that should be learned, at least in part, from books. Teodorico expresses this opinion in this way:

> It behooves practitioners of surgery . . . to frequent the places where skilled surgeons operate, and to attend their operations diligently, and to commit them to memory . . . because all things which are necessary to the art cannot be included in books, cannot easily be foreseen, and many of these frequently happen to the operator. . . . [However,] they must needs be well-read, and even if they be aided sometimes by experience, yet frequently will they fall into error and into confusion. I scarcely think that anyone can understand surgery without schooling [in texts]. (Campbell and Colton 1955, 4–5)

An Italian author of a Latin surgical manual, Guglielmo da Saliceto (1210–1277), who wrote Latin treatises on surgery in the 1270s, went so far as to argue that surgery was a *scientia* ("science," or learned body of knowledge) that could be learned entirely from books, without ever practicing. The new genre of Latin rational surgical manuals was spread to France at the end of the 13th century by Lanfranc (d. 1315), a student of Guglielmo da Saliceto, who fled Italy to go first to Lyon and then to Paris, and Henri de Mondeville (ca. 1260–ca. 1320), a pupil of Teodorico Borgognoni, who taught at Montpellier and Paris. Both physicians composed surgical manuals in Latin, and like their predecessors, they based their identities as surgeons on their knowledge of the learned textual tradition and clearly hoped to see the teaching of surgery institutionalized within the universities as a theoretical subject alongside the study of medicine.

The last of the great medieval authors of a Latin surgical manual, Guy de Chauliac (1298–1368), wrote his massive *Inventarium sive Chirurgia Magna* (*The Inventarium or Great Surgery*) around 1363. Guy earned his degree in medicine at Montpellier and studied surgery in Bologna before beginning his own medical practice and spent most of his career serving as physician to three different popes in Avignon. Although he addressed his work to surgeons, Guy appears to have been less concerned than his predecessors with strictly defending the rationality of surgery. He did not hesitate to relate cases where he had learned procedures from empirics and readily discussed the importance of his own training through practice. Nonetheless, the *Inventarium* surveyed the principle textual authorities and the historical development of the rational study of surgery to his day and provided a comprehensive, systematic overview of the

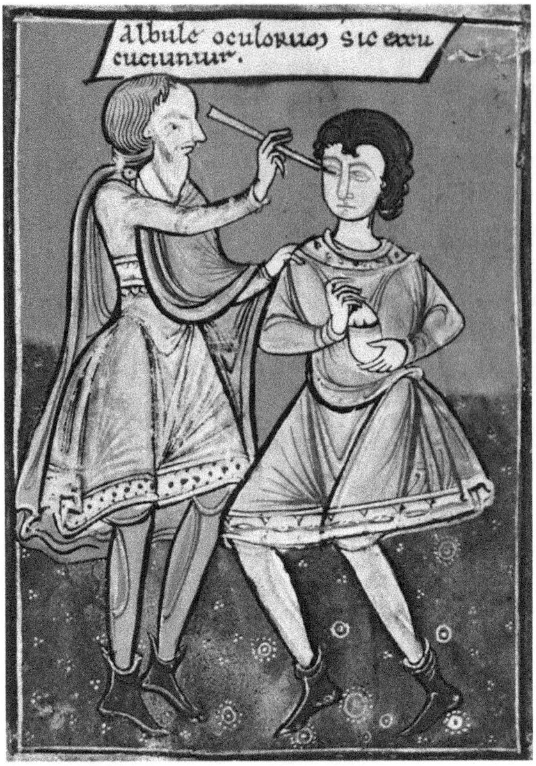

This illustration, from an early 14th-century copy of Roger Frugard's manual on surgery, depicts the procedure for couching a cataract. The long needle would be inserted into the eye to dislodge the clouded lens. (The British Library)

discipline and as such marks the culmination of the medieval tradition of rational surgery.

Vernacular Surgery Texts and Craft Practice

In their effort to promote surgery as a rational, textual subject worthy of being taught in the universities, many authors of Latin surgical manuals were dismissive of the activities of craft surgeons and de-emphasized the value of empirical learning. For example, drawing a distinction between those surgeons trained through apprenticeship and the new rational surgeons, Henri de Mondeville emphasized that "a surgery that is learned only by practice and that is carried out lacking any prior theoretical instruction, like the surgery of peasants and illiterates, is a purely mechanical effort, neither theoretical in a proper sense nor a proper science or art" (McVaugh 2006, 61). Guy de Chauliac, by contrast, sought out opportunities to observe the practice of craft surgeons and report on their successful cures. Indeed, increasingly in the 14th century learned surgeons appear to have yielded the practice of dangerous invasive procedures to the empirical specialists. In particular, the rational surgeons increasingly avoided operating for cataracts, hernias and bladder stones, leaving those procedures to a variety of traveling craft operators, who were not necessarily familiar with the written tradition of surgery. The learned physician-surgeons would have had a good reason for doing this—as Henri de Mondeville complained when noting the difficulties faced by surgeons, "the surgeon has to perform manual operations, and any mistake in his treatment leaps to the eye or touch and is bound to be set down to him; but mistakes made by physicians are not obvious to the senses and can be ascribed to 'nature' or 'the governing force of the body'" (McVaugh 2001, 332). In this regard, it might have been more advantageous for the physician-surgeon to have prescribed drugs and other treatments for cataracts and other conditions and left the manual operations to the lower-status empirics.

Nor is it possible to believe that empiric surgeons of the later Middle Ages were unaware of the tradition of rational surgery. Indeed, during this period, the proliferation of translations of surgical manuals into vernacular languages (spoken languages of the people: French, German, and English among others), including Guy de Chauliac's *Inventarium*, meant that many more people had access to the rational surgeries. Likewise, during this period, original works on surgery were also being produced in vernacular languages. The production of so many surgical manuals in the vernacular attests to the increasing demand for technical books on surgery and a growing community of surgeons who were literate in vernacular languages, if not in Latin.

9

Mental Health

The concept of psychiatry did not exist until the 19th century, and premodern views of psychopathology do not easily coincide with our own. Mental disorders or conditions that caused an individual to appear as though they were not in control of their own faculties, or in their "right mind," posed a particular challenge for premodern societies. Conditions causing psychoses, delusions, and fits were not always viewed as belonging in the sphere of the doctor, but rather were thought to be brought on by divine or supernatural powers, and thus more properly falling under the control of priests. When viewed from this perspective, it was not necessary to offer a physiological explanation for the onset of the symptoms. Medical authors, however, were often interested in the relation between the physical body and the way in which it influenced behavior and the expression of emotions, impaired the faculties of cognition, or inhibited voluntary control over one's action. They looked for theoretical explanations for mental disorders that would conform to their own understanding of the body and disease and that would dictate a rational therapeutic response. Neither group gained a monopoly over the treatment of such conditions, and as a result, responses to mental illness in early civilizations combined both religious and medical efforts.

THE MIND AND ILLNESS IN MESOPOTAMIA AND EGYPT

There is no evidence that the Mesopotamians or the Egyptians associated the brain with memory, intelligence, or emotions. Indeed, in the process of embalming, the brain was the only major organ the Egyptians removed and discarded, suggesting that they did not view it as significant. Emotions and the mind seem, rather, to have been associated with the heart in both cultures. The Egyptians specifically linked the faculties of the mind with the *ib* ("heart," sometimes also translated as "mind"), the seat of consciousness. For example, the Ebers papyrus connects the *ib* with memory, noting that "as to [when] his *ib* [mind] is drowned:

this means that his *ib* is forgetful like one who is thinking of something else" (Ghalioungui 1963, 129).

The Mesopotamians used a number of different terms to describe conditions that we might associate with epilepsy but which they also linked to a variety of mental disorders. Furthermore, it is not clear from their terminology whether the terms distinguished between different conditions or were used to speak of the same condition. The Akkadian word *bennu*, for example, is used to describe the following symptoms: "If a man is quivering all the time when lying down, shouts like the shouting of a goat, roars, is apprehensive, shouts a lot all the time, (then it is) the Hand of *bennu*, the demon deputy of (the moon-god) Sîn" (Stol 1993, 6). The Sumerian term, *miqit samê* ("what has fallen from heaven"), refers to similar symptoms: "If a sick man's neck turns to the right, time and again, while his hands and feet are paralyzed, his eyes are now closed, now rolling, saliva flows in/from his mouth, he makes . . . sounds" (Stol 1993, 8). These terms are often used interchangeably (along with terms like *miqtu*, "hand of god or goddess" and others) to denote conditions, whether epileptic or not, associated with spasms and falling down. Other phrases used to denote the same symptoms are associated with conditions that seem to verge on madness, such as "Spawn of (the god) Sulpaea":

> If a seizure seizes him at sunset and, as it seizes him, a wailing voice shouts to him and he himself responds every time, (if) he time and again shouts: "my father, my mother, my brothers, my sisters, (are) dead," . . . and stops (shouting) every time, . . . after having cried he falls asleep and does not get up: (if), as the seizure leaves him he does not know that he has cried: [he is suffering from] "Spawn of Sulpaea"; it will not go away. You burn him with fire in his illness. (Stol 1993, 15)

This example reveals that these conditions are not clearly linked with what we might consider epilepsy but rather reflect a range of possible mental illnesses. While "hand of god" (sometimes "hand of goddess") is often associated with seizures, it sometimes also has other symptoms so that the sufferer, "curses the gods, he speaks insolence, he hits whom (ever) he sees," or "he has [?] of heart-break, time and again, and forgets his (own) words, time and again" (Stol 1993, 25). Thus, this array of symptoms variously associated with seizures and linked by a number of, often interchangeable, terms appear to indicate some understanding of mental illness.

Those suffering from these various conditions were viewed in a negative light within Mesopotamian society. The Code of Hammurabi specifically mentions the condition *bennu* (possibly epilepsy) indicating that it was viewed as detrimental in slaves: "if a seignior purchased a male (or) female slave and when his month was not yet complete, *bennu* attacked him, he shall return (him) to his seller and the purchaser shall get back the money which he paid out" (Meek 1969, 177). The birth of a child having epileptic-like seizures was also viewed as an ill omen and as we have seen, those with Spawn of Sulpaea deemed incurable might be burned or in some cases, buried alive. Indeed, common curses such "may a bad *bennu* fall upon you" or wishing that your enemies might suffer "a *miqtu* that does not go away" are also indicative of the social reaction to these kinds of conditions.

MENTAL HEALTH AND HUMORAL MEDICINE IN ANCIENT GREECE AND ROME

The Hippocratic author of *On the Sacred Disease* specifically considered the problem of epilepsy. As in the Mesopotamian world, epilepsy was viewed as a disease caused by divine powers in the early Greek world, but the Hippocratic author argued that epilepsy and all mental disorders had naturalistic causes that could be explained in terms of an imbalance in the body's humoral physiology.

> Madness comes from its [the brain's] moisture [caused by excess phlegm]. When the brain is abnormally moist, of necessity it moves, and when it moves neither sight nor hearing are still, but we see or hear now one thing and now another, and the tongue speaks in accordance with the things seen and heard on any occasion. But all the time the brain is still a man is intelligent.
>
> The corruption of the brain is caused not only by phlegm but by bile. You may distinguish them thus. Those who are mad through phlegm are quiet, and neither shout nor make a disturbance; those maddened through bile are noisy, evil-doers, and restless, always doing something inopportune. These are the causes of continued madness. (Jones 1923, 175–177)

This position meant that mental health could be explained in the same terms as physical health and that mental illnesses could be treated by the same methods used to treat other diseases, namely with diet, regimen, drugs, and phlebotomy.

Greek natural philosophers and medical authors also offered theories about the ways in which race and gender might influence an individual's mental state and personality. In another Hippocratic text, *Airs, Waters, Places*, mental dispositions are explained in terms of the environmental and seasonal influences on a population. For example, the author argues that the different climates in Europe and Asia are largely responsible for the physical form of the inhabitants as well as their personal character; the mild and uniform seasons of Asia makes the men weaker, while the dramatic seasonal changes in Europe make men there stronger: "For the frequent shocks to the mind impart wildness, destroying tameness and gentleness. For this reason, I think, Europeans are also more courageous than Asiatics. For uniformity engenders slackness, while variation fosters endurance in both body and soul; rest and slackness are food for cowardice, endurance and exertion for bravery" (Jones 1984, 133). In this sense, a people's mental dispositions were shaped by their complexion (or individual balance of humors) and also by the influence of external factors on individual development. Slightly later, Aristotle (384–322 B.C.E.) would argue similarly that the female of the species tends to be dominated by the quality of cold whereas the male is dominated by the quality of heat. He maintained that these qualitative differences, beyond the humoral complexion, incline women to being timid and slow-witted (traits associated with the quality of coldness), whereas men were brave, outgoing and intelligent (traits associated with the quality of heat). Galen of Pergamum (129–ca. 216 C.E.) further refined these thoughts about the role of humoral physiology in determining an individual's mental dispositions and in explaining mental illness, offering a more systematic consideration than his predecessors of the ways in which an individual's humoral and qualitative composition would shape both body features and character traits.

THE MIND AND MENTAL HEALTH IN AYURVEDIC MEDICINE

The ancient Hindu scriptures contain several descriptions of characters suffering from mental illness—stories of madmen (*unmattaka*). The *Ramayana*, for example, relates the story of Lord Rama and his family, many of whom suffered from what we might define as depression; his grandfather was depressive after the death of his wife and eventually starved himself to death, and his father suffered bouts of depression after accidentally killing a blind man and later when he was separated from his children, from which condition he eventually died. Lord Rama himself suffered from depression while searching for his abducted wife, Sita, becoming despondent, pensive and forgetful, crying out in anguish, fainting, and experiencing loss of appetite, before finally committing suicide. Similarly, in the *Mahabharata*, the protagonist, Arjun, suffers from depression when he realizes that he will have to kill his relatives in battle, experiencing a dry mouth, unsteady thoughts, and wet palms. He is eventually alleviated of his symptoms after being counseled by Lord Krishna.

The Ayurvedic texts also consider mental health from the perspective of medical theory. These texts located the *manas* ("mind") and the *citta* ("consciousness") in the heart; they are responsible for directing the senses and controlling cognition. By contrast the eternal *atman* (self/ soul), which is shaped by the *karman* ("deeds," good or bad actions from previous lives), is only conscious by virtue of its connection with the senses. In order to maintain health, the individual needs to balance the needs of body, mind, and soul. Mental illnesses can arise from a number of physiological factors, including the blockage or destruction of pathways from the heart that convey the *manas* and the disruption of the *doshas*, brought on by an inappropriate diet or sudden mental shocks from extreme emotions. On the other hand, the medical texts also allow that mental illness could arise from the wrath of the gods or demonic possession.

The observations about the relationship between the mind and body led the authors of Ayurvedic medical texts to develop notions of individual personality types shaped by their *prakriti* ("personal temperament") or the preponderance of the different *doshas* in their body at the time of generation. The *Susruta Samhita* describes seven personality types according to which dosha (or combination of *doshas*) was predominant at birth. A person of the *vata* temperament (having a preponderance of *vata*), for example, is impulsive, restless and prone to wakefulness, while a person with a *kapha* temperament is known for self-control and unselfishness. Individuals from the different temperamental types can be recognized by their distinct bodily features, reflecting the close association between mind and body; in the *Susruta*, we learn that a person of the *vata* personality is distinguished by his unshapely body, rapid movement, and shifty eyes, while the *kapha* type often has curly hair and well-proportioned limbs.

Vagbhata's *Astangahrdaya* (*The Heart of Medicine*), written around 600 C.E., brings together many of the theories about mental illness from the early Ayurvedic tradition. He identifies six categories of *unmada* (insanity or madness) with natural causes; insanity caused by derangement of one of the three *doshas* (*vata*, *pitta*, or *kapha*), as an effect of another disease, by the anxiety from facing an unbearable loss, or as an effect of poison (including the effects of alcohol). These conditions are likened to epilepsy, which the medical texts indicate should be treated with the same methods used for those suffering from *unmada*. Patients would initially be treated with purgatives or enemas to clear the blocked pathways along which the *manas* flows. One such potion called for cooking cow's urine with ghee and some other herbs and spices, which the author declared to be "the best thing for banishing insanity, demons, and epilepsy" (Wujastyk 2003, 247). Other remedies called for making pastes and ointments that could be applied to the eyes or nasal passages, as well as burning various substances as fumigants to restore the appropriate equilibrium of the *doshas*. Vagbhata also suggests treatment through different forms of what we might call shock therapy, including flogging the patient and then throwing him into a dark pit or room, covering her with mustard oil and then tying her down stretched out in the sun, or having police grab him and threaten him with corporal punishment in the name of the king! In cases where *unmada* was caused by demonic possession, Vagbhata suggested similar cures but noted that they should be supplemented with various rituals and prayers to appease the demons, depending upon the nature of the demon causing the illness.

MENTAL ILLNESS IN TRADITIONAL CHINESE MEDICINE

Chinese literature and folklore offers useful insight into how people viewed mental illnesses in traditional China. Legends of the wandering holy man Daoji (d. 1209) highlight the ways in which he transgressed the rules of his own Buddhist religious tradition, earning him the appellation of "Crazy Ji" and leading to his removal from a monastic community. A later account of the life of Daoji relates:

> Crazy Ji's original name was Daoji. He was wild and did not pay attention to small details of conduct. He used to drink wine, eat meat [in violation of monastic dietary rules against drinking wine and eating meat], and drift about the marketplace. People thought he was mad, for which reason they called him "Crazy Ji." (Shahar 1998, 50)

In another account we learn, "Crazy Ji was getting wilder and wilder; often he would go to the Cool-Spring Pavilion and turn somersaults in it, falling flat on the ground. He would enter the Summoning-the-Monkey Cave and invite the monkey to somersault with him; or else, he would lead a group of children to the wine shop, where he would sing mountain songs" (Shahar 1998, 61). His madness, expressed as nonconformity and religious eccentricity, was viewed as a marker of his piety, and members of the laity revered him as a saint and spread stories about his remarkable healing powers. Daoji is just one among many "crazy monks" (*dian seng*) or "mad monks" (*feng heshang*) described in Chinese literature. These monks were generally recognized for their unusual behavior, including breaking religious rules, wearing rags that barely covered their bodies, having irregular speech, behaving erratically, and eating strange things. Despite their wildness, the laity often revered these wandering monks, who were separated from the monastic establishment, as holy fools and miracle workers. The stories largely reflect an undercurrent of lay hostility toward the Buddhist monastic establishment, but at the same time, they offer a perspective on Chinese beliefs about madness. In these contexts, no stigma was attached to those who displayed the symptoms of what we might recognize as mental illness.

Another folkloric tradition in China suggests a widespread popular belief in the supernatural or demonic origin of mental disease. Malign fox demons were particularly common culprits in causing mental disorders, going back at least to the period of the Han dynasty (206 B.C.E.–220 C.E.). One story from the late eighth century C.E. tells of a well-mannered 10-year-old boy, who was suddenly struck by an illness that completely transformed his personality. The father summoned a Taoist healer who, declaring that "this boy suffers from a sickness which is caused by a fox demon," brought about a cure and then cautioned that henceforth he would need to treat the boy every day to maintain his health, to which the father agreed. The story continues:

> Though the boy was cured of that disease, still he lacked a sufficient quantity of soul, wherefore he uttered every now and then insane talk, and had fits of laughter and wailing, which they could not suppress. At each call of the doctor, the father requested him to attend to this matter too, but the other said: "This boy's vital spirits are kept bound by a specter, and are as yet not restored to him; but in less than ten days he will become quite calm; there is, I am happy to say, no reason to feel concerned about him." And the father believed it. (Veith 1963, 148)

Nonetheless, the boy continued to suffer from this condition, and the father called in another doctor and then a third. These three doctors began to fight, and the father, rushing back into the sick room, found three foxes on the ground, panting and exhausted, and realized that they were the three doctors, who had first caused and then tried to prolong the disease in a scheme to get his money. In his anger, he beat the foxes to death, and thereafter the boy no longer suffered from his mental affliction. Beliefs like those expressed in this story about the demonic or supernatural cause of madness portrayed the sufferer as an innocent victim of an outside force, and attached no stigma to the individual afflicted with mental illness, although it is likely that a burden of shame fell on the family of the patient in traditional China. Treating mental illness caused by angry ghosts, demons, or other supernatural beings often required some form of exorcism. This entailed rituals of curative magic, which were sometimes associated with violence, including beating patients and exposing them to cold and uncomfortable living conditions to drive the supernatural beings from their bodies.

Traditional Chinese medicine does not clearly distinguish between psychological and physiological conditions, and there was no specialized branch of medical theory devoted to psychiatric medicine. This does not mean that Chinese medicine did not recognize psychiatric disorders—indeed, the aforementioned accounts from Chinese literature and folklore show that they did—but mental illnesses were not formally set apart from somatic disorders in the textual medical tradition as they were in other cultures. Medical authorities spoke of seven emotions (joy, anger, grief, worry, fear, desire, and fright) and the need to regulate them by avoiding displays of excess emotion for the sake of maintaining health. Furthermore, the internal organs are linked to different emotions: for example, the heart with the emotion of joy, the kidneys with fear, the liver with anger, the lungs with grief, and the spleen with worry. Excessive emotions could harm the organs and lead to derangement of the flow of qi in the body and thus to disease, or conversely, diseases of the internal organs could engender excessive emotions. As a result, psychological and emotional disturbances were viewed as important symptoms of physiological illnesses, not necessarily as independent mental disorders.

The *Huangdi Neijing*, however, does discuss two major types of madness brought on by a *yin-yang* imbalance: *dian* (an overabundance of *yin*) and *kuang* (an overabundance of *yang*). A patient with the *kuang* form of madness is described as manifesting the following symptoms:

> He will discard his clothes and run about, mount heights and sing, or get to the point of not eating for several days. He will leap walls and ascend rooftops. In short, all the places he mounts are beyond his ordinary abilities . . . he will talk and curse wildly, not sparing relatives or strangers. Not wishing to eat, he will run about wildly. (Chiu 1981, 75)

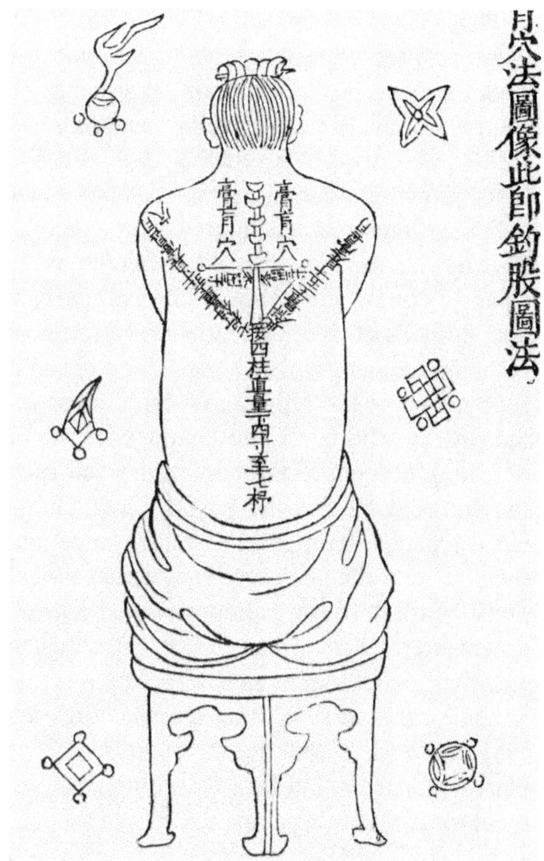

This is a woodcut illustration from a copy of the *Tongren Shuxue Zhen Jiu Tujing* (*Illustrated Manual of the Bronze Man Showing Acupuncture and Moxibustion Points*) by Wang Weiyi, published in 1443. The image depicts the method for locating the vital points for acupuncture. The point of intersection in the middle of the back was considered a panacea against a variety of conditions, including madness and memory loss. (Wellcome Collection)

The *kuang* form of madness, therefore, is associated with an excited and agitated state in which the patient is in constant motion and displays misanthropic tendencies. By contrast, the *Nanjing* (*Classic of Difficult Issues*) describes those with the *dian* form of madness as being passive, apathetic, and even staring blankly in a catatonic state. Later medical authors related these conditions to seasonal and other environmental causes. Sun Simiao (581–682), for example, pointed to a pathogenic (disease-causing) *feng* (wind): "When *feng* enters the cardinal conduit of *yang* polarity, *kuang* ensues; when *feng* enters the cardinal conduit of *yin* polarity, *dian* ensues" (Ng 1990, 36).

Physicians who considered *kuang* and *dian* predominantly advocated treating them with the same therapies they would use for somatic diseases, namely with drugs and acupuncture. Some physicians, however, felt that these cures were sometimes insufficient for relieving emotional or mental disorders. Zhu Zhenheng (1281–1358), who believed that *dian* and *kuang* were caused by excessive emotions, proposed countering those emotions with their opposites so as to neutralize the excess and cure the madness; for example, a person suffering from pathogenic (disease-causing) joy would be encouraged to feel anger or worry. The physician Chang Ts'ung-cheng (1156–1228) was perhaps even more famous for his unorthodox methods of treating madness. In one case, he was called in to treat a woman who had frequent violent screaming fits and on whom drugs had been ineffective. He had two of her female assistants dress in outlandish clothes and sent them to the patient, who burst into laughter for the first time in months; on the following day, he sent them to the patient dressed as animals, again inducing laughter; on the third day, he had them wolf down a huge feast in front of the woman, which led the patient to recover her own appetite for food. In another form of shock therapy, he had a person with a mental illness tied to a large wheel and had assistants spin it until the patient vomited a greenish fluid and finally asked to be let down, after which he was cured! The naturalistic cures offered by physicians indicate their belief that mental disorders were not caused by supernatural forces, but in some cases of shock therapy, the cures resemble the kinds of cures offered by religious healers seeking to exorcise the possessing fox demons. Perhaps the patients (or their families) had more faith in these more dramatic forms of treatment for mental illnesses.

MENTAL ILLNESS IN ISLAMIC MEDICINE

The Arabic word *majnun* ("possessed" or "madman") was the most commonly used designation in early Islamic society for an individual who would be described as "mentally ill" today. Labeling an individual as *majnun* was usually a social decision, and physicians had only a small role in making the diagnosis. Islamic literature, such as the collection of tales in *The Thousand and One Nights*, portrays some cases of madness as positive conditions from which the sufferer would not wish to be cured. In particular, those whose madness was inspired by God, such as the wise fool or holy fool, who speak the truth and dedicate their lives to serving God despite the risks, might be revered as holy mystics, so people believed that: "The madman knows best his own soul. True discourse must be heard from a madman" (Dols 1992, 349). Indeed, the Prophet Muhammad was often accused of being a madman for his willingness to speak the truth. On the other hand, under the law, the insane were viewed as having the same legal status as children, unable to have independent control over their own decisions or to own property and thus requiring legal guardians who would see to their protection. Therefore, being labeled as *majnun* was not always positive.

Spirits known as *djinn* were frequently mentioned in the Quran as causing madness in humans by possessing an individual's body and driving him mad—thus the term *majnun* means both "possessed" and "madman." Such possession could be thwarted by Prophetic and religious healers and by prayer. One text prescribes the use of magical talismans, prayers, and massages for those with epilepsy, apoplexy, and hysterical fits, so that

> the devil should be massaged out from the important organs to the less important ones and eventually out of the body through the lower extremities. The massage develops in most cases to violent beatings, which may be carried out with the hand, with a stick, show or even with a holy object, like the wooden shoe of the Madjthub. It is easier to drive out devils when the bodily condition of the possessed person is at the lowest. It is a common belief that the *djinn* prefer well-built, corpulent patients. This explains why the patients are fed so badly. Neglect of cleanliness leads to the same result. (Dols 1992, 237)

The medical authors followed their Greek forebears in offering naturalistic explanations for the causes of mental illnesses. Ibn Sina (d. 1037, known as Avicenna in the Latin West) dismissed the belief that *djinn* caused melancholia in his *Canon of Medicine*, saying, "If it were caused by the *djinn*, it happens by changing the temperament to black bile, for melancholia's cause is the dominance of black bile. Thus, the cause of that black bile may be *djinn* or something else" (Dols 1992, 81). While not denying the possibility of a supernatural cause for melancholia, he sought to frame it in terms of humoral physiology and thus made clear that mental illnesses would be amenable to cures by natural medicines.

Although many Islamic medical authors discussed the diagnosis and treatment of mental disorders, Ibn Sina's *Canon of Medicine* came to be viewed as the most authoritative Arabic text on this subject and is generally reflective of Islamic efforts to clarify distinctions between categories of madness. He regularly grounded his understanding of mental disorders in humoral pathology and aimed to identify distinct syndromes based on clusters of symptoms that revealed the underlying pathology. Among other conditions linked to brain dysfunction, he discussed phrenitis, lethargy, forgetfulness, epilepsy, apoplexy, and lovesickness. Of all the mental disorders he considered, melancholia and mania were the most emblematic. These conditions were viewed as chronic and nonfebrile mental disturbances that expressed two different states; mania generally reflected excited psychotic behavior, while melancholia was associated with a depressed state. Under each of these categories, he recognized different subcategories of the disease. For example, rabies was viewed as a form of mania, while lycanthropy (a condition in which the victim behaves like a rooster and cries like a dog, wanders among tombs in a graveyard at night, and has a yellow complexion, and a dry mouth) was a form of melancholia.

Considering mental illness to be the result of humoral imbalances, Islamic physicians resorted to the same kinds of treatments as they might apply to physical disorders. The careful regulation of diet and regimen was crucial for the *majnun* and various drugs might be prescribed, and bloodletting or cautery could be applied to restore sanity. Even conditions deemed incurable might be palliated through the judicious use of these treatments. Bathing with scented oils, massage, and sexual intercourse were also suggested as beneficial for those suffering from different forms of madness. In medieval Islamic society, some hospitals were developed specifically for the purpose of providing care to the insane. In most cases, however, family members provided for the care of the mentally ill at home, perhaps resorting to hospitals and physicians for medical advice and prescriptions. In this way, despite the efforts of physicians to medicalize the diagnosis and treatment of mental illness, the family and society continued to play the primary role in attending those suffering from mental disorders.

MENTAL ILLNESS IN MEDIEVAL EUROPE

The scholastic theologian Thomas Aquinas (1225–1274) succinctly summarized what he believed were the three possible causes that might lead people to fall into trances or display unusual mental behaviors:

> First, from a bodily cause, as is clear from those who through some infirmity are out of their minds. Second, through the power of demons, as is seen in those who are possessed. Third, from the divine power. It is in this sense that we speak of ecstasy, when one is elevated to a supernatural level by the divine spirit, with the abstraction from the senses. (Caciola 2003, 33)

Aquinas's thoughts reveal the diverse views of mental illness in medieval society. His writings indicate that he did not view mental disorders as a specifically medical problem, but rather as a social concern that was most appropriately handled by members of the clergy. Indeed, it appears that during the Middle Ages the task of diagnosing and treating mental illness fell mostly into the hands of the family and the local priests, and only rarely were medical professionals called in to offer testimony (e.g., in legal cases) confirming or repudiating diagnoses of mental disorders made by laymen.

Among theologians like Thomas Aquinas, perhaps the primary concern when faced with people manifesting mental disorders was to determine whether it was brought on by divine or demonic possession. Divine madness was viewed positively and was attributed to a divine ecstasy triggered by divine possession or the touch of God; these individuals were often seen as holy fools or even revered for their sanctity and their words were interpreted as revealing God's intentions. By contrast, demonic possession was a sign of the sufferer's weakness and sinfulness and such a person would be distrusted. The difficulty, according to Aquinas and other theologians, was how to determine whether the individual possession was of divine or demonic origin. Both kinds of possession manifested the same external signs, including shrieking and shouting, alienation of the senses, antisocial behavior, entering trancelike or catatonic states, crying, or other displays of grief or despondency. Some suggested that external, bodily signs could be considered to help solve the dilemma, but in general the local community, often with the assistance of the local priest, would make the determination based on a variety of individual factors indicating whether or not they trusted the afflicted.

The treatment of the mentally ill typically remained in the hands of the family and the local community. Families could seek religious cures, and numerous shrines had reputations for offering cures to epileptics and others suffering from mental disorders. In extreme cases, priests might intervene to exorcise demons from the possessed. For example, one man, who displayed signs of mental illness, was brought to a monastery, where the monks tried several methods to exorcise the demon until, "one day [a monk] put the psalter over the head of the possessed man, with him screaming and frothing . . . and after an hour he came to his senses . . . crying out that he had been liberated from the devil" (Caciola 2003, 233). At times, people resorted to harsh methods for treating insane family members, as in the case of a woman in the city of Ferrara, who was said to fill the whole city with terror:

> She gave terrible bites with her teeth to the hands and feet of anyone who was able to catch her. She hurled insults and curses at everyone, mixing in terrible slanders. She threw her body about in almost unspeakable and foul ways. She even tried to burn down her house. . . . [Her family] became impatient and fed up with this, and since they could find no other solution, they tied her up with a strong chain like a dog, and concealed her in a corner of a certain house, so that she could not harm anyone. (Caciola 2003, 46)

By the 14th century, hospitals started to segregate the insane from other patients and some hospitals were even established solely for the insane. The mentally ill were often chained up or confined in separate rooms in these hospitals, to isolate them from society, and people could pay to house their mentally ill family members in these institutions. In most cases, however, the mentally ill remained in their own communities and were cared for as holy fools or otherwise incorporated into society as much as possible.

Despite the fact that people in medieval Europe did not typically turn to medical practitioners to treat the mentally ill, learned physicians wrote extensively about how to distinguish and treat different forms of mental disorders. Following Galen, medieval physicians explained mental illness in terms of an imbalance of humors, distinguishing four main categories based on the specific humor that was in excess: frenzy, mania, melancholy, and lethargy. Mental illnesses were, therefore, treated in the same way that other humoral imbalances would be treated—with dietary changes, bloodletting, or drugs—but some physicians advocated other forms of treatment like using soothing words and baths, or trying different means to frighten the patient and shock them into normal behavior, and occasionally trephination (cutting a small hole in the skulls) was prescribed to release heat and other harmful substances accumulating on the brain. Mania, for example, was thought to be caused by excess yellow bile that dried and heated the brain causing uncontrollable activity, shouting, and violent behavior; it was to be treated with its qualitative opposites, moistening and cooling medicines that would counteract the excess yellow bile.

In the 13th and 14th centuries, physicians became particularly interested in the disease *amor heroicus* (lovesickness). Those who suffered from this obsessive, unrequited love could be recognized by their desiccated and jaundiced appearance, mood swings, characteristic pathetic sighing, loss of appetite, and difficulty sleeping; untreated, it could lead to death. During the Middle Ages, early discourse on *amor heroicus* tended to localize it in the brain, and mainly emphasized its effects on aristocratic men, who were brought low and even feminized by their excessive desire for the beloved. Later physicians also considered women's susceptibility to this condition, arguing that they were less rational and more desirous of intercourse and, therefore, less able to ward off their amorous desires. Cures were often designed to soothe the body and distract the mind; baths, music, travel, good food, and wine were all recommended, and some physicians even suggested therapeutic intercourse with someone other than the object of obsession.

Another mental illness that received increasing interest in the later Middle Ages was the condition of melancholy. Marsilio Ficino (1433–1499) in his *De vita libri tres* (*Three Books on Life*) offered medical and astrological advice for how to maintain health and prolong life. In particular, he was concerned with the afflictions peculiar to students and scholars, who spend their time in deep contemplation and fail to be sufficiently active. These factors combined to make students especially prone to developing an excess of black bile, which would lead to melancholy. He noted that astrological factors (the influence of Mercury and Saturn) already tend to dry out and cool the brain, and,

> Furthermore, because of the frequent movement involved in thinking, the spirit also is continually broken by such movement. . . . It all comes down to this, that with the mind and heart bent on contemplation, the stomach and the liver fail. Then, especially if you are eating rich or hard foods poorly cooked, the blood becomes cold, thick, and black. Finally, with an excessive swiftness of the limbs, and with neither the remaining stuff nor the hard glutinous stuff being separated, dusky vapors are exhaled. All these make for a melancholy spirit, a sad and fearful soul. . . . Of all scholars, those devoted to the study of philosophy are most bothered by black bile, because their minds get separated from their bodies and from bodily things. They become preoccupied with incorporeal things, because their work is so much more difficult and the mind requires an even stronger will. To the extent that they join the mind to bodiless truth, they are forced to separate it from the body. Body for these people never returns except as a half-soul and a melancholy one. (Boer 1980, 7)

In addition to being inactive, even lethargic, Ficino claims that melancholics appear sad due to their quiet, pensive natures and often share many of the symptoms associated with lovesickness. Overwhelmed by his deep thoughts and the belief that his uncle Claudius had killed his father, married his mother, and usurped his throne, Hamlet displays all of the signs of a melancholic. He contemplates death and displays an erratic, pensive nature, with dramatic mood swings, leading some of the characters to diagnose him, wrongly, as suffering from lovesickness! Yet, as a melancholic, despite the fact that the ghost of his father provided a direct imperative to kill Claudius, for most of the play, Hamlet is unable to move himself from thought into action and kill his uncle.

10

Drugs and Remedies

From the earliest times, people in all societies have recognized the physiological effects of imbibing various local plants, minerals, and other substances. They would have soon recognized those that were toxic, those that caused purgation, and those that might have narcotic effects. As people noted these physiological effects, they also began to attribute medicinal virtues to the substances that caused them. Furthermore, some substances without easily recognizable physiological effects were still deemed to have medicinal virtues because of their monetary value, or perceived magical and religious affinities. Increasingly, people began to prepare compound medicines by mixing multiple ingredients in different amounts, tailored to the individual and the disease. In this chapter, we will examine the activities of apothecaries and doctors and the theories that directed their preparation and application of medicinal substances.

THE PHARMACOPEIA OF ANCIENT MESOPOTAMIA

The *Epic of Gilgamesh* relates how the hero, Gilgamesh, went on a quest to find a cure for his friend, Enkidu, who was suffering from a deadly illness. He learned about a secret healing plant that was supposed to ward off decay and rejuvenate all who consumed it, and he swam to the bottom of deep waters to recover it. After returning to shore, Gilgamesh fell asleep, and a snake ate the healing plant and gained the power to rejuvenate itself by sloughing off its old skin. Upon awakening, Gilgamesh wept, recognizing that he had lost this most precious plant that offered the power to cure the ills of mankind.

Gilgamesh's quest reveals the Mesopotamian recognition of the healing attributes of plants, whose powers were unknown to most men. The *asu*, however, was known for his use of drugs to cure disease; his pharmacopeia included a range of plants (seeds, roots, leaves, bark, resin, and flowers), parts of animals (including dung), and some minerals. Many of these substances produced observable effects (acting as emetics, purgatives, or expectorants), suggesting to the *asu* that they were working, even if modern physicians are doubtful of their therapeutic efficacy. Obtaining the exact ingredients was believed to be very important for the success of the remedy. One *asu* makes this clear in a letter to his lord, requesting new herbs:

> The daughter of Mustalu who was coughing but not spitting out has started to expectorate after I gave her [appropriate] potions; but . . . now she is constipated. I gave her a potion for constipation to drink, and she is taking it, (but) there is no *sarmadu* herb and drawn wine available. Let my lord send (some) so that I can have her drink, lest she develop "Hand of Curse." The princess who had repeated attacks of fever has now calmed thanks to the dressing and potion. As to the herbs of which I spoke to my lord, let my lord not forget about them. (Biggs 2005, 12)

These medicinal substances would be prepared in various ways depending on the illness (e.g., being crushed, cooked, or dried) and then put into a drink (water, milk, beer, or wine) to create a healing potion or mixed with other substances (e.g., honey, ash, or flour) to create a poultice for external application on wounds or burns.

The Mesopotamian *asu* also provided medicines for cosmetic reasons, such as combating hair loss or turning gray hair black. Cures listed under headings such as, "If a man's head in his youth is full of grey hairs, to darken the grey hair . . ." listed a range of ingredients such as the gall of a black ox or the fat of a black raven, suggesting that the color of the substance used would be transferred to the hair. In one remedy, the *asu* is told to crush those or similar substances in oil of the cypress from a cemetery and then explains, "the charm seven times thou shalt recite . . . , [under] the stars thou shalt set it, (on) his head press it, bind on for seven days and he shall recover" (Thompson 1924, 12). These remedies suggest the importance of magical affinities in the selection of ingredients and in the application cures. The need to recite a charm along with the specifications for the conditions in which the compound should be applied should remind us that magic and medicine were closely united in Mesopotamian society.

THE EGYPTIAN PHARMACOPEIA

Providing medicinal substances was the most common form of treatment recommended in the Egyptian medical papyri. Indeed, Egyptian doctors were renowned in neighboring countries for their pharmaceutical expertise. The *Odyssey*, for example, indicates the high esteem of Egyptian pharmaceutical lore among the Greeks in one passage where an Egyptian woman provides a drug to ease pain: "potent gifts from Polydamna the wife of Thon, a woman of Egypt, land where the teeming soil bears the richest yield of herbs in all the world: many health itself when mixed in the wine, and many deadly poison. Every man is a healer there, more skilled than any other men on earth—Egyptians born of the healing god himself" (Fagles 1996, 131).

The Egyptian *swnw* used a variety of plant, animal, and mineral substances in his efforts to prepare drugs. In many cases, we are unable to identify exactly what substance the Egyptian doctors meant, whether because we cannot link a specific plant to the name, or because the substance is simply too fantastical (e.g., "excrement-of-the-gods"). Many of the prescriptions are simple, with only one drug taken, but the majority are compound medicines with anywhere from half a dozen to a dozen drugs, and in one case, as many as 37 different substances! The ingredients are typically mixed with different delivery vehicles including water, milk, beer, and wine to make healing potions. Even here, however, several distinctions are made so that the *swnw* might use, for example, warm beer, flat beer, sweet beer, fresh milk, spoiled milk, warm milk, milk-of-a-woman-who-has-borne-a-son, well water, spring water, salt water, or water-in-which-the-phallus-has-been-washed. Medicines were often given orally as pills, gargles, or potions, or applied externally as ointments or poultices. They could also be provided by fumigation, directing the steam or smoke from the cooking or burning medicine into the affected area. Finally, many drugs were administered rectally or vaginally as an enema or suppository.

Prescriptions are often accompanied with an explanation for their magical efficacy, or with an explanation justifying their use in terms of disease theory. In many cases, medicines were applied to purge the pathological *wekhedu* (a morbid or disease-causing principle believed to originate in the anus) from the body. The Ebers papyrus offers a remedy, using an unknown herb (*senutet*):

> Beginning of remedies to cause mucus to go down from the pelvis. A herb—*senutet* is its name—growing on its belly like the *kadet*-plant. It produces a flower like the lotus. If one finds its leaves [looking] like white wood, then one should fetch it and rub it on the pelvis. Then it (the mucus) will go down immediately. Its fruit is given on bread to [those with] *wekhedu* to cause (it) to go down from the pelvis. (Nunn 1996, 128–139)

In fact, the ancient Egyptians were continually worried about the possibility of decay brought on by *wekhedu*, especially in the anus, and many prescriptions (indeed, one entire medical papyrus) are devoted specifically to remedies for refreshing or cooling the anus and "to drive out excrement." Indeed, one Greek historian, Herodotus, observed that Egyptians regularly sought to use emetics and laxatives, noting that "for three days in succession in each month they physic themselves, hunting health with emetics and purges, because they think that from the food that nourishes mankind come all their diseases" (Grene 1987, 163). Various parts of the castor oil tree were considered especially useful as laxatives, as one remedy makes clear: "When a person who suffers from constipation chews a little of its [the castor oil tree's] berry along with beer, then the disease will be driven out of the sick one's body." In addition to castor oil, Egyptians used a variety of substances as laxatives including dates, figs, coriander, cumin, wormwood, or malachite combined with other ingredients (Bryan 1974, 16).

Egyptian pharmacology was also important for cosmetic and domestic applications. Remedies were provided to combat hair loss or gray hair, to drive away wrinkles, remove moles, or even to cure sweaty feet. The Egyptians were also masters of making eye paints, which they offered to gods (painting the eyes of the statues of gods with them) or as cosmetics. Eye paints were prescribed by the *swnw* not only for aesthetic purposes, but also as medicines to treat a variety of eye diseases. Indeed, the Ebers papyrus has a section devoted to remedies for *wekhedu* collecting with blood in the eyes, which describes a number of eye paints that can be applied around the eyes or directly on the eyes. Finally, the *swnw*'s pharmacopeia also had other uses around the household to give clothes a pleasant fragrance or to drive away vermin. One text suggests this remedy to keep mice away from clothes: use cat's fat and smear it on everything possible!

GREEK AND ROMAN PHARMACOLOGY

The Hippocratic authors left no single pharmacological book or herbal manual describing various drugs, their preparation, and application. Indeed, the favored therapy in Hippocratic medicine was the regulation of diet and regimen, and the use of drugs takes on a secondary role in therapeutics. When Hippocratic texts prescribe drugs, they are most often simple remedies (those composed of a single ingredient), which are most often prescribed for their effects as purgatives or emetics. For example, black hellebore is prescribed as a purgative while mixtures of wine and honey are offered to ease coughs and act as expectorants.

A number of specialized herbals were written in the Roman period. One of the earliest of these, the *Compositiones* (*Prescriptions*) by Scribonius Largus (ca. 1–50 C.E.) describes 271 recipes that mix plant, mineral, and animal ingredients found in regions around the Mediterranean or imported from further east. The text is divided into three parts with the first part giving remedies for diseases organized from head-to-toe, followed by a section with antidotes against poisons, bites, and stings, and a final section on plasters and wound dressings. Plant products (including carrots, aloe, fenugreek, and ginger) are most common, but he also prescribes the use of animals and minerals—his remedy for a constant headache is to touch an electric ray or torpedo fish, since the constant shocks would help suppress the pain.

One of Scribonius's contemporaries, Pliny the Elder (23–79 C.E.), also wrote about the medicinal uses of plants, animals, and minerals in his *Natural History*. Pliny drew his information largely from other Greek and Latin sources on pharmacology, and he covers a much wider range of ingredients than Scribonius. His large text describes the therapeutic properties of each ingredient, some of which seem to suggest magical powers. For example, he notes the remedies that can be derived from rosemary:

> A local application of the fresh root heals wounds . . . and hemorrhoids. The juice both of the shrub and of the root cures jaundice and such conditions as call for cleansing. . . . The seed is given in drink for chronic complaints of the chest and with wine and pepper for uterine trouble . . . an application also clears away freckles. . . . The herb itself is applied with vinegar to scrofulous sores, and with honey is good for a cough. (Jones 1956, 73)

And, from the elephant,

> The blood of an elephant, particularly that of the male, checks all the fluxes that are called *rheumatismi*. Ivory shavings with Attic honey are said to remove dark spots on the face, and ivory dust whitlows. By the touch of the trunk headache is relieved, more successfully if the animal also sneezes. The right side of the trunk used as an

amulet with the red earth of Lemnos is aphrodisiac. The blood too is good for consumption, and the liver for epilepsy. (Jones 1963, 63)

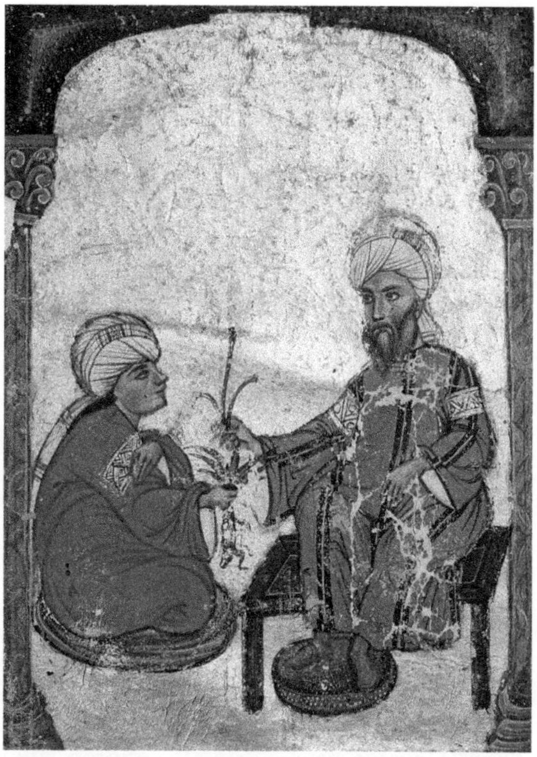
This scene from an Arabic translation of Dioscorides's *Materia Medica* from 1228 depicts Dioscorides teaching herb lore to a student. (Werner Forman/Universal Images Group/Getty Images)

Pliny also describes various medical conditions and their treatments. These conditions range from poisoning, to ulcers and fistulas, eye diseases, fevers, coughs, and warts. Pliny's work was valued for its breadth of coverage, but it is highly disorganized and later generations of physicians complained about his willingness to include rumors and hearsay in his accounts.

Perhaps the most successful pharmacological text from Greco-Roman antiquity was the *De Materia Medica* by Dioscorides of Anazarbus (ca. 40–90 C.E.). This herbal, divided into five books, describes the medicinal properties of over a 1,000 substances, including around seven hundred plants, as well as minerals and animal products. He also explains the proper means of harvesting and storing plants for medicinal use. Throughout, Dioscorides claims that he had actively sought out and tested the recipes he describes:

> [I], . . . having an unceasing desire to acquire knowledge of this matter, and having travelled much (for you know that I led a soldier's life), have by your advice gathered together all that I have commented hereupon . . . But I beg that you, and all who may peruse these commentaries, will not pay attention so much to the force of our words, as to the industry and experience that I have brought to bear in the matter. For with very accurate diligence, knowing most herbs with mine own eyes, others by historical relations agreeable to all, and by questioning, diligently enquiring of the inhabitants of each sort, we will endeavor . . . to describe the kinds and forces of every one of them. (Gunther 1959, 2)

Still, many of his remedies may seem rather strange or unappetizing: "House mice, being cut asunder, are applied profitably to those who are stung by scorpions . . . [and] being eaten roasted they do dry the spittle in the mouths of children" (Gunther 1959, 308). His herbal became the main source for pharmaceutical knowledge for the next 15 centuries, and it was translated from the original Greek into many languages including Latin, Arabic, and English, and many later editions included numerous colorful illustrations of the plants described.

Most of the medicines described in the Greek and Roman herbals were fairly simple, typically composed of a single substance but at most consisting of only a few ingredients. The complexity of drug preparation increased as the selection of ingredients rose, especially in the larger cities in the later Roman Empire. The most visible example of this was the development of the compound medicines that could serve as antidotes for snakebite and other poisons. Pliny relates the story of king Mithridates VI of Pontus (120–63 B.C.E.), who developed a poison antidote composed of 41 ingredients, which was later named "Mithridatium." In the first century C.E., Nero's personal physician, Andromachus, revised the formula to include 64 ingredients, adding viper flesh and increasing the proportion of opiates; he dedicated his recipe for "theriac" (also known as "treacle" in English) to Nero. In the next century, Galen further revised the recipe for theriac, which he prescribed for the emperor Marcus Aurelius, to include 77 ingredients listed in his *De theriaca ad Pisonem*. In later centuries, theriac was used not only as an antidote for poisons, but also as a powerful panacea, prescribed for a wide range of conditions until the 19th century.

PHARMACY IN AYURVEDIC MEDICINE

Pharmaceutical remedies provide an important cornerstone of Indian medicine. The Ayurvedic texts emphasize the importance of the *pañcakarman* ("five procedures") therapy for restoring the appropriate levels of the *doshas* in the body. The five procedures are the administration of emetics (*vanuna*), purgatives (*virecana*), enemas (*basti*), errhines (*nasya*, to promote sneezing), and bloodletting (*raktamokshana*). In theory, emetics are used to evacuate excess *doshas* orally, especially for ailments caused by *kapha* (phlegm); purgatives are used to eliminate *doshas* and malas (sweat, urine, and feces) from the lower parts of the body and especially in ailments caused by *pitta* (bile); rectal and vaginal enemas are used in cases of fevers, diarrhea, constipation, and flatulence; and errhines are used for ailments of the head, neck, ears, nose, and throat. These therapeutic actions are only supposed to be undertaken after the patient has undergone oleation (the application of medicated oils externally and internally) and sudation (sweating). The preliminary measures are taken to eliminate impurities from the body that might block the *srotas* (channels) in the body and hence cause illness and disrupt the healing action of the drugs.

The *Susruta* alone mentions over 700 medicinal herbs, not to mention mineral and animal products, and later texts add many others. The medicinal properties of these substances were classified according to the six basic *rasa* (tastes): sweet, sour, salty, pungent, bitter, and astringent.

> Sweet taste increases all *dhatus*, *ojas*, semen and breast-milk; is beneficial for eyes, hair and complexion . . . if it is used regularly alone and in excess, it produces the following diseases—cough, dyspnoea, [flatulence], vomiting, sweetness in mouth, loss of voice. . . . Sour is digestive for food as well as *dosha*, *ama* or inflammation; stimulates digestive fire, pacifies *vatta*, is carminative, produces burning in bowels, is externally cold, moistening and mostly relishing; in spite of having such properties, if it is used regularly alone and in excess, it produces tingling of teeth, blinking

> of eyes . . . causes suppuration in wounds, injuries, burns, bites, fractures and dislocations. . . . Astringent taste is anti-diarrheal, healing, stiffening, cleansing, scraping, absorbent and pressing and dries up moisture; in spite of having such properties, if used for a long time alone and in excess, it produces cardiac pain, dryness of mouth, flatulence, loss of speech, [stiff neck], quivering in body parts, tingling sensation, contraction, convulsion. (Sharma 1999, 389–391)

However, the taste of each substance was often interpreted as a combination of two or more of the basic flavors, requiring careful efforts to produce compound drugs with the appropriate balance of flavors. Substances were further classified as "hot" or "cold" depending upon the feeling that they produced in the body.

There are several methods for preparing drugs in Ayurvedic medicine. Medical texts discuss the knowledge necessary for growing and properly harvesting medicinal plants to maximize their efficacy. Once collected, plants would be prepared as drugs in a variety of forms (as pastes, juices, cold infusions, hot infusions, or decoctions), and the correct form to prescribe needed to be determined "with due regard to the strength of the patient and seriousness of the disease [since] all these preparations are not equally useful in all cases" (Sharma and Dash 1976, 85). In addition to producing these extractions, infusions, and decoctions, plants were also ground into powders or mixed with oils or other liquids to produce pastes or plasters, or prepared as pills or suppositories. Given the religious restrictions enforced by Brahmans in Hindu society, it is perhaps surprising that the *vaidya* did not restrict his prescriptions in accordance with taboos against the use of animal products in drugs and even prescribed alcoholic drinks.

Siddha Medicine and Alchemical Remedies

A system of medicine developed in the Tamil-speaking regions in south India that was different in some respects from Ayurvedic medicine. Known as Siddha medicine, this system was taught by the legendary Siddhas, "Perfect Ones," who were portrayed as combining the practices of yoga and alchemy. It is strongly influenced by tantric thought and distinguishes itself from Ayurveda by its emphasis on the examination of the pulse and by the greater use of metal-based and alchemical remedies. The classical Sanskrit texts devoted to *rasayana* ("the way of the *rasas*," or alchemy) date from about the 10th century C.E. and treat the production of healing or rejuvenating elixirs, as well the practices of transmutational alchemy. These texts view mercury as the essence (*rasa*) of all other substances, and, therefore, it was the prime alchemical reagent studied and an important medicinal substance. The Siddha medical and alchemical texts also hold the substance called *muppa*, which seems to have been similar to the "philosopher's stone" pursued by Western alchemists, in particular reverence since it was believed capable of bringing about both physical and spiritual transformations. The Siddha pharmacopoeia, therefore, makes greater use of mineral and metallic ingredients than Ayurvedic medicine, but it also attaches importance to the use of medicinal plants.

THE TRADITIONAL CHINESE PHARMACOPEIA

Early Materia Medica

Works on materia medica spread among the people of China even prior to the Han dynasty (206 B.C.E.–220 C.E.), but most have been lost. Like the *Wu-shih-erh ping fang* (*Fifty-Two Prescriptions against Fifty-Two Ailments*), unearthed in the Mawangdui tombs from ca. 168 B.C.E., these texts likely contained lists of various pharmaceutical products that could be applied for different conditions. Although these texts list individual remedies and sometimes offer a theoretical justification for their use, they do not attempt a systematic consideration of pharmacy.

The earliest extant treatise to provide a theoretical classification of the ingredients in the materia medica was the *Shen Nong Ben Cao Jing* (*Shen Nong's Classic of Materia Medica*), produced sometime in the first century C.E. It lists 365 drugs of plant (252), animal (67) and mineral (46) origin, which were classified into three grades or potencies: superior, average and inferior. Superior drugs (120 kinds, including ginseng), were deemed nontoxic and were used as tonics for long-term treatment to produce an invigorating effect. By contrast, the average drugs (120 kinds, including Chinese angelica) were toxic in some cases and could be used as tonics to help resist disease or expel unhealthy pathogens from the body. Finally, the inferior drugs (125 kinds, including croton), many of which were recognized as toxic, were prescribed in drastic cases to help expel harmful materials from the body and were not meant to be taken for prolonged periods. The properties of each drug were carefully described as in the case of ginseng, which was said to have, "the quality of tonifying the five viscera (*zang*), relieving mental stress . . . ending palpitation, removing pathogenic Cold and Heat, improving acuity of sight, enlightening and benefitting the brain, [assisting] longevity and pleasing and relaxing the mood when taken over a long period" (Zhenguo, Ping, and Peiping 1999, 64). In addition to classifying the drugs and describing their therapeutic properties, the text also addresses problems of harvesting, processing and storing the various ingredients and how they can be combined in compound medicines, including explanations for adding ingredients that could diminish the toxic side effects of others. The *Shen Nong Ben Cao Jing* was recognized for its utility and quickly became the primary pharmaceutical text in China.

Alchemy and Pharmaceutical Chemistry

The spread of Taoism had an important influence on the development of alchemical medicine in ancient China. Taoist doctrines encouraged a return to a simpler way of life and the pursuit of harmony with nature, and for some, this pursuit led to a search for immortality. Taoist thought had greatly influenced the development of herbal medicine, but it also encouraged the study of alchemy. The Taoist adept, Ge Hong (ca. 281–341 C.E.), known also by his pseudonym, Baopuzi, was perhaps the most eminent alchemist to turn his interest toward medical applications in his pursuit of drugs to prolong life. He worked mostly with cinnabar (the principle ore of mercury) and other mineral and metallic substances (sulfur, realgar, saltpeter, alum, mica, iron, tin, and gold) in alchemical experiments, but he also studied medicinal plants. He summarized his alchemical experiments in the *Bao Pu Zi Nei Pian* (*Bao Pu Zi's Inner Treatise*), which included many alchemical drugs for the purpose of producing longevity, like this one:

> The Lesser Divine elixir: Take three pounds of real cinnabar, six pounds of white honey, stir together, expose to the sun, and cook until it can be shaped into pills. Every morning take ten of these pills about the size of a hempseed. In less than a year, whitened hair will become black, lost teeth will regrow, and the skin of your whole body be moist and rejuvenated. Those who take it will not age, and old men will regain their youths, enjoy Fullness of Life, and become immortal. (Ware 1966, 95, 188)

Tao Hongjing (452–536 C.E.), another Taoist physician, also aimed to combine the alchemical tradition with medical pharmacy. In addition to writing several works on alchemy, Tao Hongjing wrote a commentary on the *Shen Nong Ben Cao Jing* in an effort to correct the mistakes he found in it. His *Ben Cao Jing Ji Zhu* (*Collective Notes to the Classic of Materia Medica*), quoted the original *Shen Nong Ben Cao Jing* in red ink with a supplementary commentary in black ink printed alongside in order to facilitate interpretation and help highlight corrections. He also added 365 drugs to those already described in the *Shen Nong Ben Cao Jing* (730 altogether) and revised the classification system so that they were first divided into categories based on their origin (jade and stone, plant, insect and animal, fruit, vegetable, cereal, and others) before further organizing them according to their medicinal grades (superior, average, and inferior). Tao Hongjing's classification system became the standard method for organizing drugs in Chinese medicine for more than 1,000 years.

Standardizing Materia Medica and Regulating the Drug Market

Shortly after the national unification under the Tang dynasty (618–907 C.E.), the imperial government perceived the need for an official pharmacopeia. Emperor Gaozong asked the physician Su Jing to evaluate previous pharmaceutical manuals and produce a revised and corrected materia medica. Starting in 657, Su Jing led a group of over 20 scholars, and augmented Tao Hongjing's *Ben Cao Jing Ji Zhu* with more than 100 new drugs. Completed in 659, the *Xin Xiu Ben Cao* (*Newly-Compiled Materia Medica*), later known as the *Tang Ben Cao* (*Materia Medica of the Tang*), was the first government sponsored pharmacopeia in the world and became the standard pharmaceutical reference manual in China for the next 300 years. The original version included several volumes of illustrations, which are unfortunately now lost. Among other things, this book contains the first recorded description of a silver electuary (made of tin, silver foil, and mercury) for dental fillings.

The imperial court of the Song dynasty (960–1279 C.E.) was also extremely concerned with the regulation of pharmacological texts, especially given the rapid proliferation of these texts allowed by the introduction of woodblock printing. In response, the court established the Bureau for the Re-Editing of Medical Books to oversee the revision and printing of classical medical textbooks. The Bureau was also charged toward the end of the 10th century C.E. with the production of the *Taiping Sheng Hui Fang* (*Peaceful Holy Benevolent Formulas*), a formulary listing 16,834 prescriptions for compound medicines that drew together and standardized material from previous texts on pharmacology. The Song government also implemented a large-scale investigation of drugs from around the country, which resulted in the publication of the *Ben Cao Tu Jing* (*Illustrated Classic of Materia Medica*) in 1061, the first extant illustrated pharmacopeia from China. The book contained folk remedies and proven herbal drugs with 933 illustrations to assist in their proper identification.

The Song imperial court also organized the first official institute to oversee the manufacture and sale of drugs in 1076 and by 1103 six new dispensaries had been established in different parts of China. These drug-processing workshops were responsible for collecting, testing, manufacturing, and selling drugs, and for dispensing medicines to the poor in times of medical emergency. The Institute also printed its own formulary that included 788 prescriptions (far more manageable than the list in the *Taiping Sheng Hui Fang*) in the *He Ji Ju Fang* (*Prescriptions Collected by the Pharmaceutical Institute*).

PHARMACY IN THE ISLAMIC WORLD

Islamic pharmacy relied heavily on the Greek tradition, especially on the works of Dioscorides and Galen's treatise *On the Powers of Simple Drugs*. These works were increasingly available in Arabic translation from the 10th century onward. However, the Greek materia medica were limited in that the plants they described were frequently unknown in many parts of the Middle East, although local related species could sometimes be identified. At the same time, the wide geographic range of the Islamic world (from Spain, across North Africa, and into the Middle East) and the extended trade routes that reached as far as India and China meant that Islamic authors came into contact with many new drugs that had not been described by their Greek forebears. So, while the Greek texts offered a theoretical framework within which to consider drug therapy, Islamic authors wrote numerous original pharmacological treatises.

One of the most common genres of pharmacological literature were the synonymic lists of drugs, providing equivalent names in different languages such as Greek, Latin, Syriac, Persian, Hindi, Berber, and Spanish, to aid in the proper identification of plants. For example, Maimonides (d. 1204), one of the most famous Jewish scholars writing in Arabic, composed a list containing 408 well-known drugs with their synonyms, like this entry on *ratina* ("resin"):

> This is the resin which the people of the Maghrib [Berbers] call *rajina* and the people of Egypt *qulfuniya*. It is also called *zaft al-ghadhawa*. It is the resin of the male pine or of the dry terebinth. On the contrary, the resin called κολοφωυια in ancient Greek is the resin of the small pine which is not *al-qulfuniya*. (Levey 1966, 8)

In addition to clarifying the local names for plants described in the Greek texts, these lists might offer suggestions for possible substitutes.

Islamic authors also wrote original treatises on materia medica. These typically presented drugs in alphabetical order for ease of reference and generally include a description of the plant, a discussion of its preparation and therapeutic use, and a summary of the opinions about the drug from various authorities. Probably the best-known manual of this kind is Ibn al-Baytar's (d. 1248) *Comprehensive Book on Simple Drugs and Foodstuffs*, which lists over 1,400 drugs. Al-Baytar reports his own observations about the medicinal value of many of these drugs and also draws upon over 260 written sources, augmenting the Greek and Roman pharmacopeia with many new items discovered through practice and in exchanges with India and China, including camphor, musk, senna, and cotton (which was prescribed for use in wound dressings).

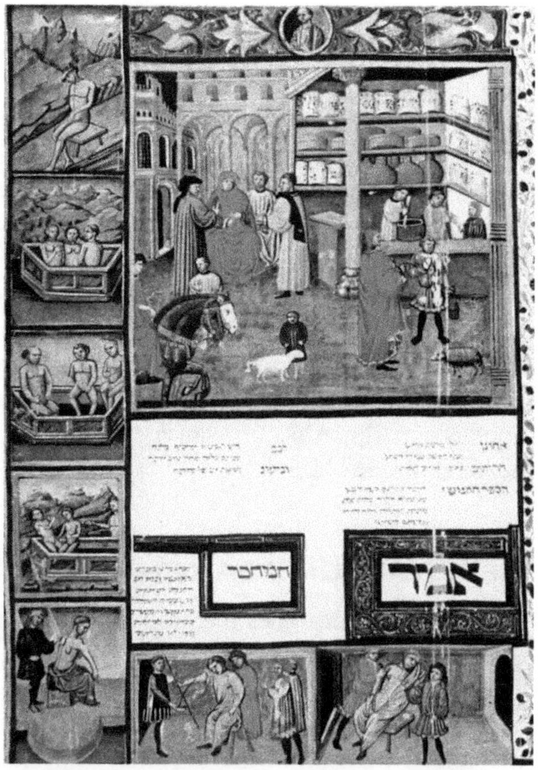

A page from a Hebrew edition of Avicenna's *The Canon of Medicine*, ca. 1440. The central scene depicts a university-trained physician (in his academic gown) meeting patients during his office hours. In the foreground, another physician meets a messenger carrying a basket used to transport a urine sample. Physicians claimed to be able to diagnose a patient's condition from their urine, without having to see him or her in person. Both physicians are conveniently located next to an apothecary's shop with its shelves lined with containers for medicinal herbs, where patients could fill their prescriptions. During the Middle Ages, some physicians had arrangements with local apothecaries to share profits from drug sales. Smaller images around the edge depict other forms of therapeutics, including balneology (baths), cupping, bloodletting, and surgery (perhaps to lance a boil). (National Library of Medicine)

Several Arabic pharmacological treatises focused exclusively on poisons. These texts consider the dangers of bites by various insects, snakes and mad dogs, as well as the stings of scorpions, and the poisonous properties of various minerals and plants. A typical example was the *Kitab al-sumum* (*Book on Poisons*) by Ibn Wahshiyah (fl. before 912), which describes a number of poisons and venoms. For example, he observes that some people use a particular species of blister fly deceitfully as a poison, mixing it with food or drink. Anyone, he says, who imbibes the fly in this way will experience burning in his throat, a violent stomachache, abdominal swelling, and sometimes the suppression of urination and bowel movements, concluding that "this animal is fatal in one day and no later." He suggests a number of antidotes, including the following: "To save the poison victim quickly, the best remedy is to suck milk from the breast of a woman many times. He sucks, stops, sucks, and stops continuously until his belly symptoms disappear. If he is anointed with pure violet oil, it is useful for him" (Levey 1966, 9–10).

Islamic authors also wrote formularies, which provided recipes for mixing compound medicines. Such texts were usually organized according to the kind of compound produced (pill, syrup, powder, gargle, emetic, suppository, poultice, etc.) and described the conditions for which it could be used. Formularies could be appended to other medical texts or circulate independently, like al-Kindi's (d. after 870) *Aqrabadhin* (*Prescriptions*), and they appear to have been produced frequently for use in hospital dispensaries, such as the formulary by the Jewish apothecary, Ibn Abi al-Bayan (d. ca. 1240), who practiced in the famous Nasir hospital in Cairo, Egypt.

MEDIEVAL EUROPEAN PHARMACOLOGY

In medieval Europe, the task of preparing and selling drugs was typically undertaken by apothecaries. These tradesmen were often involved in the spice trade and thus able to import exotic substances from all over Europe, the Mediterranean, and the Near East. Although they held a lower status and did not have the theoretical training of the university physicians, apothecaries would also often dispense medical advice and thus served as another class of medical practitioner. The competition among the different kinds of medical practitioners did not always create tensions, and in some places, apothecaries and physicians entered into mutually beneficial agreements whereby the physician would meet patients in the apothecary's shop and then write prescriptions that could be filled on the premises and for which the physician might receive a percentage. Increasingly, physicians, especially those in university towns, sought to establish their authority to regulate the preparation and sale of drugs. Several physicians reported on the dangers of different medicines, especially laxatives and opiates, and questioned whether apothecaries should be allowed to prepare such drugs without supervision, let alone sell them without a physician's prescription. For example, a physician in Montpellier, Bernard of Gordon (active in the late 13th and early 14th centuries), recalled a case in which he was called to treat an apothecary who had accidentally suffered an overdose of theriac due to his own negligence:

> It happened that a certain apothecary had sold a toxic substance and some remained behind the nail of his thumb. When he began to pick his nose with his thumb, his color began to change and he fainted repeatedly. When he took three drams [of the antidote, theriac], his condition became more serious. I was called around midnight and I saw that the amount of theriac had been too high. I made him vomit and after he had purged his stomach sufficiently, I gave him one dram of theriac and he was cured. (Demaitre 1980, 76)

Bernard's point here is that apothecaries are not careful in their drug preparation, and they do not understand the theory that dictates appropriate dosage for different remedies. Despite the learned physicians' fears, however, apothecaries regularly prepared and sold drugs and offered medical advice throughout Europe.

One reason that university physicians sought to regulate the activities of apothecaries was that they increasingly emphasized the theoretical and technical difficulties of drug preparation in their new pharmacological literature. In particular, physicians aimed to incorporate Galenic theories about simple medicines that categorized them by their primary qualities (hot, cold, wet, or dry), which served as a rational explanation for their actions on a patient's humoral imbalance. In its simplest sense, a patient would be given a medicine qualitatively opposed to the disease, for example, a cold medicine to counteract the effects of a hot disease. However, the theory as it developed was far more complicated. Following Galen and the pharmaceutical writings of Arabic authors like al-Kindi, university physicians argued that medicinal simples (single substances) could be graded in four "degrees" according to the strength of their primary quality. Arnald of Villanova (ca. 1238–ca. 1310), working at the medical school of Montpellier, elaborated upon this theory and its application in making compound medicines.

> There are many reasons for the compounding of medicines; namely, strength of the disease, contrariety of diseases, contrary disposition of members [parts of the body], . . . [and] violence of the medicine. For certain violent diseases such as leprosy, apoplexy and epilepsy can rarely if at all be cured by simple medicines. Compounds must therefore be used, so that their force may more easily bring about the cure of a violent disease. A compound medicine is also necessary in the case of contrary diseases present in one and the same body, such as a fever [hot disease] and leucophlegmancy [cold disease], where we must employ a medicine compounded from both hot and cold, so that it can act against the opposite diseases. . . . A compound medicine must also be made up in the case of contrary qualities present within the bodily members, as when the stomach is chilled but the liver is heated. Finally, violent medicines, such as scammony, hellebore, and the like, cannot be given simply, but must have others admixed with them to diminish their violence. (McVaugh 1975, 14)

Taking these factors into account, Arnald developed theories for how to mix substances composed of different degrees and different qualities to produce a compound medicine appropriate for the nature of the disease(s) afflicting an individual patient. In theory, this meant that the physician needed to recognize the degree of the patient's complexional imbalance (e.g., a disease might be caused by excess phlegm, cold and wet, in different degrees, depending on its strength) and then mix suitable simples to achieve the appropriate degree to counteract the disease (e.g., a drug hot in the first degree and dry in the second degree). The theory sparked extensive debate and justified physicians' efforts to regulate apothecaries, but in practice, it was too complicated and even Arnald's prescriptions suggest that he did not always follow it. In practice, physicians and apothecaries were more likely to tailor prescriptions for compound medicines according to the wealth of the patient (e.g., suggesting less expensive ingredients for poor patients), or the availability of substances, than follow the complex mathematical theory. Nonetheless, this is an early effort aimed at applying mathematical theory in mixing compound drugs.

11

War, Health, and Medicine

Prehistoric humans developed a number of weapons, including fire, spears, and stone clubs, for use as protection against animals and other human tribes. Over time, other weapons were developed that could be used at greater ranges (such as the sling and the bow and arrow), and as humans learned how to work metals, they replaced traditional stone tools with bronze weapons that could be easily sharpened, including swords, axes, and bronze tips for spears, javelins, and arrows. Early cave paintings from the Paleolithic period (35,000–12,000 B.C.E.) indicate that humans had begun to employ strategies and tactics that would best use their weapons in combat, creating the first organized warfare. As humans organized into cities and began to deploy larger armies, they began to adopt more systematized policies for composing and deploying their forces, training and arming different groups that might serve as specialized foot soldiers, cavalrymen, archers, or other positions. Each unit would be recognizable based upon its specialized armor and weaponry.

Being wounded in combat was, in many ways, the least of the dangers faced by soldiers in any premodern army. The difficulties of transporting the food necessary to maintain a fighting force in the field meant that soldiers were often left to fend for themselves, scavenging what food they could find from the lands through which they moved, and hunger was ever present. Of even more concern, the sanitary conditions of military life meant that armies were often troubled by a wide range of different diseases so that a soldier's chance of dying from illness was at least as great as dying from a wound in battle. Civilians faced similar health dangers as invading armies moved through their lands, stealing and destroying crops, raiding and burning villages, and besieging cities.

WEAPONS AND WOUNDS

What type of wound was a soldier likely to encounter in battle? The most common weapons used were arrows, sling bullets, swords, axes, maces, spears, and

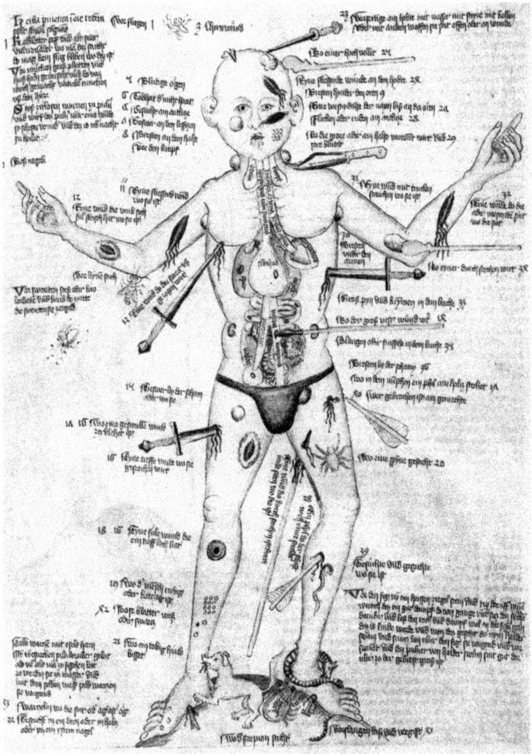

The "wound man" illustration, like this one from around 1420, was common in surgical manuals. Wound-man images depict the numerous wounds a human body could suffer, including sword and knife cuts, crushing blows from clubs, arrow wounds, bites from insects and animals, and various rashes or burns. Some wound-man illustrations, like this one, also provided a schematic view of internal organs. (Wellcome Collection)

javelins. These weapons produced different kinds of wounds, and treatment varied considerably according to the type of injury. Slashing weapons, especially very sharp swords or heavy axes, could produce traumatic amputations (of limbs or heads), but more often they produced flesh wounds, which many surgical authors considered the least dangerous of wounds, so long as they did not contact the bone or cut through nerves and tendons. Piercing wounds from thrusting weapons like swords, arrows, javelins, and spears were usually considered more deadly. For this reason, Roman soldiers were often trained to use their swords as thrusting rather than slashing weapons; as one Roman author noted: "a cut, with whatever violence it may come, does not often kill . . . but, on the other hand, a stab, thrust in two inches deep, is fatal" (Salazar 2000, 12). Weapons like clubs, maces, and war hammers were designed for delivering heavy blows that could crush armor and fracture bones.

The excavation of a mass grave near the Towton battlefield in England has allowed archaeologists to examine the variety of wounds soldiers typically experienced in battle (Boylston 2000, 357–380). The Battle of Towton took place during the War of the Roses between King Henry VI of the house of Lancaster and Edward Earl of March of the house of York on March 29, 1461, with over 100,000 combatants and approximately 28,000 deaths. Examination of skeletal remains reveals that many individuals sustained multiple injuries from a variety of projectiles and hand weapons. Blows appear to have been clustered around the head and face, with fewer injuries to the limbs and torso. These findings suggest that the limbs and torso were not targeted as often, that the individuals were wearing armor in those places, or that wounds in those regions were slashing or piercing flesh wounds that did not penetrate to leave marks on the bones. Many of the wounds are quite brutal, with one skeleton revealing that the soldier's jaw had been sliced from his face by a sword that cut through the roots of a molar and almost certainly severed his tongue. Other remains reveal previous injuries that had healed, showing that not all battle wounds were fatal. Interestingly, it appears that some remains show damage to the teeth that would likely have resulted from archers using their teeth to string their bows.

Surgical manuals reveal the kinds of operations battlefield surgeons would have needed to perform in order to attend to this array of wounds. With most wounds, the control of hemorrhage would have been the surgeon's most immediate concern. The application of pressure to the wound was the first recourse, but sometimes the surgeon would need to resort to more extreme measures. The Roman author Celsus (ca. 25 B.C.E.–ca. 50 C.E.) describes two other methods that could be used to stop hemorrhaging:

> But if even these [other procedures] are powerless against the profuse bleeding, the blood-vessels which are pouring out blood are to be seized, and round the wounded spot they are to be tied in two places and cut across between so that the two ends coalesce each on itself and yet have their orifices closed. When circumstances do not even admit of this, the blood-vessels can be burnt with a red-hot iron. (Spencer 1953, 81)

This account by Celsus is one of the earliest of the application of a vascular ligature, and it was not an easy procedure to perform, especially on a battlefield. Once the initial bleeding was under control, wounds would be bandaged or closed with sutures.

Closing abdominal gashes required extra attention as attested by the numerous accounts of the operation. Galen (129–ca. 216 C.E.) graphically explains the procedure: "first one needs to put away the prolapsed intestines into their proper place," which "needs a dexterous assistant," then "grasping the entire wound with his hands from the outside, he needs to push it inwards and press it together and present it to the one who is suturing little by little, and then also compress moderately that which has been sutured, until it has been sutured accurately" (Salazar 2000, 51). Sometimes the intestines themselves were sliced and needed to be sutured, as in the case described by the medieval European physician and surgeon Guglielmo da Saliceto (1210–1277):

> When I saw him lying with his intestines gashed, I was very worried, but I immediately caused hot wine to be brought (since there was no time to wait for something else) and warmed and bathed the intestines in this, while feces continued to come out from the various slashes. After I had washed them I drew the parts of the intestines together with a skinner's stitch, and put over the suture joining the lips of the wound a goodly quantity of [my adhesive] powder, which glued it together quickly; then after sewing them up I tried to reduce them but could not. So I took a razor and widened the wound to the necessary extent, and they went back in right away; then I united the parts of the *sifach* [peritoneum] and the external skin all together with a single stitch. I continued to watch over his treatment thereafter . . . and he recovered; eventually he had a wife and children and lived for a long time. (McVaugh 2006, 114–115)

In ancient India, surgeons used a more exotic cure, described in the *Susruta Samhita*:

> Large black ants should be applied even to the perforated intestines in such a case and their bodies should be separated from their heads after they had firmly bitten the perforated parts with their claws [i.e., jaws]. After that the intestines with the heads of the ants attached to them should be gently pushed back into the cavity and reinstated in their original situation therein. The bulged out intestines should be rinsed with grass, blood, and dust, washed with milk and lubricated with clarified butter and gently re-introduced into the cavity of the abdomen with the hand with its finger nails cleanly paired. The dried intestines should be washed with milk and lubricated with clarified butter before introducing it into their former and natural place in the abdomen. (Bhishagratna 1911, 272–273)

Using the vicelike grip of a large ant's mandibles to clamp a wound closed may sound shocking, but entomologists have confirmed that several species of ants might be used for this kind of procedure!

Head injuries also presented a particular challenge to the battlefield surgeon. If the surgeon suspected a fracture based on the injured soldier's symptoms, he needed to bare the skull (expanding the flesh wound if necessary) and scrape it to ascertain how deep it was. Paul of Aegina (ca. 625–ca. 690 C.E.) recommended that if the fracture was difficult to distinguish, the surgeon should pour a solution of black writing ink onto the skull and scrape the bone on the following day when the fracture would be visible as a black line. In cases where the crack in the skull was deep and did not disappear with scraping, surgeons needed to use trephination, cutting the skull to remove any bone fragments that pressed upon the brain. The Hippocratic text, *On Wounds in the Head*, describes how to saw through the bone in detail, including the advice that, "while trephining, you should frequently take out the saw and plunge it into cold water to avoid heating the bone, for the saw gets heated by rotation, and by heating and drying the bone cauterizes it and makes more of the bone around the trephined part come away than was going to do" (Withington 1944b, 49).

The extraction of arrows would also have required specialized training and equipment. One Roman surgeon emphasized that soldiers should be told, "to put up with the arrows until they can have them removed by a person who can do so properly," because, "it can escape even an altogether experienced man that the point [of the arrow] is concealed" (Salazar 2000, 47–48). As he suggests, one of the real dangers in extracting arrows was if the shaft should come away leaving the arrowhead behind, making it difficult for the surgeon to find and remove. Otherwise, the surgeon needed to determine whether the arrow should be simply pulled out through the side it had entered or pushed through the body, perhaps making an incision on the other side of the body through which it could be extracted. The Islamic surgeon, Abu al-Qasim al-Zahrawi (fl. ca. 1000, known as Albucasis in the Latin West), described an especially difficult case he had treated.

> I once drew out an arrow from one of the officers of the State, that had struck him in the middle of the nose and was inclining a little to the right, and the whole arrow was buried. I was called to treat him three days after he had received the arrow wound; and I found the arrow wound very narrow. I explored it with a fine probe but

> did not find it; but the patient felt a pricking and a pain beneath the right ear, and I hoped that the pricking was due to the arrow. So I applied a poultice to the spot, a poultice with power to draw out and cause suppuration, desiring that the place should swell and that a sign to indicate the arrow should appear so that I could cut down upon it. But nothing happened at that place to indicate that the arrow had come through to there; so I persevered with poulticing it for many days; yet nothing fresh manifested itself and the wound healed up meanwhile, and the patient despaired for a time of its extraction. Then one day he felt the arrow inside his nose, and he told me of this; so for a number of days I applied a caustic medicine to the wound until it opened. I explored it, and felt the slim end of the arrow which is fastened to the shaft then I enlarged the opening of the wound by the use of the caustic until the tip of the arrow was plainly visible to me. About four months passed. Then when the wound was enlarged and I was able to introduce forceps into it I pulled on it and moved it, but it would not come out. And I went on skillfully and gently trying for it with various instruments until one day I caught hold of it with a pair of strong forceps . . . and drew it out; then dressed the wound. The medical men judged that the cartilage of the nose would not be restored, but I restored it and the wound healed up and the patient made a complete recovery nor did he suffer any harm. (Spink and Lewis 1973, 610–614)

Clearly, the extraction of arrows was not a simple task, requiring specialized tools, patience, and no doubt a great deal of pain for the patient!

In extreme cases, war wounds might necessitate the amputation of limbs. This might occur when a slashing wound had already nearly severed the limb, when crushed bones were too severely damaged to be set, or when gangrene set in, threatening to destroy the entire limb and claim the wounded soldier's life. The surgical manuals typically indicate that amputation was only done to remove lower joints; when gangrene had spread above the elbow or knee, one Islamic physician advised, "there is nothing of any avail in this case but to leave it, and for the patient to resign himself to death" (Savage-Smith 2000, 316). The operation entailed applying a ligature to the limb above and below the site to be cut, and then, following the operation, the wound would be cauterized and styptics would be applied to stanch bleeding. Evidence regarding the survival rate for this operation is mixed, but the risks were severe as another Islamic physician reported: "I once saw a group of thieves in the hospital whose hands and feet had been cut off. Their limbs became spasmodic because of the amputation, and not a single one of them escaped death" (Savage-Smith 2000, 316). On the other hand, the physician al-Zahrawi recorded examining a patient in Spain who had previously amputated his own foot after it was infected with gangrene. When this man requested that the physician amputate his diseased hand, al-Zahrawi refused, fearing that the operation could lead to the patient's death; he later discovered that the patient had cut off the hand himself and recovered!

As the previous allusion to gangrene suggests, death from the initial wound was not all a soldier might need to worry about. Chances of infection were great, and it is likely that more soldiers died from infected wounds than those who succumbed to injuries during the battle itself. Gangrene posed a significant threat, but so did other wound infections. Surgeons expected a degree of inflammation around the wound, which would typically be accompanied by fever, and suppuration. Depending upon how widely the inflammation spread or whether it exuded a "good" or "bad" pus, the surgeon stood ready to intervene as necessary with medicines or to drain off "bad" pus from abscesses around the wound. An account in the Edwin Smith papyrus offers an example of how an Egyptian *swnw* would approach postoperative care of a shoulder wound:

> You should say concerning him: "One having a gaping wound in his shoulder, its flesh being laid back and its sides separated, while he suffers with swelling (in) his shoulder blade. An ailment which I will treat." You should bind it with fresh meat the first day. If you find that wound open and its stitching loose, you should draw together for him its gash with two strips of linen over that gash; you should treat it afterward (with) grease, honey, (and) lint every day until he recovers. If you find a wound, its flesh laid back, its sides separated, in any member of a man, you should treat it according to these directions. If, however, you find that his flesh has developed inflammation from that wound which is in his shoulder, while that wound is inflamed, open, and its stitching loose, you should lay your hand upon it. Should you find inflammation issuing from the mouth of his wound at your touch, and secretions discharging therefrom are cool like *wenesh*-juice you should say concerning him: "One having a gaping wound in his shoulder, it being inflamed, and he continues to have fever from it. An ailment with which I will contend." If, then you find that man continuing to have fever, while that wound is inflamed, you should not bind it; you should moor (him) at his mooring stakes [i.e. continue with a regular diet and do not administer any medicines], until the period of his injury passes by. (Breasted 1930, 417–424)

Recovering from these kinds of injuries would be difficult in any circumstances, but for a soldier in an army on the march, the onset of wound infections would have frequently been fatal.

DISEASE AND HUNGER IN WAR

One Egyptian text describes the life of a soldier on campaign:

> He is called up for Syria. He may not rest. There are no clothes, no sandals. His march is uphill through mountains. He drinks water every third day; it is smelly and tastes of salt. His body is ravaged by illness. The enemy comes and life recedes from him. He is told, "Quick forward, valiant soldier! Win for yourself a good name!" He does not know what he is about. His body is weak, his legs fail him. If he leaps and joins the deserters, all his people are imprisoned. He dies on the edge of the desert, and there is none to perpetuate his name. (Archer, Ferris, Herwig, and Travers 2002, 12)

Although it was likely written specifically to emphasize the inglorious aspects of being a soldier, this account makes clear that military life entailed far more than simply fighting in battles. Long marches with little food or water and the ever-present threat of disease could exact a far deadlier toll on an army than battles.

Epidemic diseases including smallpox, cholera, diphtheria, typhus, dysentery, and numerous other febrile and diarrheal diseases regularly afflicted armies in the premodern world, claiming many a soldier's life. Indeed, diseases like the "bloody flux" (as dysentery was known) were often endemic. Poor nutrition, contaminated water supplies, inadequate camp sanitation, sleeping on cold or marshy ground, and close quarters weakened soldiers' immune systems, ensuring that any epidemic could spread swiftly through the ranks. And, nobody was immune to these depredations; for example, the army of King Henry V of England (1413–1422) suffered severely from dysentery throughout his Agincourt campaign, and the king himself finally died from the bloody flux in 1422 at the young age of 35, likely having contracted it while besieging the town of Meaux during a later campaign in France.

Early in the first century C.E., the Romans started to build hospitals (*valetudinaria*) in the permanent military forts on the frontiers of the Empire for the treatment of sick and wounded soldiers. These forts were typically many days behind the actual battle lines, so injured soldiers would be treated in the field, and the seriously injured would likely die before they could be transported back to the hospitals. However, the *valetudinaria* provided a space where wounded soldiers could receive postoperative care and soldiers afflicted with the inevitable camp diseases that followed armies could recuperate. A Roman hospital was typically constructed with the need to limit the spread of disease in mind. They were usually designed as a large rectangular building, having a main corridor running around the building with cubicles opening off of both sides where the patients could sleep away from draughts and noise. Additionally, the hospitals would have a large hall with good illumination that could serve as an operating room or reception area. Romans also made sure that the hospitals were supplied with plenty of fresh water and constructed sewers and latrines to remove waste. The staff of a Roman hospital typically included one or two doctors (*medici*), along with a range of other health care providers, including bandagers, students, and drug dispensers.

Frontier military garrisons during the Han dynasty (206 B.C.E.–220 C.E.) in China were similarly equipped with medical supplies and physicians. Each garrison was expected to maintain a careful register of troop illnesses like this one:

> Gao Zidang, private soldier of the 24th beacon unit, fell sick with headache on the seventh day of the fourth month and was unable to raise his four limbs; Zhou Liang, private soldier of Bingting beacon unit, fell sick and suffered cold damage on the fifth day of the fourth month; Jiang Tan, private soldier of the second beacon unit, fell sick on the sixth day of the fourth month and suffered swelling and fullness of the heart and belly; . . . Su Shang, private soldier of the thirty-seventh beacon unit, fell sick with arrow wounds to both flanks on the first day of the third month, and is slightly better; . . . Shangwu, private soldier of the thirty-first beacon unit, fell sick with headache on the eighth day of the fourth month, he had cold and heat, drank five doses of drug and has not yet recovered. (Guihua 2005, 91)

These somewhat monotonous records show that armies were susceptible to wounds, illness, and disease even when not actively on campaign. Other records indicate that these garrisons were usually well supplied with the ingredients necessary to mix drugs to treat many different diseases including chronic coughs, diarrhea, "accumulation" in the heart and belly, "cold damage," and for "curing itching."

SIEGE WARFARE

Warfare hit civilians especially hard. The *chevauchée*, a tactic of warfare employed during the European Middle Ages (and similar to the tactics of invading armies in general), employed mobile mounted soldiers to range across enemy territory and spread terror by burning crops and homes, stealing livestock, and killing peasants without mercy. Faced with these tactics, many peasants abandoned their farms in despair and fled into nearby woods to hide and wait for the army to pass. Other peasants might choose to flee and seek protection behind the walls of a nearby city.

Huddling behind the walls of a city may have provided protection against the immediate depredations of an invading army, but it brought entirely new problems if the army should choose to besiege the city: besieged cities were ideally suited for the spread of famine and disease. Cities facing a potential siege tried to gather a good supply of food and water behind their walls before the besieging army could arrive, with the intention of being able to defend the walls from the attackers and have sufficient resources to outlast the besiegers. This tactic often worked well since most armies could not carry enough food to be able to sustain a siege for more than a few weeks. In the end, it was not uncommon for both the besieging army and the besieged to grow hungry from lack of food.

Henry V's siege of Rouen, one of the wealthiest and most beautiful cities in France, gives some sense of what a siege may have been like. Learning of Henry's advance, the city stockpiled food, gathered from the surrounding countryside, and destroyed any food they could not bring into the city so that there would be no easy supplies for Henry's army; once he arrived at Rouen at the end of July 1418, Henry needed to ship food across the English Channel and up the Seine River to feed his army. Rouen also received numerous refugees from the countryside, confident that its massive walls and stockpile of supplies would allow it to hold out against the attacking English army, at least until a French army could come and relieve the siege. No relieving army arrived, however, and Henry was able to import enough food to maintain his army, while supplies in the city were running low; by mid-October the people in the city were eating horseflesh, and by December they were eating cats, dogs, rats, and even mice. Finally, the leaders of Rouen decided to expel the poor from the city to reduce the number of people they needed to feed; they drove more than 12,000 noncombatant refugees, including old men and nursing mothers, out of the city gates. King Henry did not wish to allow the city of Rouen to stretch their supplies and extend the siege in this way and refused to let the poor refugees pass beyond his siege lines, driving them back toward the city. When the leaders inside the city did not reopen the gates and allow the refugees to return, they were forced to huddle in the ditches outside the city walls where they were left to starve in the depths of winter. Many of Henry's English soldiers were horrified by the plight of the poor refugees now trapped beneath the walls and some even chose to share their food with them. One soldier described the scene in these terms:

> There one might see wandering here and there children of two or three years old begging for bread as their parents were dead. These wretched people had only

sodden soil under them and they lay there crying for food—some starving to death, some unable to open their eyes no longer breathing, others cowering on their knees as thin as twigs. A woman was there clutching her dead child to her breast to warm it, and a child was sucking the breast of its dead mother. There one could easily count ten or twelve dead to one alive, who had died so quietly without call or cry as though they had died in their sleep. (Seward 1978, 176)

Conditions were little better within the city, and on New Year's Eve, the defenders sent envoys to parlay with Henry. The pleaded with the English king to allow the refugees to flee from beneath the walls, to which Henry replied, "I put them not there," and demanded that the city surrender. Finally, faced with famine behind the walls, even after having expelled 12,000 people from the city, Rouen agreed to surrender.

Along with famine, besieged cities might also succumb to an outbreak of epidemic disease. The Greek historian Thucydides documented the Spartan siege of the city of Athens during the Peloponnesian War (431–404 B.C.E.) where this was the case. Faced with a superior invading Spartan army, the Athenian leader Pericles (ca. 495–429 B.C.E.) advised that the people of Attica withdraw behind the walls of Athens and avoid a direct battle with the Spartans. He argued that since the Athenians would still have access to their harbor, they would be able to resupply the city with food by sea, while the Spartan army would run out of food and be forced to withdraw. At first, the plan seemed sound, but an epidemic broke out within the city, and many people, including Pericles, died. Thucydides explains that the calamity of the disease was aggravated by the overcrowding behind the walls and that the high mortality and confines of the city meant that the Athenians were unable to observe the usual burial customs. Seeing the smoke from the funeral pyres and learning of the spread of plague within the city, the Spartans finally withdrew, fearing that they might become infected, but this was no victory for Athens.

The dangers of famine and disease aside, defenders faced many other threats during a siege. Attacking armies often used powerful siege engines (like catapults and trebuchets) to try to batter down the walls or throw large stones into the city. Perhaps the most immediate concern for defenders was when their enemies used these devices to throw incendiary devices over the walls to spread fires, an extreme danger in any premodern city. It was also common for armies to catapult dead and diseased animals, and even the severed heads and limbs of captured enemies, into cities. These actions served the twofold purpose of inciting fear within the city and also of spreading disease—an early form of biological warfare.

12

Medical Institutions

Beyond the work of doctors treating individual patients, larger institutions such as charitable groups, religious organizations (e.g., churches and monasteries), and governments (both locally and on a national level) engaged in funding large-scale programs for attending to the health and welfare of the general populace. The activities of these institutions could take the form of building projects that would promote sanitation and public health or fund the construction and maintenance of hospitals that could provide charitable care to the poor. In other cases, the sanction and support of civil and religious authorities was necessary to regulate medical activities and to encourage certain forms of medically related research, especially that related to the study of human anatomy. These activities sponsored by the state or by religious organizations reflected ideals of the general populace and general attitudes about how best to see to the health needs of the larger population. Nonetheless, we should also recognize that many of these state or religiously sponsored activities were not necessarily concerned with preventative medicine and medical research, for the same reasons as we may expect today; indeed, they were often motivated by goals that were not necessarily associated with an interest in providing health.

GOVERNMENTAL AND RELIGIOUS INSTITUTIONS IN MESOPOTAMIA AND EGYPT

Irrigation Systems

One of the most significant needs of early civilizations, especially those in the relatively dry climates of Mesopotamia and Egypt, was to ensure a sufficient supply of water to sustain crops that would feed the growing urban populations. This task required the development of irrigation systems that could deliver water to crops in the right amounts at the right times. Furthermore, irrigation systems needed to be designed that could reduce the threat of flooding and that could store water for use during the dry season. Evidence reveals that irrigation systems were being built in both Mesopotamia and Egypt as early as the sixth millennium B.C.E., when individual farmers were likely able to take measures to see to their own water needs. As the civilizations grew, however, the need to develop more complex irrigation systems often required large investments in labor and capital, which might in turn have necessitated increased governmental oversight to fund and coordinate their construction.

The Nile River was the source of life in ancient Egypt. It receives no tributaries during its course through Egypt, and it therefore provides the only regular source of fresh water in the region. Fortunately for the inhabitants of ancient Egypt, the flow of the Nile is exceedingly predictable, beginning in June with the snowmelt in the highlands of Africa, rising to a peak in late September or early October and then receding by the end of November. This regularity allowed ancient Egyptians to plan for one crop season per year, which would be planted in the soil watered by the floods. They dug simple canals that would reach to the high point of the Nile's flood, with sluices at their mouths that could regulate how much water was directed from the river into the fields. Water would be left in the fields for months to saturate the ground thoroughly and then would be drained off through another system of canals prior to planting the crops. By 1500 B.C.E., the Egyptians were making use of a *shadouf*, a simple tool composed of a long pole suspended in the middle by braces with a weight on one end and a bucket on another, which could be used to raise water from a lower level to canals at a higher level, further enhancing the irrigation system.

The regularity of the flooding meant that the ancient Egyptians were not especially concerned with developing systems for water storage since the summer floods provided sufficient water for a crop season. However, they were always concerned with determining how high the river would reach in its flood since this dictated how far to dig the canals. For this reason they built a series of "nilometers," spaced along the river, which allowed them to monitor the height of the Nile at various points and thus predict with some accuracy the high water mark. Furthermore, records in palaces and temples recorded the level reached by the flood each year to aid in these predictions. Aside from these efforts at prediction, the Egyptian irrigation systems were fairly simple and did not require a vast number of laborers to build and maintain, suggesting that they were likely designed and built at a local level, without the intervention of the central government. Indeed, the fact that no written laws concerning water regulation exist in the legal codes of ancient Egypt suggests that the water management system was not complex or contentious enough to require significant governmental intervention.

Mesopotamia, the land between the Tigris and Euphrates rivers, faced very different conditions from Egypt. Whereas the flooding of the Nile was gentle and predictable from year-to-year, the Tigris and Euphrates rivers were far less regular and were liable to run dry or bring sudden flash floods. Faced with these concerns, the Mesopotamians needed to develop an irrigation system that would protect against sudden floods and that could create areas for water storage. Furthermore, the Mesopotamian irrigation systems were more prone to the danger of salination (the accumulation of salts in the soil caused by repeated irrigation) than in Egypt. Increased soil salinity would prevent crops from growing in the fields (sometimes for 100 years or more), and Mesopotamian history records several salinity crises that necessitated the abandonment of previously arable land. As might be expected, the unpredictable supply of water prompted numerous disputes over water rights, as attested in the surviving legal records.

The more significant technical challenges of designing and coordinating an irrigation system, and the prevalence of legal disputes over water, required greater centralized governmental oversight than in Egypt. Whereas individual farmers or local communities might coordinate to build and maintain their irrigation systems in Egypt, in Mesopotamia, city-states passed laws requiring farmers to contribute labor to build and maintain canals and also dictated where canals would be built. Perhaps the earliest example of this process is from around 2400 B.C.E. under the king Entemenak of Girsu. The city-states of Girsu and Umma along the Euphrates had disputed water rights and Umma, upstream of Girsu, had regularly breached canals dug by the people of Girsu to irrigate their crops. In order to provide water for Girsu, Entemenak oversaw the digging of a vast canal to the Tigris River that was thereafter able to provide irrigation for the city's fields; by about 1700 B.C.E., this canal was so large and important that it was known simply as "the Tigris." Similarly, the Assyrian ruler, Sennacherib (704–681 B.C.E.), oversaw the construction of a massive irrigation system and also built a massive aqueduct to supply water to his capital city of Nineveh. Reflecting the extreme importance of irrigation in Mesopotamian society, Sennacherib boasted that it was he

> who digs canals, opens irrigated fields, and makes irrigation ditches murmur (with water); who established prosperity and abundance in the wide crop-lands of Assyria; who put irrigation water in the fields of Assyria where, from days of old, no one had seen, no one had known, those who preceded me had not made, canals and irrigation in Assyria. (Russell 1987, 535)

These activities make clear the important role of kings and the state in developing irrigation systems in ancient Mesopotamia.

Embalming in Ancient Egypt and Knowledge of the Body

Governmental and religious institutions in ancient Egypt supported conditions that allowed for the opening of the body, although this was not usually done for the purposes of gaining medical or scientific knowledge. Embalmers in ancient Egypt displayed extensive technical expertise in opening the body and preparing it for mummification. They were able to remove internal organs through relatively small incisions, including the brain, which was extracted through the nose after perforating the ethmoid bone. The lungs, stomach, liver, and intestines would then be transferred to four separate canopic jars; the heart, deemed the site of intelligence in the body, was not removed. The body cavity would then be washed out with oils and preserving fluids, stuffed with straw and linen, and the incisions would be covered (in one mummy, the incision was closed with sutures). Finally, the body would be covered in natron, a natural salt, which was also put into the cavities, and left to dry out for roughly 40 days before being wrapped.

These procedures attest to the embalmers' general knowledge of major anatomical structures and of methods of preservation. It is not clear, however, whether the embalmers passed their anatomical skills to doctors. Herodotus (ca. 484–ca. 425 B.C.E.), a Greek historian, who wrote extensively about the beliefs and practices of other cultures, observed that in his time, the embalmers were regarded as ritually unclean and were thus unlikely to have communicated extensively with doctors or that surgeons would have been able to practice their skills by helping to prepare mummies. Thus, although embalmers fulfilled an important state-sponsored function, the anatomical knowledge they gleaned was likely of little value to medical practitioners.

INSTITUTIONAL SUPPORT FOR HEALTH AND MEDICINE IN ANCIENT GREECE AND ROME

The Museum and the Library in Alexandria, Egypt

After the death of Alexander the Great (356–323 B.C.E.), his vast territories were divided up among his leading generals. One of his Greek generals, Ptolemy, seized control of Egypt, and thenceforth his family ruled as the pharaohs, establishing a Greek dynasty in the country that ended with the death of queen Cleopatra VII (69–30 B.C.E.) and the Roman conquest in 30 B.C.E. The city of Alexandria served as the capital city of the Ptolemies and grew to be one of the most populous cities in the ancient world. The early Ptolemies were great patrons of the arts and sciences. Perhaps their most important activities in this regard were the foundation of the Museum (a temple of the Muses) as a philosophical school like Plato's Academy and their willingness to provide financial support to any scholars willing to live and work there. They also built the Alexandrian Library, associated with the Museum, in which they gathered written works on all subjects of learning. Whenever scholars arrived in Alexandria, their scrolls would be examined, and if they contained texts not already in the Library, they would be confiscated and copied by scribes, and then the copy would be returned to the owner while the original would be added to the collection. In this way, the Library grew to become the greatest library of the ancient world. Together, the Museum and the Library served to make Alexandria the center of learning in the Mediterranean for several centuries.

The Ptolemaic patronage of scholarship and research extended to providing support for the study of human anatomy through dissection and possibly vivisection. Although such activities would likely have been prevented in the rest of the Greek world due to strict religious taboos against handling dead bodies, two medical researchers at Alexandria are especially associated with the study of human anatomy: Herophilus (335–280 B.C.E.) and Erasistratus (304–250 B.C.E.). Both men were said to have dissected the bodies of criminals, who were provided by the authority of the government, for the purposes of medical research; some ancient accounts even suggest that Herophilus and Erasistratus vivisected criminals, that is, dissected them while they were still alive! In his later works on human anatomy, Galen of Pergamum (129–ca. 216 C.E.) refers to the anatomical discoveries of

Erasistratus and Herophilus on several occasions, but by his time, it appears that the cultural taboos against cutting dead bodies had been reasserted; indeed, it is unlikely that Galen ever dissected human bodies. Nonetheless, for a brief period of time under the institutional support provided by Ptolemaic patronage, the study of human anatomy through the dissection of human bodies was made possible in the ancient world.

Roman Engineering: Aqueducts and Sewage Systems

Sextus Julius Frontinus (ca. 40–104 C.E.) served in the Roman army and later as the Provincial Governor in Britain before being appointed the Water Commissioner for Rome. He wrote about the responsibilities of this position in his *De aquis urbis Romae* (*On the Aqueducts of the City of Rome*), which provides many details of the water supply of ancient Rome and in which he boasts that his work in this regard improved the health of the city. According to Frontinus, Roman inhabitants originally obtained their water from the Tiber River or from private wells. However, in the year 312 B.C.E., the consul, Appius Claudius Crassus, who had overseen the construction of the great road, known as the Appian Way, which connected southern Italy to Rome, built an aqueduct to bring fresh water to the city from springs in the Alban hills. Other aqueducts were built so that by the first century C.E., Rome was supplied with fresh water by means of nine aqueducts, with different systems for supplying drinking water and water for use in gardens or industry. The Roman system of aqueducts was designed to produce a constant gravitational flow of water, with settling tanks (*piscinae*) along that line that served to trap the silt and could be used to raise the water to higher elevations. Water flowed continuously from the aqueducts to a number of public fountains in the city, providing fresh water to inhabitants, and the overflow from the fountains was allowed to wash the streets and flush the sewers.

By the first century C.E., the maintenance of the aqueducts was a fulltime job and a position of *curator aquarum* (procurator of the water supply) of consular rank was created with two assistants of senatorial rank to oversee this work. The emperor Augustus (r. 27 B.C.E.–14 C.E.) bequeathed 240 skilled slaves to the city for the purpose of caring for the water supply systems, and this number was augmented by an additional 460 slaves bequeathed by the emperor Claudius (r. 41–54 C.E.), attesting to the amount of labor involved and the value given to this work by the imperial leaders. It was in his role as the procurator of the water supply that Frontinus came to write his book on the aqueducts of Rome. He describes their construction and the difficulties faced by those in his position. One problem in particular was the illegal siphoning of water from the system:

> My investigations show that they [employees of the water Catchment Board responsible for maintaining the water supply] have been diverting water from public conduits for private use. There is also a significant number of landowners tapping the conduits that by-pass their property. As a result, the public supply is brought to a standstill by private citizens just to water their gardens . . . I found irrigated fields, shops, garrets even, and every house of ill repute in Rome, with fixtures to ensure constant running water. (Amulree 1973, 245)

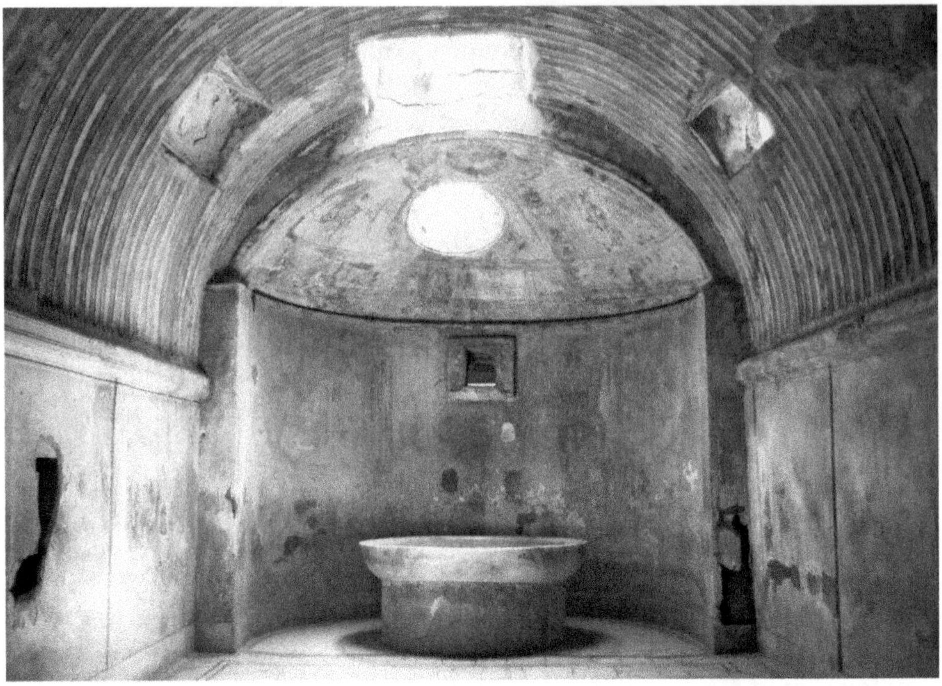

Interior of the *caldarium* (hot water bath) located in the Forum Baths of Pompeii, Italy. The central marble *labrum* (basin) was filled with colder water for those who became too hot. Water was heated in an underground furnace and directed through pipes into the appropriate rooms. Other rooms in the bath house would contain a *tepidarium* (warm water pool) and a *frigidarium* (cold water pool). Hot air was often channeled through empty space under the floors to heat the floor tiles. Large bathing houses might also contain a *palaestra* (exercise area). (Allan T. Kohl/Art Images for College Teaching)

The Romans were concerned with individual hygiene and starting in the second century C.E., they built public baths (*thermae*), often at the expense of Rome's richest citizens and emperors, making them available to the poorest Romans. These bathhouses usually had furnaces for heating water, and they even engineered methods for sending hot air under the floors to provide a form of central heating to the rooms. They would typically have many different rooms for cold baths (*frigidarium*) and hot baths (*caldarium*), with changing rooms for men and women and rooms where people could contract the services of barbers and masseuses. Although people went to them for the purpose of hygiene and for their health, the bathhouses were in many ways the center of urban life, and people would regularly meet in them to socialize at the end of the day. One Roman, whose apartment was located above one such establishment, complained of the noise that rose from the many bathers, people exercising before their baths, and all of the food vendors, barbers, and others, hawking their wares to the bathhouse clientele.

One of the other great marvels of Roman engineering was their sewer system. The *Cloaca Maxima*, the main conduit of the Roman sewage system running from the Forum to the Tiber River, dates to around the sixth century C.E., when it was constructed to drain local marshes. In the following years, a network of conduits was connected to it, and it served to drain storm water and sewage. The government also paid for the construction of public latrines and cesspits that were emptied at various times; a census reveals that there were roughly 150 public latrines in Rome during the reign of Emperor Constantine (r. 306–337 C.E.). Some of these latrines were free, but some charged a small fee. Romans did not have toilet paper, but would often supply each bathroom with a sponge on a stick for the use of its patrons that could be rinsed out between uses in a bowl of water. The maintenance and care of the sewer system was also undertaken by the state, and governmental officials were appointed to oversee these projects.

INSTITUTIONAL MEDICINE IN ANCIENT INDIA

During the reign of King Ashoka (ca. 273–232 B.C.E.), the third king of the Mauryan age, centralized royal administration was increasingly exerted over the empire, and the government became greatly involved in the spread of medical care, among other things, to the general population in India. At the start of his reign, King Ashoka was renowned for his military conquests and cruelty. He famously had many of his brothers murdered in his rise to power and later maintained an extensive prison filled with a wide range of torture devices, which he employed upon criminals and enemies. About eight years into his reign, however, Ashoka witnessed the aftermath of a war he had waged, the loss of life and social turmoil that it caused, and was deeply affected by the experience. As a result, he resolved to abandon his program of conquest and dedicate the remainder of his life to applying Buddhist principles to the administration of his territories. He outlined his new principles in a series of edicts carved on stone pillars that were distributed throughout his empire (they have been found in over 30 sites within India, Nepal, Pakistan, and Afghanistan). In the Rock Edicts, Ashoka apologized for the suffering his wars had caused and declared that he would look upon his subjects as his children and make their welfare his main concern in the future.

Many of the edicts are aimed at enacting judicial reforms but also encouraged the practice of religion (he promoted Buddhism but sought the protection of all religions and encouraged harmony between them) and moral reforms. To ensure that his reforms were carried out, he traveled the empire on inspection tours, and he expected his officials to do likewise. Many edicts indicate that Ashoka believed the state should have an important role in fostering the provision of health care to his people; the second rock edict in particular proclaims that everywhere within his empire, the state should make provision for the medical care of humans and animals. According to the edicts, the state should see to the importation or cultivation of medicinal herbs and fruits in all parts of the empire, as well as dig wells for fresh water along main roads, and plant groves of trees along the roads to provide shade for humans and animals. These public works activities aimed at the provision of health care for his subjects encouraged the idea in India that the care of the sick should be a social responsibility.

Under later Mauryan kings, the state developed a bureau dedicated to directing the settlement of uncultivated land and to controlling the distribution of water. Land and water were regarded as properties of the king, and the state developed irrigation canals and water storage cisterns and demanded revenues in the form of taxes and rents for such services. These state-funded irrigation projects provided water for agriculture and also for the growing cities throughout the empire. Although centralized government control was not always as powerful after the death of Ashoka, in later centuries, kings continued to emphasize the importance of public irrigation projects dedicated to maintaining the economic vitality of the state and the welfare of the people. Specialized hydraulic engineers were charged with the construction and maintenance of irrigation and water storage facilities, and it appears that treatises on the science of hydrology circulated widely in south India by the 14th century C.E. These texts provided information on the different kinds of irrigation canals and how and where to dig wells and construct storage cisterns. They also emphasized the importance of planting trees along the banks of canals to arrest soil erosion and breaches due to flooding. In other parts of India, hydraulic engineers also built irrigation works on a massive scale, damming rivers and creating large artificial lakes to serve as water reservoirs, many of which still exist today. One of these reservoirs, the Colagangam constructed under Rajendra I (r. 1012–1044), was 16 miles long.

Ashoka also generously supported the development of Buddhist monastic communities (*sanghas*). Buddhist monasteries had played a significant role in the development of medicine in India since the fifth century B.C.E., especially in regards to the rise of the written medical tradition and as centers of medical education. Although most often they offered a refuge for travelers, they also came to serve as important institutions for the provision of health care. The *Caraka Samhita* describes such early medical institutions as "halls for health," or what we might consider hospitals, which were dedicated to providing care to the sick, emphasizing that in the interests of patients, the hospital should be constructed "out of the path of smoke, sunlight, water, or dust, as well as unwanted noise, feelings, tastes, sights, and smells. It should have a water supply, pestle and mortar, lavatory, bathing area, and a kitchen" (Wujastyk 2003, 36). In addition to the general construction of the halls for health, the author of the *Caraka* describes the personnel, tools, and medicines with which it should be equipped. He intended that these halls be furnished so as to treat not only a patient's physical ailments, but also maintain her emotional and mental health by providing a serene and pleasant environment. To this end, attendants were expected to be skilled at medicine and also be able to sing, play musical instruments, recite verses, and tell stories to entertain the sick. Although it represents an idealized picture of what an Indian hospital might look like, it does reflect the early appearance of health care institutions in the Indian subcontinent.

HEALTH AND THE STATE IN CHINA

The state played an especially important role in the regulation of health from an early point in Chinese history. As we have seen in other chapters, the central Chinese government took control over medical education as early as the second century B.C.E., creating imperial universities and administering qualifying examinations for medical students. Likewise, the state took responsibility for the standardization of pharmacopeias and other medical texts by the seventh century C.E. and established state run pharmaceutical dispensaries that were charged with overseeing the manufacture and sale of drugs to ensure their quality throughout the empire. Through these efforts, the central imperial government in China took an active role in regulating the provision of medical care that was not matched in other premodern societies.

The earliest institutions providing charitable health care in China were those associated with Buddhist monasteries, as in India. During the Tang dynasty (618–907 C.E.), the state gradually assumed control over the Buddhist health care institutions; in the eighth century state run orphanages and infirmaries for the destitute were established and then in the mid-ninth century, Buddhist monasteries and lands were nationalized, and the revenues from those properties were used to fund charitable hospitals. The emperors of the Song dynasty (960–1279 C.E.) continued to establish free hospitals for the care of the sick poor in major cities in the empire. These state run charitable institutions were expensive, however, and by the late Ming dynasty (ca. 1500–1644), emperors ceased to sponsor these medical services, and private charities stepped in to pay for hospitals for the poor.

Increasing urbanization during the Song period also encouraged state sponsorship of a number of other activities that provided for the general health and welfare of city dwellers. In particular, the authorities in the Song dynasty implemented measures to enhance public health and hygiene in cities. In the capital city of Hangchow in the 13th century C.E., for example, numerous canals were dug to allow for transportation and irrigation in and around the city. Furthermore, an artificial lake was created and carefully maintained to serve as a reservoir for pure drinking water, and earthenware conduits were built to bring fresh water from the lake into the city. Public authorities also paid for street sweepers and garbage removal (garbage was removed by boats on the canals and left on wasteland outside the city), and groups of night soil collectors gathered waste from cesspools, which was either taken from the city or used as fertilizer in gardens and vegetable plots. By comparison with European cities in this period, Hangchow was a very clean city, a fact that Marco Polo commented on in some amazement, noting that travelers, "both on horseback and on foot [can walk] through all the lands of it without soiling the feet" (Wright 1962, 42). Although these public efforts to maintain the city's cleanliness were not necessarily taken strictly for the purposes of maintaining health in the city, they would have served an important role in reducing the risk of epidemic disease.

HOSPITALS IN THE ISLAMIC WORLD AND MEDIEVAL EUROPE

In the Islamic world, the most visible institution dedicated to the provision of health care was the hospital. The earliest Islamic hospitals emerged in the late eighth or early ninth century in Iraq and were modeled on the Nestorian Christian hospices, charitable institutions that provided shelter to travelers and the poor and also assumed the task of providing medical care to the infirm. However, the

Islamic hospitals, or *bimaristans* as they were called, increasingly took on a more specifically medical function in Islamic society than had been the case in the Christian hospices; whereas Christian hospices were typically governed by monks and served a religious function, the Islamic hospitals were most often overseen by elite physicians and were secular in character.

The *bimaristans* were typically founded by acts of royal patronage to provide free medical care to the poor and were often symbols of the charity and prestige of the ruler. By the 12th century, any large Islamic town in the East or North Africa would have a hospital, making them significant medical institutions in Islam. Despite their wide geographic distribution, however, their influence as a source of medical relief was limited; people living in the countryside did not have access to hospital care, and hospitals could only receive a small number of patients in comparison to the size of the urban populations they served.

Hospitals made their greatest impact in the Islamic world, therefore, not as sites of treatment but rather as centers for the dissemination of learned medicine. *Bimaristans* attracted the elite physicians from the Islamic world, such as Abu Bakr Muhammad ibn Zakariya al-Razi (d. ca. 925, known as Rhazes in the Latin West), and positions in the hospitals would provide markers of prestige and financial security. Physicians would visit and treat patients in the hospitals in addition to maintaining their own private clients (al-Razi, for example, counted many high-ranking officials among his private patients). Many of the physicians drawn to the hospitals were also scholars involved in the translation of ancient Greek and also Ayurvedic medical texts, and many wrote their own books on medicine. In this way, the hospitals developed renown as centers for medical learning and attracted students from all over the Islamic world. Indeed, it appears that many hospitals had libraries and larger rooms set aside as lecture halls, and students would often accompany the physicians on their rounds.

In addition to their role in disseminating learned medical knowledge, the *bimaristans* were complex institutions, prepared to meet a variety of medical needs. Hospital staffs included numerous physicians, surgeons, oculists, bonesetters, and pharmacists, as well as orderlies charged with providing basic care, and administrators who were not involved in treating patients but would oversee the general functioning of the hospital. Hospitals were divided into a number of wards, reserved for people suffering from different conditions (e.g., wings were set aside for the mentally ill, those with eye ailments, those recovering from surgery, patients with specific gastrointestinal disorders, etc.), with separate halls for male and female patients. Furthermore, they had rooms for the pharmacy as well as kitchens, living quarters for the staff, latrines and storage areas. These divisions allowed hospitals to accommodate a range of conditions, from those who might require only brief stays to those who would need more long-term medical care.

By contrast, hospitals in Western Europe during the Middle Ages continued to provide primarily religious aid and shelter for the poor and for pilgrims; medical assistance was often only a secondary concern. Indeed, many medieval European hospitals banned those suffering from fever, plague, or other contagious diseases for fear of spreading such afflictions to other patients and most did not have

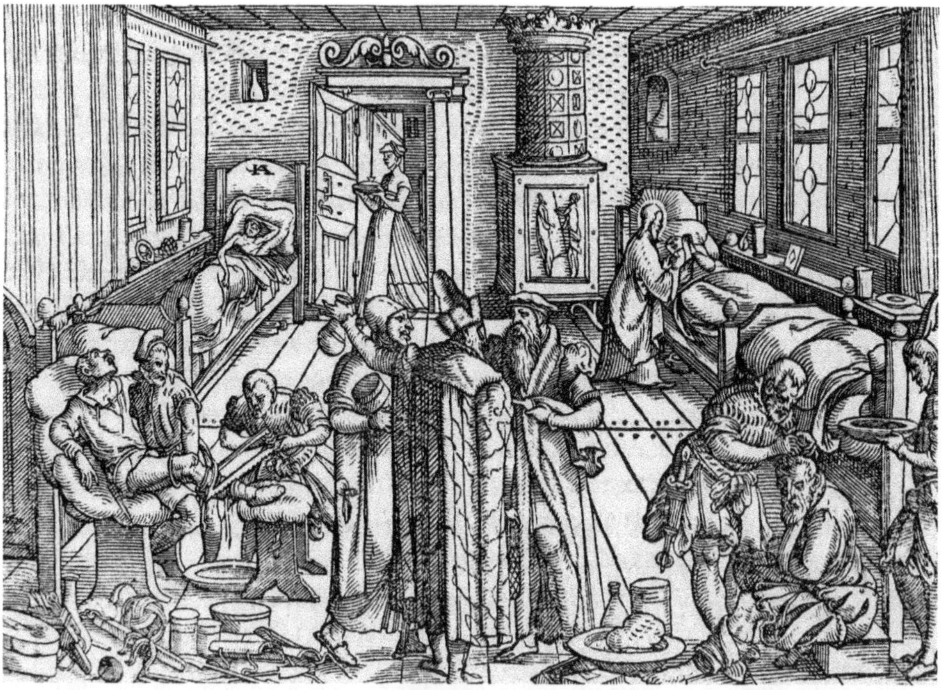

This 16th-century hospital scene emphasizes both the medical and religious goals of hospitals. It shows patients in bed receiving medical care. In the foreground, three physicians with their backs to the patients debate the significance of the signs they see in the urine flask, which one of them holds. Meanwhile, surgeons are actively engaged in treating patients, performing an amputation on the left and a trepanation on the right. A nurse also appears through a doorway bringing food. In the background, Christ (recognized by his halo) cares for a sick patient. This image was clearly intended to aggrandize the work of surgeons over physicians; surgeons, like Christ, are seen actively caring for patients, while the physicians are depicted as being more interested in theoretical debates than treating the sick. (Wellcome Collection)

permanent physicians on staff, although some of the religious leaders who staffed hospitals had medical knowledge. Only during the later medieval period did some European hospitals increasingly start to set aside beds specifically for the sick poor and maintain physicians on staff, but even then the care was provided within a religious context, and hospitals did not become the centers of education that they were in the Islamic world. Even the leprosaria, special houses founded to provide aid to lepers, did not serve a primarily medical function but rather aimed to provide charitable assistance to those deprived of shelter and livelihood as a result of their condition. Many urban hospitals, like the Hôtel-Dieu in Paris, from the mid-13th century onward maintained special wards for pregnant women who had nowhere to live or who wished to give birth in secret, and some even kept a midwife on staff, but again the charitable assistance was as much aimed at preventing infanticide in cases where women might wish to hide their sexual sins or where they could not afford to raise a child as it was at providing medical care.

THE BLACK DEATH AND PUBLIC HEALTH IN MEDIEVAL EUROPE

The arrival of the Black Death in Europe in 1348 galvanized the interest of civic authorities in developing state run public health efforts. Initially, some towns, especially in Italy, established temporary committees to coordinate public health responses to the spread of the plague, which included isolating those infected with the disease or evicting them from the city, imposing quarantines, and even outright banning refugees arriving from plague infested areas. Such measures required the administrative and financial support of the government; doctors alone would not have had the authority or power to enforce these regulations. By 1400, many towns had established permanent health boards that were composed of lay officials who were supported by medical advisers.

Health boards continued to enact and enforce quarantines and to close borders, but increasingly took additional actions to curb the spread of epidemic diseases. Cleaning the city to prevent the collection of materials that might produce the harmful airs, or miasmas, thought to spread disease became one of the main responsibilities of the health boards. Thus, in addition to seeing to the removal of sewage, health boards passed regulations requiring butchers, tanners, and other industries known for producing waste that could rot and produce foul smelling miasmas to dispose of their wastes in appropriate ways. In some cases, they also claimed the right to inspect the quality of meats, wine, and fish in the market for the good of the city.

In a perhaps more sinister role, health boards in some cities also created regulations to control the behavior of those deemed dangerous. Prostitutes were frequent targets of public health officials, who viewed them as a significant cause of the spread of infection. Likewise, beggars, "ruffians," and "loafers" were also viewed as potential carriers of plague. As a result, public health regulations often targeted these socially undesirable individuals under the guise of combating the spread of plague. In Venice, we find the following regulations, for example:

> Just as was done with prostitutes, it is necessary that male and female ruffians who are in the city be known to all, because they are the source of many evils. That is, others are persuaded by their example to live in their disgraceful fashion. So the [Venetian health board] by the power given them by the senate, have deliberated and decided that all these ruffians who are staying in the city must wear the color yellow. Thus they will be recognized by everyone. Violators will be whipped from San Marco to the Rialto, and then banished forever from the territory. (Carmichael 1986, 125)

Clearly, health boards acquired a wide-reaching authority to exert its influence on many areas of civic life.

13

Disease and Healing in the Arts

ENCOUNTERS WITH THE DOCTOR IN ART AND LITERATURE

Although it is not uncommon today for people to dismiss the practices of premodern medicine as superstitious and as having little more than a placebo effect at best, it is important to recognize that healers were often portrayed positively in art and literature across cultures in the premodern world. Some portrayals depict examples of the idealized or miraculous healer, serving as a model that average doctors might be expected to emulate, while others illustrate the more mundane, even messy aspects of medical practice. Considered together, these stories and visual depictions of healers provide useful insight into the status of healers in society, the general level of confidence in their curative abilities, and typical complaints about their failings.

In some cases, physicians were portrayed as having extraordinary, even miraculous, healing powers. One widely circulated legend in medieval Europe told of the medical activities of the brothers Cosmas and Damian, Christian physicians of the third century C.E. According to the legend, the brothers were learned in the art of medicine and were renowned for their willingness to treat patients, without accepting any reward for their services, symbolizing their Christian charity. The story most often told about Cosmas and Damian, which was the subject of many paintings in medieval and Renaissance Europe, recounts how they successfully transplanted the limb of a dead Ethiopian onto a white patient whose own cancerous leg they had removed. In conjunction with their charitable healing, this and other miraculous cures attributed to the brothers provided evidence of their sanctity and, after their martyrdom, they were recognized as the patron saints of physicians and surgeons throughout Europe. This story emblematizes a belief in the close connection between healing and faith in Christian culture and offers a model for the ideal Christian physician, trained in naturalistic medicine and motivated by religious piety to apply his knowledge charitably.

In China, legends about the physician Hua Tuo (ca. 145–208 C.E.) offer a similar account of a selfless healer, who could bring about spectacular cures by means of naturalistic medicine. According to stories, Hua Tuo turned down offers from eminent figures to assume a more lucrative career in government service, choosing rather to travel in the provinces curing peasants and seeking medical knowledge. He gained such renown for his medical skills (especially in acupuncture and surgery), however, that Cao Cao, ruler of a kingdom in northern China, demanded that Hua Tuo come to court and serve as his personal physician to treat his chronic headaches. Hua Tuo came and through the use of acupuncture alleviated the king's headaches, but he refused to remain at court, intending rather to return to his work in the provinces, and out of spite, Cao Cao had him killed. The legends say that while in prison awaiting execution, Hua Tuo wrote down his medical techniques, including his recipe for *mafeisan* (an anesthetic powder he used during surgery), but "when Hua Tuo was about to be executed, he brought out a scroll with writing on it and handed it over to the jailer, saying, 'This can preserve people's lives.' Fearful of the law, the prison subaltern would not accept it, nor did Hua Tuo force it upon him. Instead, he asked for a fire in which he burned the scroll" (Mair 1994, 694). The loss of Hua Tuo's contribution to medical knowledge was regretted ever after.

More mundane physicians were depicted in art and literature as having mastered an extensive theoretical knowledge about the body and disease that was increasingly embedded in a sophisticated textual tradition. The mastery of this text-based knowledge distinguished the learned physicians from the wide range of other healers, whose knowledge of healing was grounded in empirical learning and craft practice with little emphasis on theoretical medicine. Therefore, physicians were often portrayed in close association with their books or in the act of teaching students. Physicians were also portrayed in the act of diagnosis, taking the pulse, or studying the patient's urine. Successful use of these diagnostic techniques was supposed to require extensive textual training, and many texts were written about them. Some of the texts even included illustrations of "urine wheels," showing the different colors of urine a physician may encounter and explaining which disease they may portend; these are similar to the pages of illustrations of tongues common in Chinese medical literature, which explain how to recognize signs of disease by examining the tongue. Indeed, the examination of urines came to be so closely associated with textual medical training that the urine flask came to be the symbol of scientific medicine in the European Middle Ages, similar to how the stethoscope and white lab coat are symbols of scientific medicine in the West today.

Healers were also often depicted in art in the act of mixing medicines or treating patients. Certain practices, as with the portrayal of diagnostic techniques, were often associated with those physicians trained in the textual medical tradition. For example, the application of moxibustion and acupuncture in China required significant training, and those depicted doing so would likely have been learned physicians. In other cases, healers might be shown in the act of surgery or with their surgical tools. Surgical skill was often highly regarded in Greek and Roman art and literature. In the *Iliad*, for example, when Menelaus was injured by an arrow, the soldiers immediately found one warrior, Machaon, the son of Asclepius, known for his surgical skills: "the god-sent healer reached the captain's side and quickly drew the shaft from his buckled belt—he pulled it clear, the sharp barbs broke back. . . . When he saw the wound where the tearing arrow hit, he sucked out the blood and deftly applied the healing salves that Chiron, friend of Asclepius, gave his father long ago" (Fagles 1990, 152). Greek and Roman doctors are similarly depicted in art engaged in surgical operations. By contrast, in China and medieval Europe, surgery was usually considered the province of lower status craftsmen and avoided by physicians. Indeed, in the artwork of the medieval West, it was not uncommon to see physicians portrayed as being so closely associated with the symbols of their textual training that they appeared uninterested in the actual task of treating patients! Surgeons and barber-surgeons, on the other hand, were often shown engaging in treating patients by performing surgical operations, letting blood, and cupping (healers were often shown with their cupping flasks), a stark contrast to images of physicians with their books and urine flasks, engaging in theoretical debates while their patients suffered quietly in the background!

In the general prologue to his *Canterbury Tales*, Geoffrey Chaucer (ca. 1343–1400) offers a typical portrait of the physician in medieval culture—one that may have seemed familiar in most of the cultures we have examined. Chaucer praises his "doctor of physic" for his deep knowledge of astrology and the written medical tradition:

> Nowhere in all the world was one to match him
> Where medicine was concerned, or surgery;
> Being well grounded in astrology
> He'd watch his patient with the utmost care
> Until he'd found a favorable hour,
> By means of astrology, to give treatment.
> Skilled to pick out the astrologic moment
> For charms and talismans to aid the patient,
> He knew the cause of every malady,
> If it were "hot" or "cold" or "moist" or "dry,"
> And where it came from, and from which humor.
> He was a really fine practitioner.
> . . .
> Well-read was he in Asclepius,
> In Dioscorides, and in Rufus,
> Ancient Hippocrates, Hali, and Galen,
> Avicenna, Rhazes, and Serapion,
> Averroës, Damascenus, Constantine,
> Bernard, and Gilbertus, and Gaddesden. (Wright 1985, 11–12)

Chaucer, a dedicated satirist, did not raise doubts about the efficacy of the physician's cures, however, and did not portray him as being too in love with theory to treat patients; indeed, he notes that the good doctor regularly attended the sick during the Black Death. From where did his doctor's motivation to treat the sick come? Not from a pious desire to treat the poor, such as displayed by Cosmas and Damian and Hua Tuo (indeed, Chaucer's physician "read but little in the Bible") but rather because he was able to earn such high fees from those he treated, as Chaucer notes: "In medicine gold is the best cordial. So it was gold that he loved best of all" (Wright 1985, 11–12). Greed motivated the physician even more than love of theory!

THE BODY IN MEDICAL ART

Medical texts in China and the medieval West often include a number of medical illustrations, revealing the importance of the visual representation of the medical body in both cultures. Sanskrit medical texts from the Ayurvedic tradition in premodern India, by contrast, were normally not illustrated and do not include anatomical sketches, line drawings for surgical guidance, or any other visual depictions of the medical body; representations of the medical body in the Ayurvedic tradition do not appear in the Indian subcontinent until the 18th century (Wujastyk 2009). The medical illustrations from Chinese and Western cultures evolved to reflect a number of distinct genres, each with different aims. In some cases, the pictures may have been designed merely to be aesthetically pleasing or humorous, like the images of people representing different humoral types in medieval Europe—a series of four pictures showing the personality of a man whose temperament was controlled by each of the four humors. In addition to providing aesthetically pleasing pictures, however, many illustrations also served a more didactic purpose.

One of the most common genres of medical illustration portrayed the human body to reflect upon the interaction between the microcosm and the macrocosm. In Western art, the "zodiac man" usually displayed a human with the signs of the zodiac placed over the parts of the body with which they were thought to exert an influence (Capricorn on the head, Pisces with the feet, Cancer with the chest, etc.) In these figures, the point is to show the human body as the microcosm and how it relates to the wider universe, the macrocosm. One example from Chinese art, the *Neijing Tu* (*Diagram of the Inner Realm*), found on a stone stele in the Baigunguan Temple in Beijing, displays the body as a macrocosm. The head is shown as a mountainous landscape with rapids descending from it and continuing down the spinal column to the ocean below the abdomen, the torso contains a forest, and the abdominal region has an ox pulling a plough through fields where crops are being sown. Human figures are also arrayed in the picture, such as a white-haired old man in a yoga pose in the head and a pretty girl by a spinning wheel in the upper abdomen. Carefully interpreted as a whole, the *Neijing Tu* reveals certain Taoist medico-alchemical concepts of the body, the relationship between the microcosm and the macrocosm, and the quest to prolong life and attain immortality. Slightly different versions of the *Neijing Tu* exist, but all reflect the same basic concepts.

Other medical images are designed to offer guidance on treatment. In the West, where bloodletting was a primary therapeutic action, figures of the "bloodletting man" were common, depicting a human body with the major veins marked, sometimes with notations indicating specific locations where one could let blood. Some images did double duty, combining the "zodiac man" and "bloodletting man" figures. These figures were similar to depictions of the "wound man" and "disease man," which again showed the human body either with text describing diseases with arrows indicating the parts of the body they afflicted or with images of the kinds of gruesome wounds a body could receive. In China, images of the body were depicted not to indicate bloodletting points but rather to mark out sites for the application of acupuncture and moxibustion. In many cases, these images were even updated to reflect changes in theory or practice. For example, the famous Tang physician Sun Simiao (581–682 C.E.) was concerned that older illustrations may contain errors and show the wrong points for acupuncture and sought to create newer more accurate drawings to teach practitioners.

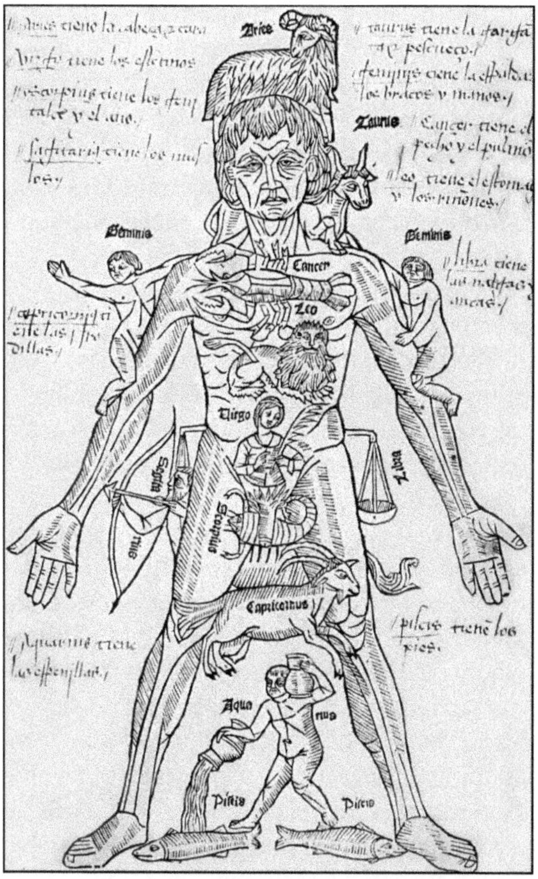

A "zodiac man" illustration from a medieval European manuscript. The zodiac man was a typical genre of illustration in medieval manuscripts in which the signs of the zodiac were drawn over the parts of the body they were believed to influence. These charts reflect the prevalent belief in the role of astrological influences on individual health. (National Library of Medicine)

The study of human anatomy developed in different ways in China and the West, but in both cases, it was linked to the depiction of anatomical structures in art. Opening dead bodies was seldom practiced in ancient China due to traditional beliefs about the sacredness of the body and taboos about disfiguring bodies for any reasons. During the Song dynasty (960–1279 C.E.), however, some texts recount efforts to dissect dead bodies for the purposes of studying human anatomy. In the first case, from around 1045, the bandit Ou Xifan was executed and, at the command of the local governor, his body was delivered to physicians so that it could be dissected and drawings could be made of the internal structures (some versions of this recount that his body was dissected along with those of some 50 fellow bandits). Later, the physician Yang Jie (1068–1140) produced a volume of anatomical drawings also based upon the dissection of executed criminals who were delivered for this purpose by the local governor. It is significant that in both of these cases, the dissection took place with the express intention of producing illustrated textbooks of human anatomy. Unfortunately, copies of the books that were produced do not exist today, and their illustrations are lost. The study of the human anatomy did not receive extensive attention in later periods of Chinese history, which no doubt reflects the continued taboos against opening dead bodies and also the fact that a detailed understanding of human anatomy was not deemed necessary for the proper application of traditional Chinese medicine. Nonetheless, images of internal anatomy continued to circulate in medical texts, perhaps copies of those originally drawn from the dissection of criminals. In these images, internal organs are not depicted as distinct entities, with a recognizable shape or form, and were usually intended to depict the *zang* and *fu* organs in relation to specific acupuncture points. As such, they would not have been especially useful for learning sufficient anatomical detail for success in surgery, but they would have helped elicit principles of theoretical importance for physicians interested in knowing the number of orifices in the throat or the position of the liver in relation to important acupuncture points.

Whereas the practice of human dissection was limited in other ancient cultures, it came to be considered a necessary component of a physician's medical training in the medieval European universities. Starting in Bologna shortly after 1300, many universities began to perform public dissections of two or three human bodies (criminal bodies, preferably at least one male and one female) once per year (usually in winter to minimize the effects of putrefaction) for the purposes of teaching human anatomy. The dissection would be held in a church or a temporary lecture hall, hastily built for the occasion, and would take place over the course of about one week, during which time the dissectors would focus on revealing the organs of the three main body cavities (abdomen, thorax, and head). The labor of the procedure itself was divided among three main participants: a senior student, who would read a relevant passage from an anatomical text concerning the structure about to be revealed, a surgeon, who would do the actual cutting, and a professor of medicine (a physician), who would point out the structure and add additional commentary as a means of teaching the material discussed in the text. Pictures of a university dissection scene became common in the later Middle Ages, and they serve to emphasize a number of points, including social distinctions between the theoretical learning of the physician and the manual craft practice of the surgeon. These illustrations of physicians studying anatomy thus came to signify their theoretical training, just like the images of the physician holding a urine flask.

A number of anatomical texts were written that included illustrations of the structures of internal anatomy, the most famous being that by Mondino de' Liuzzi (ca. 1270–1326), the *Anathomia corporis humani* (*Anatomy of the Human Body*). The most common illustrations were the five figure series, pictures of squatting men, each of whom depicted a major anatomical structure: artery man, vein man (similar to the bloodletting man figures), nerve man, skeleton man, and muscle man. These illustrations were typically highly schematic and did not necessarily seek to provide an accurate depiction of the body parts (e.g., skeleton man would often have the wrong number of ribs, while muscle man was usually shown with a characteristic donut shaped muscle around the stomach). Other illustrations depicted a body with the major organs on it, usually including the lungs, heart, stomach, liver, kidneys, and intestines. While these illustrations often did more to distinguish the major organs from one another and give rough attention to their shape than the Chinese organ illustrations, they were still highly schematic.

Given the fact that students would have had little opportunity for hands-on examination of the bodies during the dissection lessons, it is unlikely that they learned much anatomical detail during them, so medical students were mostly expected to learn anatomy by reading textbooks. Likewise, the illustrations they could view in these texts would not have conveyed enough detail to offer practical guidance for surgery. However, as with the Chinese illustrations, they were detailed enough to help answer significant theoretical questions of interest to the physician, who did not otherwise need to have an exceedingly detailed knowledge of anatomy for successful practice. In 1543, Andreas Vesalius (1514–1564) published his *De Humani Corporis Fabrica* (*On the Fabric of the Human Body*), a lavishly illustrated anatomical textbook, which revolutionized the study of anatomy and anatomical illustration. Vesalius's pictures aimed at providing accurate depictions of the shape of organs and their positions within the body, drawing a sharp contrast in terms of the detail and goals to previous anatomical illustrations from the Middle Ages and those produced in China.

GLOSSARY

acupuncture
The therapeutic practice common in traditional Chinese medicine in which needles are applied at specific sites on the body to redirect the flow of qi and restore health.

ashipu
The exorcist, or priest, who treated the sick in ancient Mesopotamia with charms, drugs, and magical cures.

asu
The physician in ancient Mesopotamia, who treated the sick with charms, drugs, and magical cures.

Ayurvedic medicine
Ayurveda literally means "knowledge for longevity." This is the medical tradition in India based on the oral traditions passed on by practicing healers from the Vedic period (ca. 1500–500 B.C.E). Ayurvedic medicine emphasizes rational or naturalistic medical knowledge but also incorporates magical healing traditions.

bloodletting
The therapeutic practice used in several premodern cultures, but most common in the humoral tradition practiced in Greece, Rome, the Islamic world, and medieval Europe. Small amounts of blood would be let from various parts of the body (typically by cutting open veins but also through applying leeches) in order to remove unhealthy humors from the body and thus restore a healthy humoral balance.

chirurgicus
The surgeon in medieval Europe.

cupping
The therapeutic practice in which the doctor would put a piece of burning material into a little metal or glass cup so that when applied to the skin, the flame would be extinguished and create a vacuum, holding the cup to the skin. The suction was believed to help draw internal humors to the site, to help rectify localized humoral imbalances in the body and restore health. The practice of "wet" cupping (as opposed to "dry" cupping) entailed scarifying the skin to cause bleeding before applying the cup, so that harmful excess humors could be drawn out of the body.

dhatus
The seven basic structural constituents (tissues and fluids) of the body in Ayurvedic medicine: *rasa* ("plasma" or "chyle"), *rakta* ("blood"), *mamsa* ("muscle" and "flesh"), *meda* ("fat"), *asthi* ("bone"), *majjan* ("marrow" and "nerve tissue"), and *shukra* ("semen").

doshas
The concept in Ayurvedic medicine of humors or substances in the body required for its proper functioning. They are *vata* (wind or air), *pitta* (bile or fire), and *kapha* (phlegm or water). They are transported through the body through a network of channels or tubes called *srotas*.

Hippocratic Corpus
The body of approximately 60 texts written from 450 to 350 B.C.E. and ascribed to Hippocrates. These texts are often mutually contradictory and reflect different dialects, indicating that they were not likely written by a single individual. It is not clear which, if any, of these texts may have been written by the real Hippocrates.

humoralism
The theoretical system originating in Greek medicine that envisions the body as a being composed of four humors: blood, phlegm, black bile (melancholy), and yellow bile (choler). According to humoral theory, disease arises when the humors are out of balance in the body. Humoralism was central to the medical practices in Greece, Rome, the Islamic world, and the medieval West.

***iatros* (pl. *iatroi*)**
The physician in ancient Greece.

malas
The main waste products of the body produced as a result of digestion in Ayurvedic medicine: feces, urine, and sweat. The maintenance of health requires that these be effectively eliminated from the body.

moxibustion
The therapeutic practice common in traditional Chinese medicine in which mugwort tinder (moxa) is used to cause a burn on specific points of the body, typically to help redirect the flow of qi in the body and restore health.

naturalistic medicine
Medical beliefs that explain health and disease as a rational and natural process in which gods and supernatural beings are not involved.

physicus
The university-trained physician in medieval Europe, as distinguished from the *medicus*, or doctor who may or may not have earned a university degree.

qi
The concept in traditional Chinese medicine translated as "vapor," "breath," or "energy" and recognized as the vital principle that flows through meridians or pathways in the body and is essential for promoting growth and the healthy operation of the body.

swnw
The physician in ancient Egypt.

systematic correspondence
The concept present in many premodern medical theories by which the actions of the universe (macrocosm) are connected to and exert and influence on the functioning of the human body (microcosm).

vaidyas
Physicians in Ayurvedic medicine.

wu xing
The concept in traditional Chinese medicine of the "five phases" or "five elements" (wood, fire, earth, metal, and water), which compose the universe and the body.

BIBLIOGRAPHY

Amulree, Lord. "Hygienic Conditions in Ancient Rome and Modern London." *Medical History* 17 (1973): 244–255.

Archer, Christon I., John R. Ferris, Holger H. Herwig, and Timothy H. E. Travers. *World History of Warfare*. Lincoln: University of Nebraska Press, 2002.

Bhishagratna, Kaviraj Kunjalal. *An English Translation of the Sushruta Samhita Based on Original Sanskrit Text. Vol. 1, Sutrasthanam*. Calcutta: Forgotten Books, 1907.

Bhishagratna, Kaviraj Kunjalal. *An English Translation of the Sushruta Samhita with a Full and Comprehensive Introduction, Additional Texts, Different Readings, Notes, Comparative Views, Index, Glossary and Plates. Vol. 2, Nidana-Sthana, S'Arira-Sthana, Chikitsita-Sthana and Kalapa-Sthana*. Calcutta: Forgotten Books, 1911.

Biggs, Robert D. "Medicine and Public Health in Ancient Mesopotamia." *Journal of Assyrian Academic Studies* 19, no. 1 (2005): 1–19.

Bloomfield, M. *Hymns of the Atharva Veda*. Whitefish, MT: Kessinger Publishing, 2004.

Boer, Charles. Marsilio *Ficino's Book of Life*. Woodstock, CT: Spring Publications, 1980.

Boylston, Anthea. "Evidence for Weapon-Related Trauma in British Archaeological Samples." In *Human Osteology in Archaeology and Forensic Science*, edited by M. Cox and S. Mays, 357–380. London: Greenwich Medical Media, 2000.

Breasted, James Henry. *The Edwin Smith Surgical Papyrus*. Vol. 1. Chicago: University of Chicago Press, 1930.

Bryan, Cyril P. *Ancient Egyptian Medicine: The Papyrus Ebers*. Chicago: Ares Publishers Inc., 1974.

Caciola, Nancy. *Discerning Spirits: Divine and Demonic Possession in the Middle Ages*. Ithaca, NY: Cornell University Press, 2003.

Campbell, Eldridge, and James Colton, trans. *The Surgery of Theodoric, ca. A.D. 1267*. Vol. 1. New York: Appleton-Century-Crofts, Inc., 1955.

Carmichael, Ann G. *Plague and the Poor in Renaissance Florence*. Cambridge, MA: Cambridge University Press, 1986.

Chadwick, J., and W. N. Mann, trans. *Hippocratic Writings*, edited by G. E. R. Lloyd. New York: Penguin Books, 1950.

Chiu, Martha Li. "Insanity in Imperial China: A Legal Case Study." In *Normal and Abnormal Behavior in Chinese Culture*, edited by A. Klein-Man and T.-Y. Lin, 75–94. Dordrecht: D. Reidel Publishing Co., 1981.

Cholmeley, H. P. *John of Gaddesden and the Rosa Medicinae*. Oxford: Clarendon Press, 1912.

Cruse, Audrey. *Roman Medicine*. Stroud, Gloucestershire: Tempus Publishing, 2004.

Demaitre, Luke. "The Care and Extension of Old Age in Medieval Medicine." In *Aging and the Aged in Medieval Europe*, edited by Michael M. Sheehan, 3–22. Toronto: Pontifical Institute of Mediaeval Studies, 1990.

Demaitre, Luke. "The Idea of Childhood and Child Care in Medical Writings of the Middle Ages." *Journal of Psychohistory* 4 (1977): 461–490.

Demaitre, Luke. *Leprosy in Premodern Medicine: A Malady of the Whole Body*. Baltimore, MD: Johns Hopkins University Press, 2007.

Demaitre, Luke E. *Doctor Bernard de Gordon: Professor and Practitioner.* Toronto: Pontifical Institute of Mediaeval Studies, 1980.

Dols, Michael W. *The Black Death in the Middle East.* Princeton, NJ: Princeton University Press, 1977.

Dols, Michael W. *Majnun: The Madman in Medieval Islamic Society*, edited by Diana E. Immisch. Oxford: Clarendon Press, 1992.

Edelstein, Emma J., and Ludwig Edelstein. *Asclepius: Collection and Interpretation of the Testimonies.* Vols. 1 and 2. Baltimore, MD: Johns Hopkins University Press, 1998.

Edelstein, Ludwig. *Ancient Medicine: Selected Papers of Ludwig Edelstein*, edited by Owsei Temkin and C. Lilian Temkin. Baltimore, MD: Johns Hopkins University Press, 1967.

Fagles, Robert, trans. Homer, *The Iliad.* New York: Penguin Books, 1990.

Fagles, Robert, trans. Homer, *The Odyssey.* New York: Penguin Books, 1996.

Finucane, Ronald C. *Miracles and Pilgrims: Popular Beliefs in Medieval England.* London: J. M. Dent & Sons, Ltd., 1977.

Furth, Charlotte. *A Flourishing Yin: Gender in China's Medical History, 960–1665.* Berkeley: University of California Press, 1999.

Ghalioungui, Paul. *Magic and Medical Science in Ancient Egypt.* New York: Barnes & Noble, Inc., 1963.

Gies, Joseph, and Frances Gies. *Life in a Medieval City.* London: The Folio Society, 2002.

Green, Monica H. *Making Women's Medicine Masculine: The Rise of Male Authority in Pre-Modern Gynaecology.* Oxford: Oxford University Press, 2008.

Grene, David, trans. Herodotus. *The History.* Chicago: University of Chicago Press, 1987.

Guihua, Xie. "Han Bamboo and Wooden Medical Records Discovered in Military Sites from the North-Western Frontier Regions." In *Medieval Chinese Medicine: The Dunhuang Medical Manuscripts*, edited by Vivienne Lo and Christopher Cullen, 78–106. London: Routledge, 2005.

Gunther, Robert T. *The Greek Herbal of Dioscorides.* New York: Hafner Publishing Co., 1959.

Hanawalt, Barbara A. *Growing Up in Medieval London: The Experience of Childhood in History.* Oxford: Oxford University Press, 1993.

Hanawalt, Barbara A. *The Ties That Bound: Peasant Families in Medieval England.* Oxford: Oxford University Press, 1986.

Hanson, Ann Ellis. "Diseases of Women 1." *Signs* 1 (1975): 567–584.

Hopkins, Donald R. *The Greatest Killer: Smallpox in History.* Chicago: University of Chicago Press, 1983.

Horrox, Rosemary. *The Black Death.* Manchester: Manchester University Press, 1994.

Jones, Frederic Wood. "Some lessons from ancient fractures." *British Medical Journal* 2 (August 22, 1908): 455–458.

Jones, Peter Murray. "John of Arderne and the Mediterranean Tradition of Scholastic Surgery." In *Practical Medicine from Salerno to the Black Death*, edited by Luis García-Ballester, Roger French, Jon Arrizabalaga, and Andrew Cunningham, 289–321. Cambridge, MA: Cambridge University Press, 1994.

Jones, W. H. S., trans. Hippocrates, "Airs, Waters, Places" and "Epidemics I and III." In *Hippocrates*, 1:65–137 and 139–287. Cambridge, MA: Harvard University Press, 1984.

Jones, W. H. S., trans. Hippocrates, "On the Sacred Disease." In *Hippocrates*, 2:129–183. Cambridge, MA: Harvard University Press, 1923.

Jones, W. H. S., trans. Pliny, *Natural History.* Vol. 7. Cambridge, MA: Harvard University Press, 1956.

Jones, W. H. S., trans. Pliny, *Natural History*. Vol. 8. Cambridge, MA: Harvard University Press, 1963.
Kutumbiah, P. *Ancient Indian Medicine*. Chennai, India: Orient Longman, 1962.
Lambert, W. G. "The Gula Hymn of Bulluùsa-rabi." *Orientalia*, n.s., 36 (1967): 105–121.
Lemay, Helen Rodnite. *Women's Secrets: A Translation of Pseudo-Albertus Magnus's De Secretis Mulierum with Commentaries*. Albany: State University of New York Press, 1992.
Leung, Angela Ki Che. *Leprosy in China: A History*. New York: Columbia University Press, 2008.
Levey, Martin. *The Medical Formulary or Aqrabadhin of Al-Kindi*. Madison: University of Wisconsin Press, 1966.
Lonie, I. M., trans. *The Hippocratic Treatises on Generation, on the Nature of the Child, Diseases IV: A Commentary*. Berlin: Walter de Gruyter, 1981.
Mair, Victor H., trans. "The Biography of Hua-t'o from the History of the Three Kingdoms." In *The Columbia Anthology of Traditional Chinese Literature*, edited by Victor H. Mair, 688–696. New York: Columbia University Press, 1994.
Majno, Guido. *The Healing Hand: Man and Wound in the Ancient World*. Cambridge, MA: Harvard University Press, 1975.
McLeod, Katrina C. D., and Robin D. S. Yates, "Forms of Ch'in Law: An Annotated Translation of the Feng-chen shih." *Harvard Journal of Asiatic Studies* 41 (1981): 111–163.
McVaugh, Michael R. *Arnaldi de Villanova Opera Medica Omnia*. Vol. 2, *Aphorismi de Gradibus*. Granada and Barcelona: Seminarium Historiae Medicae Granatensis, 1975.
McVaugh, Michael R. "Cataracts and Hernias: Aspects of Surgical Practice in the Fourteenth Century." *Medical History* 45 (2001): 319–340.
McVaugh, Michael R. "Incantations in Late Medieval Surgery." In *Ratio et Superstitio: Essays in Honor of Graziella Frederici Vescovini*, edited by Giancarlo Marchetti, Orsola Rignani and Valeria Sorge, 319–346. Leuvene-la-Neuve, Belgium: Fédération Internationale des Instituts d'Etudes Médiévale, 2003.
McVaugh, Michael R. *The Rational Surgery of the Middle Ages*. Florence: Sismel—Edizioni del Galluzzo, 2006.
McWilliam, G. H., trans. Giovanni Boccaccio, *The Decameron*. New York: Penguin Books, 1995.
Meek, Theophile J., trans. "The Code of Hammurabi." In *Ancient Near Eastern Texts Relating to the Old Testament*, 3rd ed. with Supplement, edited by James B. Pritchard, 163–180. Princeton, NJ: Princeton University Press, 1969.
Ng, Vivian W. *Madness in Late Imperial China: From Illness to Deviance*. Norman: University of Oklahoma Press, 1990.
Ni, Maoshing. *The Yellow Emperor's Classic of Medicine: A New Translation of the Neijing Suwen with Commentary*. Boston, MA: Shambhala, 1995.
Nriagu, Jerome O. "Occupational Exposure to Lead in Ancient Times." *Science of the Total Environment* 31 (1983): 105–116.
Nunn, John F. *Ancient Egyptian Medicine*. Norman: University of Oklahoma Press, 1996.
Oppenheim, A. Leo. "The Mother of Nabonidus." In *Ancient Near Eastern Texts Relating to the Old Testament*, 3rd edition with Supplement, edited by James B. Pritchard, 560–562. Princeton, NJ: Princeton University Press, 1969.
Park, Katharine. "Birth and Death." In *A Cultural History of the Human Body in the Medieval Age*, edited by Linda Kalof, 17–38. Oxford: Berg Publishers, 2010.
Park, Katharine. "Medicine and Society in Medieval Europe, 500–1500." In *Medicine in Society: Historical Essays*, edited by Andrew Wear, 59–90. Cambridge, MA: Cambridge University Press, 1992.

Pormann, Peter E., and Emilie Savage-Smith. *Medieval Islamic Medicine*. Washington, DC: Georgetown University Press, 2007.

Potter, Paul, trans. "On Haemorrhoids." In *Hippocrates*, 8:377–389. Cambridge, MA: Harvard University Press, 1995.

Riddle, John M. *Contraception and Abortion from the Ancient World to the Renaissance*. Cambridge, MA: Harvard University Press, 1992.

Robbins, G., V. M. Tripathy, V. N. Misra, R. K. Mohanty, V. S. Shinde, et al. "Ancient Skeletal Evidence for Leprosy in India (2000 B.C.)." *PLoS ONE 4*, no. 5 (2009): e5669. Doi:10.1371/journal.pone.0005669.

Russell, John Malcolm. "Bulls for the Palace and Order in the Empire: The Sculptural Program of Sennacherib's Court VI at Nineveh." *The Art Bulletin* 69 (1987): 520–539.

Salazar, Christine F. *The Treatment of War Wounds in Graeco-Roman Antiquity*. Leiden: Brill, 2000.

Savage-Smith, Emilie. "The Practice of Surgery in Islamic Lands: Myth and Reality," *Social History of Medicine* 13 (2000): 307–321.

Schipper, Kristofer. *The Taoist Body*. Translated by Karen C. Duval. Berkeley: University of California Press, 1993.

Scurlock, J. A. "Baby-Snatching Demons, Restless Souls and the Dangers of Childbirth: Medico-Magical Means of Dealing with Some of the Perils of Motherhood in Ancient Mesopotamia." *Incognita* 2 (1991): 135–183.

Seward, Desmond. *The Hundred Years War: The English in France, 1337–1453*. New York: Atheneum, 1978.

Shahar, Meir. *Crazy Ji: Chinese Religion and Popular Literature*. Cambridge, MA: Harvard University Press, 1998.

Sharma, Priya Vrat. *Susruta-Samhita with English Translation of Text and Dalhana's Commentary alongwith Critical Notes*. Vol. 1, *Sutrasthana*. Varanasi, India: Chaukhambha Visvabharati, 1999.

Sharma, Ram Karan, and Vaidya Bhagwan Dash. *Agnivesa's Caraka Samhita: Text with English Translation & Critical Exposition*. Varanasi, India: Chowkhamba Sanskrit Series Office, 1976.

Sigerist, Henry E. *A History of Medicine*. Vol. 1, *Primitive and Archaic Medicine*. Oxford: Oxford University Press, 1951.

Spencer, W. G., trans. Celsus, *De Medicina*. Vol. 2. Cambridge, MA: Harvard University Press, 1953.

Spencer, W. G., trans. Celsus, *De Medicina*. Vol. 3. Cambridge, MA: Harvard University Press, 1961.

Spink, M. S., and G. L. Lewis. *Albucasis On Surgery and Instruments: A Definitive Edition of the Arabic Text with English Translation and Commentary*. London: Wellcome Institute of the History of Medicine, 1973.

Stol, M. *Epilepsy in Babylonia*. Groningen: Styx, 1993.

Temkin, Owsei. *Soranus' Gynecology*. Baltimore, MD: Johns Hopkins University Press, 1956.

Thompson, R. Campbell. *Assyrian Medical Texts*. London: John Bale Sons & Danielsson, Ltd., 1924.

Veith, Ilza. *Huang Ti Nei Ching Su Wên: The Yellow Emperor's Classic of Internal Medicine*. New Edition. Berkeley: University of California Press, 1972.

Veith, Ilza. "The Supernatural in Far Eastern Concepts of Mental Disease." *Bulletin of the History of Medicine* 37 (1963): 139–158.

Ware, James R. *Alchemy, Medicine, Religion in the China of A.D. 320: The Nei P'ien of Ko Hung (Pao-p'u tzu)*. Cambridge, MA: MIT Press, 1966.

Wilson, John A. "Egyptian Rituals and Incantations." In *Ancient Near Eastern Texts Relating to the Old Testament,* 3rd ed. with Supplement, edited by James B. Pritchard, 325–331. Princeton, NJ: Princeton University Press, 1969.

Withington, E. T., trans. Hippocrates, "On Joints." In *Hippocrates,* 3:201–397. Cambridge, MA: Harvard University Press, 1944a.

Withington, E. T., trans. Hippocrates, "On Wounds in the Head." In *Hippocrates,* 3:1–51. Cambridge, MA: Harvard University Press, 1944b.

Wright, David, trans. Geoffrey Chaucer, *The Canterbury Tales: A Verse Translation with an Introduction and Notes.* Oxford: Oxford University Press, 1985.

Wright, H. M., trans. Jacques Gernet, *Daily Life in China on the Eve of the Mongol Invasion 1250–1276.* Stanford: Stanford University Press, 1962.

Wujastyk, Dominik. "Interpreting the Image of the Human Body in Pre-Modern India." *International Journal of Hindu Studies* 13, no. 2 (2009): 189–228.

Wujastyk, Dominik. *The Roots of Ayurveda: Selections from Sanskrit Medical Writings.* New York: Penguin Books, 2003.

Zhenguo, Wang, Chen Ping, and Xie Peiping. *History and Development of Traditional Chinese Medicine.* Vol. 1. Beijing: Science Press, 1999.

Zysk, Kenneth G. *Asceticism and Healing in Ancient India: Medicine in the Buddhist monastery.* 2nd ed. Delhi: Motilal Banarsidass, 1998.

PART 2

15th through 18th Centuries

Joseph P. Byrne

1

Key Factors in Health and Wellness

FACTORS IN INDIVIDUAL HEALTH AND WELL-BEING

The notion that all people are created equal is a fine political and legal standard, but in terms of health and wellness, it could not be further from the truth. Within every human community, however large or small, are a wide variety of health conditions. Some are a matter of birth and family, others depend upon the course of one's life, and still others emerge from specific historical circumstances.

Birth and Family

"We choose our friends but not our family," the old saying goes. One's bloodline provided a set of genetic traits and dispositions. In the age before our modern knowledge of genetics and disease, and compensating drugs and therapies, an inherited predisposition to alcoholism, sickle-cell anemia, poor eyesight, cancer, or crippling depression could mark one for life. In addition, one's mother provided not only genes but the prenatal environment for the child: Did she smoke, consume alcohol, eat a healthy diet? How old was she? Was she beaten or forced to perform difficult work while pregnant? Where in the birth order was the particular child? How helpful were the midwife and assistants at the birth? In each of the five cultures—the Aztecs, Chinese, Europeans, Muslims, and Caribbean slaves—this volume highlights pregnant women, new mothers, and most infants were provided special care. After all, they were the future of the family and society, whether an empire or a plantation worked by slaves.

The "accident of birth" also determined where and when one was born and into what social class. At that time, it was not that one set of environmental challenges and opportunities was "better" than another but that they were different. Rural and urban environments presented different opportunities and hazards. In Europe, for example, health care professionals and institutions such as orphanages and hospitals were urban phenomena, but the air, water, and food were often unhealthy. Infants in well-off families were often sent to nurse in the countryside where conditions were recognized as being healthier.

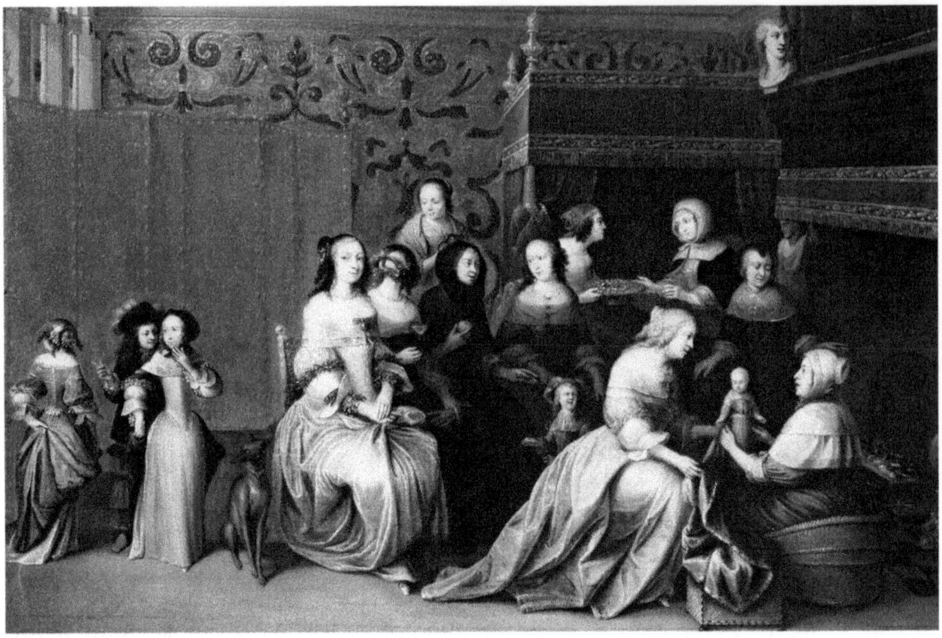

A wealthy Dutch family celebrates the birth of a child. Two gentlemen remain discretely hidden behind a screen, while the midwife presents the new family member. The painting is by Hieronymus Janssens (1624–1693). (Private Collection/Photo by Christie's Images/Bridgeman Images)

Within a society, a family's social and economic class determined opportunity. Higher status might mean one could avoid hard physical labor, have a richer and more varied diet, ride a horse rather than walk, avoid epidemics by fleeing, afford appropriate medical care when needed, live in a more safe and secure residence, and likely retain and pass along one's privileged status to one's children. For one born into the lower classes, early life might be marked by hard physical labor and hazards, poor living quarters, poor diet, hygiene, and health care options, greater exposure to disease, and few options in charting one's future.

Of course, one was also born male or female. Across cultures and classes, girls tended to be less valued than boys; abandonment and even infanticide were far more likely to have girls as their victims. In general, men had more and more varied options in life, greater access to education, and control of wealth and resources. The family identity usually passed through the males, while women left their birth family and "married into" their husband's family, often taking their husband's family name. Even today we speak of the woman's father "giving away the bride" at a wedding. A woman was above all valued for reproduction, but the children would not be hers or her birth family's but belong to the father and his birth family, sharing his name and social identity.

The Course of One's Life

The early modern girl growing into womanhood faced few choices, whatever her class. Since fathers usually determined the fates of their daughters, with relatively few exceptions, women became wives and mothers at an early age. The European, Chinese, and Islamic cultures kept especially tight reins, as the unattached young woman with neither husband nor guardian was deemed likely to be or become a prostitute. While some became nuns or household servants, the 16th-century Reformation ended the first option in much of Europe and the second always left the woman vulnerable to being fired or molested. Most women married within their birth status group. Outside of war, epidemics, and other environmental disasters, the greatest threat to the health and even lives of women in all cultures was pregnancy and childbirth.

Men tended to have more options in life than women, including some level of mobility, both social and geographic: even poor peasants could become wealthier peasants by hard work and a good marriage. Depending on class, men had many more occupational choices and could reasonably choose to remain rural or move to the nearest big town. The man's accomplishments as a hunter, warrior, apprentice, artist, or student really determined his—and his family's—status in the community. The higher one's status, the greater were his opportunities to avoid the community's hazards or have access to its resources or to move beyond it to improve his position. But there was also the matter of individual choice. We know that even the wealthiest modern Americans can choose to endanger their health by avoiding a good diet, exercise, and medical checkups, while embracing junk foods, drugs, alcohol, or tobacco. The same was true in the early modern community: the larger and less traditional the community, the greater the freedom to go against the societal norms.

For the adult male and his family, good health depended on his wealth and status, occupation, choice of residence, access to healthy foods and clean water, personal habits of eating, drinking, and hygiene, and access to and choices in health care.

The Vagaries of History

Everyone has always been subject to the occasional accident: being hit by lightning, falling from a ladder, setting oneself on fire, or eating poisonous mushrooms. Such things may happen to king or serf, mature adult or child, man or woman. But sometimes the broader forces of history impinge on people and directly affect their health and well-being.

Warriors or soldiers suddenly descend on a small community and disrupt every aspect of life. Women are molested, and protesting husbands and fathers beaten or killed. Food and animals are stolen; crops and residences are destroyed; and local holy men are murdered out of religious hatred. Typhus, dysentery, plague, and venereal disease (sexually transmitted diseases) are left behind as the predators move on.

During the Reformation, Protestant leaders closed down Catholic female monasteries and convents in areas such as England, Holland, and northern Germany where they held sway. Women who had dedicated their lives to divine service were now cut adrift. Some sought and found new places of residence among secure communities of nuns in Catholic areas. Many, however, found husbands and took on the joys and hazards of childbirth and family.

We have several autobiographies of Africans enslaved before 1800, and each recounts the horrors of suddenly shifting from lives of freedom safe within their communities to becoming first captives, then prisoners, and then slaves in a strange and far-off land.

In Peru's highlands, far from any of the dimly rumored white men whose sudden appearance along the coastlines was both exciting and troubling, a village begins to suffer from a divine curse. Red blotches and fever blanket bodies of the very old and very young, killing them very quickly. The healthy and vigorous succumb until few are left to tend the sick. The gods are angry, the shamans confused, and the community terrorized, or simply destroyed. The virus—perhaps measles or smallpox—had been carried into the place not by the strange white men down on the coast but by a friend who had been the latest in a chain of contacts.

A natural disaster? An accident? Yes, but the historic moment that brought the men of Portugal and Spain, in search of knowledge and riches, touched off a perhaps unprecedented demographic catastrophe in which each life was utterly transformed by death or survival. Historical trends and forces determined the health and well-being of millions in the early modern world.

THE EARLY MODERN WORLD

An Age of Empires

The chronological period from roughly 1500 to 1800 was an era of empires. The African Songhai Empire, which had controlled populations from the mouth of the Gambia River to Lake Chad, fell to Muslim troops sent from Ottoman-controlled Morocco in 1589, ending the last of the great empires of the Sahel. The ensuing social disruption and political power vacuum invited the rule of local warlords and even more successful exploitation by Arab and European slavers.

The Aztecs were one of many groups of natives living in what is today Mexico. By the 14th century, they had established themselves as rulers over an empire that spread from coast to coast and from modern Nicaragua to the northern desert. Led by fierce warriors who preferred to capture their enemies and sacrifice them to their gods, they shared the stone-based technology with their neighbors and readily borrowed their arts of civilized living. Their capital of Tenochtitlán was a magnificent city of canals and perhaps 80,000 residents in the highland Valley of Mexico, which the Spaniards compared favorably with Italy's Venice. Aztec doom came early in our period, when the Spanish conquistador Hernán Cortés and fewer than 600 soldiers brought their guns, horses, and deadly diseases to the Aztec world and quickly claimed it for the Spanish Crown. Henceforth, the Aztec Empire was the Spanish colony of New Spain, or colonial Mexico.

China experienced most of its Late Imperial period of the Ming (1368–1644) and Qing ("ching," 1644–1911) dynasties during these three centuries. The emperor, who was said to have the "mandate of Heaven," ruled according to ancient traditions and through a court and a classically educated bureaucracy of civil servants. Their capital was Beijing (Peking), a city purported to have had 672,000 residents in a country of 110 million. The era was one of widespread prosperity and relative peace, with a national population that doubled or perhaps tripled in size. Cities grew as commerce thrived and material wealth increased for rich and poor alike. There was an increase of social mobility, and as Charlotte Furth put it, "of urbanization, the spread of a money economy, of the loosening of status boundaries, [and] of cultural experiment" (Furth 1999, 155).

Yet in many ways, China turned in on itself. As with the classicism of the 16th-century European Renaissance, Chinese intellectuals, including men of medicine, were focused backward on their national traditions (Neo-Confucianism). Printing was revitalized among the Chinese, with more and higher-quality works appearing. Literacy and the distribution of books were far from universal, but both were spreading further than in previous centuries. The revival of traditional Chinese cultural values known as Neo-Confucianism emphasized the wisdom of the ancients as well as benevolence: doing good for the benefit of others and society. This could mean the sponsoring of useful—including medical—books and the provision of medical care for the needy.

Unlike Renaissance Europeans, however, the Chinese had little use for the bits of Western culture that washed up on their shores and made few attempts to reach out from their Middle Kingdom. Some 800 Christian missionaries from Europe entered China between 1552 and 1795, but the religion made little headway. Certain imported goods were more welcome, including peanuts, corn, sweet potatoes, cinchona (quinine), tobacco, and opium.

The Islamic World was dominated by three early modern empires: the Ottoman Turks, the Safavids of Iran, and the Mughals in India. Since each developed the use of firearms and cannon to a high degree, they are often called the "gunpowder states." The Turkish Ottoman Empire had conquered Byzantine Constantinople in 1453, bringing to a formal end the 1,000-year-old Christian empire. They continued their conquests in the Balkans, seizing Hungary and reaching Vienna by the 1680s. During the 1510s, the Turks expanded their hegemony along the Mediterranean from Syria south through Egypt to North Africa. By 1520, the sultans controlled major capitals and trade centers such as Istanbul (former Constantinople), their capital, with perhaps 200,000 people in 1500, Damascus, Cairo, and Alexandria. Their empire straddled three continents. They saw themselves as the heirs of the ancient Roman emperors and great medieval caliphs. As recent conquerors, they had to neuter their enemies and flaunt their own form of Muslim benevolence. The lives of the common folks remained largely untouched, and the vibrant intellectual life of medieval Islam remained a matter of past glory.

From 1501, the Muslim Safavid dynasty ruled an empire that lay between Mughal India and the Ottomans. It included parts or all of modern Iran, Iraq, Azerbaijan, Armenia, Georgia, and Afghanistan. Such a broad empire required a firm center point, and the rulers called themselves shahs and identified with the great ancient Persian empires. To defend their long borders, they needed at least to match their surrounding Ottoman and Mughal rivals. Under Shah Abbas, in the early 17th century, the state reorganized its military. He followed the effective Ottoman model of combining infantry with firearms, cavalry, and artillery. The Safavids' major cities included the venerable caravan trading centers of Isfahan and Herat, and their culture was closer kin to that of the steppe and mountain tribal folk of south-central Asia than to the civilizations of India or the Mediterranean (Liu 2010). Even so, much of their intellectual culture remained influenced by the Greek heritage absorbed by Islam in the 10th and 11th centuries, and this included medicine.

In India, from 1526, the Mongol dynasty of the Muslim Mughals blended their Central Asian steppe traditions with the ancient, sophisticated, and wealthy Hindu urban civilization. They created a culture with magnificent written and visual expressions—the Taj Mahal comes to mind. Since this text does not engage this region, however, we shall leave it here.

Europe from its Renaissance through its Enlightenment hosted the Habsburg Empire, Russian Empire, Portuguese Empire, Spanish Empire, Dutch Seaborne Empire, British Empire, and Napoleon's short-lived French Empire. Each was aggressive both commercially and militarily. The French and the Habsburg rulers of Spain and the Holy Roman Empire fought in Italy for control of the peninsula for six decades (1494–1555), and Louis XIV battled endlessly for domination of bits and pieces along his frontier. They developed firearms, artillery, and the techniques of using them effectively, which gave them the advantage against all adversaries but each other. In Europe, the period opened with the Spanish destroying the last Iberian Muslim state, Granada, in 1492 and subsequently sponsoring Columbus's fateful voyage. In 1494, the French army of King Charles VIII bullied its way through Italy to retake (unsuccessfully) Naples from the Spaniards. The era ended with Napoleon's opening bid for domination of the entire continent. The real gains were to be grabbed at the rest of the world's expense, however, and every empire except the Austrian Habsburgs seized a share of Asia, Oceania, Africa, or the Americas for its own. The globe shrank as European sailing ships mastered the oceans and Europeans made claims on much of the world.

From 1492, Europeans conquered and colonized most of the Western Hemisphere. Huge swathes were depopulated by disease, and entire cultures disappeared. The enormous and well-organized empires of the Aztec and Inca in Latin America crumbled before tiny Spanish armies and waves of disease. As a terrible balancing, the kingdoms along the West African coast sold some 12 million of their subjects and neighbors into European colonial transatlantic slavery. European ships also brought the riches of Southern and East Asia and Oceania to their homelands and other colonies. In exchange, they brought Christianity and Western technology, including effective firearms, navigational aids, and some aspects of Western medicine. From a world historical perspective, the era from Columbus to the French Revolution is usually considered the early modern period, the threshold to our own.

Europe's Brave New World

Contact with the world by sailing ship initiated and sustained exchanges of plants, animals, people, technologies, and ideas. Some of these were commercially traded, some stolen, some imposed by force, and some exchanged purely by accident, as with infectious diseases. African kings traded people for European weapons of war, and European tables featured exotic chocolate from Mexico, coffee from South America, tea from China, and sugar from the Caribbean, while North American tobacco was smoked to get high and avoid plague (see Osterhammel and Petersson 2005). Rapidly expanding European populations demanded more and cheaper goods, and the combination of trade in cotton and early industrial organization shifted colonial demands from luxuries to the simple pleasures of soft and easily laundered clothing.

Over the three early modern centuries, the population of Europe roughly doubled, despite the continuing cycles of bubonic plague. Due to both natural population growth and immigration, Europe's cities, especially its capitals, expanded by several times. In the absence of census data, there are many estimates: London went from perhaps 70,000 in 1500 to nearly a million in 1800, Paris from 200,000 to 550,000, and Rome from 50,000 to 150,000. Despite demands for labor, poverty increased in the resident and transient subcultures of Europe's cities. Meanwhile, educational opportunities were expanding and making literacy more common, a trend greatly aided by the invention of the printing press in the 1450s and by Protestantism's emphasis on reading the Bible. For various reasons—including war, religion, public health needs, and perhaps dreams of the old Roman Empire—Europe's political leaders, from local guild leaders to the pope and emperor, were seeking actively to increase their power and authority at the expense of traditional competitors, such as the Church and nobility. Politically, it was the age of absolutism.

Intellectually, Europe in 1500 was in the midst of its Renaissance love affair with Greek and Roman antiquity. This reinforced the ancient, largely incorrect yet revered traditions of Hippocrates, Aristotle, and Galen and their theories of health and medicine. The coincidence of global discovery and the religious, social, and political revolution known as the Reformation, however, challenged old certainties. The Catholic Church, Aristotle's geocentric universe, and Galenic medicine all came under attack, but they each proved quite resilient. By 1600, several differing denominations had revised Catholic teaching in many places, and the cultural trend was toward replacing religious opinion with natural or scientific truth. Personal experience, experimentation, and observation (empiricism) gained authority as men such as Galileo, Francis Bacon, and René Descartes outlined the proper techniques for gaining truth from empiricism (scientific method). By 1700, this new and cumulative study of nature (Scientific Revolution), including the human body, was in full swing. The backward-looking focus of the Renaissance had all but died out in favor of the intentional creation of a new, secular, and humane world based on knowledge and freed from superstition, ignorance, and human want. The ongoing advances in knowledge and technology seemed to promise enlightenment and freedom where darkness had once shrouded humanity. During the French Revolution, the people of Paris turned Notre Dame cathedral into the Temple of Reason. Could there be a better symbol of the Enlightenment's aspirations?

SOCIETAL FACTORS IN HEALTH AND MEDICINE

An individual's genes, childhood, and adult status and choices all operated within a cultural framework of possibilities and options created by nature and history. Five aspects of early modern societies that were important to the nature of health and the provision of health care included cities and urbanization (city growth), standards of living, sanitation and hygiene, patterns of endemic and epidemic disease, and state provisions for medical education and health care.

Cities and Urbanization

Throughout the early modern world, cities of varying antiquity were growing in size and importance. By 1800, about 3 percent of the world's population lived in cities, but because of their wealth and concentration of functions, they dominated the world around them. They provided political centers, goods and services, employment, religious ritual, protection, education, and social mobility. But as they grew, cities became more densely populated, dirtier, harder to feed, more poverty stricken, and disease ridden. In Europe, with plague slowly disappearing, newly common diseases included smallpox, tuberculosis, syphilis, and influenza, and imported cholera waited in the wings. Communicable diseases require certain densities of people to sustain themselves. Without a high concentration of potential victims, the germs eventually disappear as they kill their hosts, die away, or simply fail to find healthy new hosts. Cities provided these densities.

Early modern cities were also centers of animal life, and many illnesses came directly from animals. We know of swine and bird flu, of tick-borne spotted fever, of rabies, and of poisonous spiders and snakes. In 1700, wool workers contracted anthrax from sheep's wool; milkmaids, cowpox from cows; cowherds, ringworm from their cattle; caravan drivers, scabies from camels; and wranglers, glanders from horses (Mantovani et al. 1999). Like influenza, bubonic plague is a disease of animals (zoonosis) that "jumped" to humans when nearby rats died off and the fleas that carried the germs changed their diets to human blood.

Ship traffic brought many diseases into port cities and disseminated them from infected cities. A host of different pathogens and parasites could live in a ship's water supply, and in or on its rats, passengers, slaves, cargo, or crew. Once among a new population that neither understood nor was immune from the dangers, the pathogens and their carriers could thrive.

Standards of Living

In any city, the poor occupied more ramshackle quarters that could freeze during winter and swelter during summers (see, for example, Allen, Bengtsson, and Dribe 2005). Human, animal, and food waste in large amounts attracted insects and scavengers and their diseases. Water and food supplies could be tainted or poisoned in the absence of sanitary water supplies and reliable food storage (see Matossian 1989). The poorest poor might well lack permanent housing and be reduced to a single garment, which would naturally be filthy and perhaps ridden with fleas. These were a particular problem in the cooler, northern climes. Even the presence of good food did not mean that the poor could partake of it, and poor nutrition weakened immune systems and invited opportunistic diseases. Poverty also meant that one lived with a greater physical threat from one's desperate peers, from fire and accident, and from many infectious diseases—all with little or no access to reasonable health care or necessary medicines. In such situations, children and the elderly were at the greatest risk. During epidemics, some cultures, including European, provided aid to the poor, hiring public physicians or surgeons. But these were as much a means of social control as an act of humanity.

By definition, the higher classes had access to the better and best residences, nutrition, material goods, and services, including medical care. Servants could maintain a certain level of cleanliness, and in some societies, possession of rural properties could mean escape from the city's endemic or epidemic environmental hardships.

Nutrition

Healthy foods in the Christian and Islamic worlds meant those that were appropriately "hot," "cold," "moist," or "dry" according to Galen's teaching from the second century, or "hot" or "cold" according to ancient Chinese lights. Qualities or contents such as protein, fat, fiber, vitamins, carbohydrates, or calories had no meaning. Diet was largely a matter of opportunity and culture, and the vast majority of most people's diets came from carbohydrate-rich grains and tubers. Yet even staples could lead to serious deficiencies: corn (maize) could cause pellagra and a niacin deficit that could cause symptoms from diarrhea to dementia and death; too much unbalanced and unhusked rice could lead to beriberi, a vitamin B1 deficiency; and many bread grains could harbor ergot, a fungus that caused a very uncomfortable condition known as Saint Anthony's Fire. Too little vitamin C led to scurvy, a lack of vitamin A to night blindness, and a lack of iodine to goiter (Porter 2006, 39–41).

In Africa, cultural norms forbade the consumption of eggs, and tsetse flies kept many societies from herding cattle and using cows' milk. The starchy diets of taro, bananas, yams, rice, and millet were slim on vitamins and protein, resulting in chronic malnourishment even in years of plenty. Under Caribbean slavery, the Africans' diets improved but little, with the addition of small amounts of meat and fish and some local vegetables grown in private gardens. On sugar plantations, some surplus brown sugar and molasses came their way at harvest time.

But the ships that carried the gold and slaves also carried plants and seeds. Above all, plants from the Americas made their way to Europe, Africa, and China. Maize, squashes, sweet potatoes, multiple types of beans, tomatoes, and of course the potato enhanced diets around the world. This helped stabilize populations in Eastern Europe and allowed a population explosion in Ireland. Frederick the Great of Prussia had his troops force peasants to plant them when a famine struck. About the same time, France's Louis XVI tantalized his guests by hiding potato plants in a secret garden and by serving potato dishes fit for a king (Laws 2004, 7–9).

Hygiene and Sanitation

By all accounts, the Aztecs and Chinese were clean societies that valued personal hygiene and environmental sanitation. By contrast, early modern Europeans were comfortable amid filth even in the greatest of palaces. Changing one's soiled clothes and laundering them, bathing, and maintaining oral hygiene came slowly to Europeans. Poorer folk had few garments, and keeping them clean was not really an option, especially during the winter. Bathing was known, and bathhouses could be found in many parts of later medieval Europe, but the miasma theory of disease that was popularized with plague claimed that open pores allowed poisonous air into the body. By 1500, bathing was all but taboo, only to be revived with the withdrawal of plague by the 18th century. Of course a society that tolerated poor personal hygiene courted a host of personal problems from skin and eye diseases to infections and deadly parasites.

The accumulation or regular disposal of human waste materials, including food scraps, will either draw or keep at bay many types of disease-carrying pests. Toilets were only coming into fashion in Europe as our era closed, and were unknown elsewhere. In China, waste collectors made regular nightly rounds and used the material to fertilize a city's nearby fields. This presented its own health problems, but it effectively removed the objectionable stuff from the population centers. Some European cities attempted something like this with "night soil men," but it was easier to dump waste into the gutters and urban streams that flowed into larger rivers that flushed it to the unfortunates downstream. Water supplies in many urban areas were filthy and no less so in downstream rural areas. One reason for the fads of boiled coffee and tea and the mixing of rum with water was that it seemed to make the fluid safe to drink.

Patterns of Epidemic and Endemic Disease

This chapter could feature long lists of diseases that were "always there" (endemic) in a particular locale, as the common cold is for us, and a somewhat shorter list of epidemic diseases that struck for short periods and killed large numbers of people. Endemic germs tended to make people sick but quickly recover, which allowed both the pathogen and the host to survive and thrive. Endemic diseases often became embedded in a region because the local population developed forms of resistance or immunity over long periods of time or as a result of natural exposure. Africans developed a form of iron-poor blood cells known as sickle cell, which made them naturally resistant to the most common form of African malaria. Childhood measles in Europe was fairly benign and conferred natural immunity, so after maturing, people were safe from the more deadly adult version. When nonimmune adults came into a measles outbreak, or when measles carriers took the disease to a nonimmunized population, such as the Indians of South America, the result could be (and was) catastrophic.

Local environments also provided various insect vectors of disease such as fleas, flies, ticks, and mosquitoes; venomous animals such as scorpions, certain toads, black widow spiders, and black mamba snakes; large predatory animals such as tigers, bears, wolves, and people; internal parasites such as hookworms and Guinea worms; and soil-induced infectious agents such as tetanus and yaws-causing spirochetes. Control of the larger animals had been part of civilized life for centuries in most places, and poisonous snakes and reptiles were well known and avoided by locals. To neutralize most other challenges required the revolution in modern medicine and public health that took place after 1800. Even now, we often have to react with antibiotics or antivenoms. Today, we can look back and understand how diseases operated among early modern populations, but at the time, nowhere on Earth did anyone make the connections we can in retrospect. People lived with their disease regimes, blaming cases on spirits or witches, or on God's displeasure, or on some natural but unknown causes. Insofar as early modern people reacted effectively to their threats, some progress could result. Quarantines helped stifle plague revisitations; draining swamps curbed malaria; and Africans' willingness to relocate away from still waters and avoid cattle reduced their exposure to tsetse flies. Even when they did not understand how or why such measures worked, they trusted their experience.

State and Educational Provisions for Health Care

In China, the benevolent emperors supported the Medical Bureau and the publication of classics in traditional medicine. They expanded the medical content of civil service exams, ensuring that failed applicants would be well prepared to practice traditional medicine in their communities. They funded the public apothecaries that mixed drugs to exacting specifications and distributed them to those who needed them, and in the 18th century they provided public granaries to feed the hungry during droughts or famines.

In the Ottoman Empire, the sultans established hospital-like *bimaristans* in their newly won empire. Their patronage stemmed from a sense of social duty but equally from their Muslim desire to please God through good works and from their status as new conquerors to show their goodwill to the conquered. Older *bimaristans* continued to operate, and market officials continued to monitor the quality of food and drugs. While some medical innovation occurred at court, however, it tended not to flow outward into the broader society, as it did in China. In one area, some limited progress was achieved, as some efforts were made to improve public sanitation and to limit plague's spread by grudging attempts at quarantine.

Because Europe remained divided into multiple independent states, it is difficult to generalize about governmental efforts, but a few points are in order. First, governments sought greater control over their people, and this meant the gathering of information (it was the birth of attempts at accurate censuses, bills of mortality, and the science of statistics). These tools were used for military drafting, taxing, monitoring of epidemics, and the very limited provision of aid to the needy. Second, governments increasingly valued their people's good health in the face of plague and other epidemics. They valued them as taxpayers, child-bearers, workers, and soldiers. Healing trained soldiers to fight again, keeping mothers safe to have more children and increase the state's population, and preventing the wholesale slaughter of urban populations by disease led to state actions such as building military hospitals, licensing midwives, and imposing isolation and quarantine when epidemics struck. Third, states created few educational institutions but supported the idea that medical practitioners needed to be educated as well as licensed. Partially, this was at the prompting of the professionally educated or trained and organized physicians, apothecaries, and surgeons, who sought to protect their high status by maintaining a monopoly. This was a trend that continued throughout the early modern period.

Fourth, formally recognized European practitioners continued to be divided into university-educated physicians and apprenticed and trained surgeons and apothecaries. The early modern trend, however, was toward professionalization. Physicians were to undergo practical medical training in such areas as medicinal botany, anatomy, and physiology and through clinical training in hospital wards with real patients. On the other hand, schools were opening up to provide educational opportunities to apothecaries, surgeons, and even midwives, to increase their knowledge and effectiveness. Fifth, this formalized education was increasingly informed by the advances in the sciences of the Scientific Revolution and Enlightenment. By the 18th century, "empirical medicine" was not what the uneducated did but was the standard informed by the scientific method: hypothesize, test, observe, record, repeat, and share. (An "empiric" was one who practiced medicine with neither formal training or education, nor a license.) Yet many discoveries bore no fruit among the sick or injured, and some inventions, such as the microscope, were underused in advancing practical medicine.

Sixth, European medicine was gathering under its wing a number of human conditions that had previously not been considered "medical." This has happened in our day. When this author was a student, homosexuality was formally considered a mental illness and alcoholism was not. Today, the definitions have been reversed. Likewise, there was an important shift in defining some conditions. For example, lunatics went from being possessed by demons to being mentally ill, which radically changed the way they were treated. Similarly, giving birth came to be recognized as a medical procedure rather than just an act of nature. One can say that both labor and madness were medicalized by the culture and that the scope of medicine was thereby expanded.

Finally, no medical culture, however sophisticated, possessed an understanding of the foundations of most modern medicine. The discovery of fundamental physiological processes and, most importantly, of germs and their role in human health and medicine had to await the 19th century.

2

Education and Training

Though most sick and injured people have always been treated at home by experienced family members or neighbors, by 1500, societies had developed healing theories and practices that were controlled, utilized, and passed on by specially educated or trained specialists. Many cultures had a range of types of healers, including spiritual practitioners (diviners, priests, monks, magicians, witch doctors, shamans), internists (herbalists, physicians, apothecaries, empirics, folk healers, wise women), and those who manipulated the body from the outside (surgeons, barber-surgeons, dentists, midwives, bonesetters, acupuncturists, leeches). Literate societies such as the Europeans, Muslims, Indians, and Chinese usually drew a distinction between practitioners who were formally trained in theory and practice through written texts and, sometimes, schools, and those whose knowledge derived from oral traditions, experience, or apprenticeships. Nonliterate societies tended to be more accepting of varying approaches to healing, since in the end, it was success that really mattered.

WESTERN TRADITIONS

The Western medical cultures of Europe and much of the Islamic world had long been dependent on the Greek and Greco-Roman traditions of Hippocrates and Galen. Lacking codified medical traditions of their own, medieval Muslims and Christians adopted the classics wholesale.

Arab and Persian scholars and commentators had their heyday between the 9th and 11th centuries. Latin Christian medical thinkers absorbed much through translations of Islamic texts as well as bits of the originals two and three centuries later. Muslim medical students trained through reading of texts and practice gained in the *bimaristans*—which served as both hospitals and teaching facilities—that graced most large cities. European students gained formal knowledge of the Greek tradition through medical faculties associated with universities. Salerno, on the cusp of the Muslim, Byzantine Greek, and Latin worlds in southern Italy, hosted the first Christian medical school, and by 1500, dozens dotted Europe's landscape. (An excellent introduction is Lindemann 2010.)

European Medical Education

The early modern medical curriculum, whether European or Muslim, featured the ancient ideas of Galen (see Nutton 2008) and Hippocrates. Despite developments in medical education between 1500 and 1800, the core of Western medical theory remained the body's four humors and the attempt to maintain their balance. Each person's body contained four humors, usually visualized as fluids: blood, phlegm, yellow bile, and black bile. Each of these corresponded to or was associated with a vast range of phenomena from planets to personality types and bodily organs. In addition, there were four qualities—hot, cold, wet, dry—that were also associated with the humors and organs, as well as all foods and beverages, herbs and drugs, and one's age, sex, diet, level and type of exercise, and other physical attributes or conditions. A person's "complexion" was a mixture of the balancing of humors and the appropriate balancing of qualities. This was a factor of diet, activity, passion, and other generally controllable variables. Under normal circumstances, the trained physician understood how to use foods, drink, medicines, exercise, and procedures such as drawing blood to maintain or restore good health, all of which were articulated by Hippocrates and Galen.

The 16th century saw the spread of printing (from 1454) and the humanist interest in original classical texts. New, printed editions of Hippocrates and Galen replaced older, Muslim-influenced commentaries and editions, and reinforced the Greeks' influence among scholars and doctors alike. Command of ancient theory in Greek and Latin lay at the root of distinction between the formally educated physician and the other "illiterate" practitioners. While surgeons and apothecaries may have understood humoral theory in order to follow physicians' orders, they had been trained as apprentices and belonged to craft guilds that ranked with carpenters and painters. Like theologians and lawyers, university-trained physicians did not work with their hands, unless to study a flask of urine or feel a pulse. They were strictly internists who prescribed the diet, exercise, and medicines that their theory dictated. Their guilds tended to rank with those of judges, international merchants, and bankers, and their fees reflected their acquired status. Most commoners could never afford a physician's service, which is why many towns hired physicians to serve as salaried civic doctors, with the stipulation that they serve all comers.

In 1500, medical schools relied almost exclusively on classical medical texts and those derived from them. Education was largely theoretical, with experience being acquired after graduation, often as civic physicians. Anatomy as a formal subject of study was in its infancy, with educational dissections being few and far between. Since surgeons literally handled the human body, there seemed little need for it. Most physicians knew few of the qualities of healing herbs (simples) or their compounds beyond their being "hot" or "wet."

The cultural phenomena we label the Renaissance, Scientific Revolution, and Enlightenment had some effect on medical education. By 1600, the earliest anatomy and dissection theaters had been built for student physicians, and the Netherlander Andreas Vesalius had pioneered both dissection and demonstration of the corpse by the physician and the use of high-quality anatomical illustrations. Botanical gardens were established around medical schools for teaching purposes, especially important as European discovery and colonization revealed new plants with clear medicinal value. Perhaps most important was the innovation of students accompanying the professor on his hospital rounds, widely adopted only in the 18th century. This integration of the hospital with the classroom would prove to be a major step in Western medical education.

The differences between the model medical curricula in 1500 and 1800 demonstrate some of the changes the era implemented. At a typical Italian medical school in 1500, after spending several years studying the liberal arts and philosophy, the medical student spent four or five years studying Latin translations of Arabic and Greek texts including Hippocrates and Galen. Astrology was considered a necessary medical subject (mandatory in Bologna from 1405) but anatomy was not. By 1800, the model of medical education had shifted northward. German medical schools did not share a common curriculum, but the dozen or so students enrolled in a typical program spent three years studying anatomy and physiology, chemistry, and botany in year one; pathology (diseases) and *materia medica* (medicinal plants and drugs) in year two; and therapy, clinical practice, prescription writing, and in some, obstetrics, surgery, and forensic (legal) pathology. Lectures dominated years one and two, and experiential learning, the third. Similar trends reached through the Netherlands (especially Leiden) to Edinburgh, Scotland, whose highly influential medical school was founded in 1726. Its standard three-year curriculum consisted of anatomy, chemistry, surgery, botany, *materia medica*, midwifery (obstetrics), medical "theory and practice," and clinical medicine. Everything except the largely Galenic "theory" portion was new to our period, having been pioneered and established during the intervening years. The biggest differences may have been the recent inclusion of surgery and midwifery, which had been the monopoly of guild surgeons and midwives, and botany and *materia medica*, which had long been the purview of non-university-trained apothecaries. By the later 18th century, much broader expertise was expected of the university-trained physician. This was significant insofar as Edinburgh directly influenced English medical education and early American medical schools in Philadelphia and New York. Edinburgh's success may also be gauged by the fact that it graduated 219 students from the West Indies alone between 1744 and 1830 (see Broman 1996 and Sheridan 1985).

Challenges to the Galenic model of humoralism were not unknown, though they had little effect on early modern formal education in the short run. The most important was that presented by the 16th-century German physician and alchemist known as Paracelsus. Among the first generation of Protestants, he associated the established medicine with paganism and Catholicism and sought to "reform" medicine as Martin Luther had done Christianity. He and his followers shifted emphasis away from the four humors and organic treatments to inorganic chemicals that he believed dictated health and illness. Though his conclusions were as misguided and false as those of mainstream medicine, his challenge developed into iatrochemistry ("iatro-" meaning "medical"). Many wealthy clients and patrons supported Paracelsians, and their research helped open up important windows into human physiology even if their treatments and remedies proved futile. The fact that chemistry appeared on Edinburgh's curriculum is a testament to his long-range impact.

Medical Preparation in the Ottoman and Safavid Empires

The Islamic world dominated by the Ottoman Turks blended many cultures. As in Europe and elsewhere, many types of healers circulated, with roots in Arabic, Persian, Turkic, North African, and Islamic religious traditions. Homeschooling, tutors, apprenticeships, self-study, and courses taught at *bimaristans* or mosques all provided levels of practical medical knowledge for a wide range of practitioners, both male and female. Only at Istanbul's Süleymaniye complex was there a recognized school of medicine, and little about its operation has been uncovered. Formal medical education of males in Islamic countries seems to have been associated primarily with the *bimaristan*, a health and religious facility provided with royal or noble patronage. Galenic theory and hands-on training appear to have characterized education in these institutions in the same way that the education of religious scholars took place in mosques. Most learning still appears to have been based upon self-study rather than formal instruction, and some *bimaristans* included extensive medical libraries. A position on the staff of these facilities placed one at the top of the medical ladder and reflected years of practical experience in junior positions (Shefer-Mossensohn 2009, 141–143).

Such a system hardly encouraged experimentation or innovation, and little occurred across our period. People learning to become medical practitioners of whatever type accepted the classical texts and formal or informal practical experiences offered as they came. In the Islamic world, the closest thing to professors of medicine were more bureaucrats than healers, especially under the Ottomans. The once rich Muslim intellectual and scientific tradition that had produced the great medical authors and texts studied by Muslims, Christians, and Jews alike had largely dried up. In medicine, this accompanied the rise of what was called Medicine of the Prophet (Muhammad). Alongside the empirical and Galenic approaches to medicine was this body of teachings attributed to Muhammad and interpreted by religious rather than secular medical specialists. To criticize or compete with this system of explanation and practice when invoked was considered an offense against Islam. The relative dynamism of the post-Reformation West drew Ottoman Christian students in small numbers, and the little change that occurred between 1500 and 1800 was generally attributable to borrowings from Europe.

Medical preparation in the area dominated by Safavid Persia was even less innovative and organized. Their rulers expended very little in support of the *bimaristans* and their educational roles, and no more in overseeing how practitioners were trained or functioned. As in the Turkish Empire, dissections, and therefore detailed and accurate anatomy and physiology, were all but unknown. Medicine amounted to the application of Galenic principles and folk healing. While this could and did often prove effective in daily life, it nonetheless demonstrates the intellectual stagnation under Safavid rule. Since they were geographically detached from Europe, the practical advances absorbed by the Turks, for example in public health, were lost on the Persians. What seems to have had an impact arrived via missionaries and some merchants, especially from England after 1600 (Elgood 1970, 1–12, 121–128).

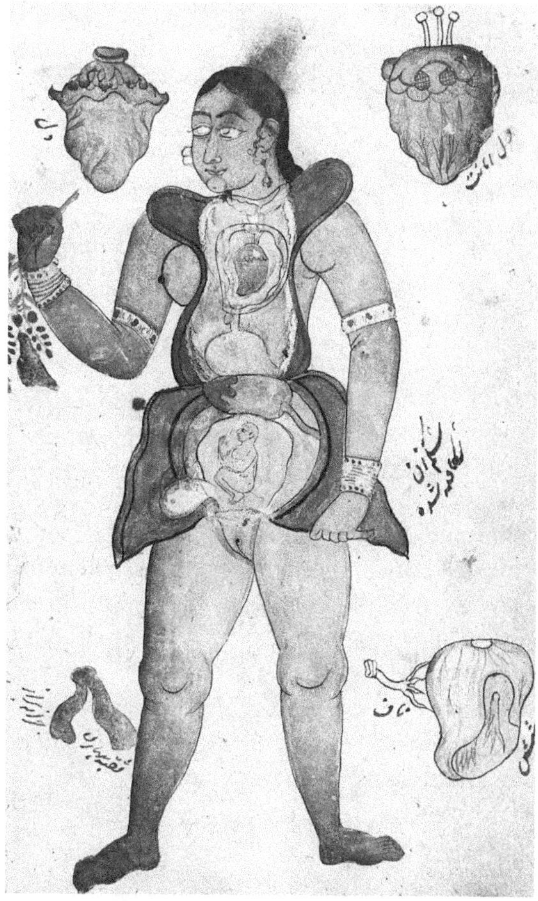

An 18th-century copy of a Safavid Persian anatomical illustration of a pregnant woman. The original was in *Tibb al-Akbar* (*Akbar's Medicine*) completed in 1701 by Muhammad Akbar. It is a Persian translation of the 13th-century Arabic *Causes and Symptoms* by Najib al-Din al-Samarqandi. Note the rather crude level of detail and depiction of anatomy, which reflects the Safavid culture's relative disinterest in the subject. (National Library of Medicine)

Patients, Suffering, and Care in the West

Insofar as the Islamic tradition centered physician education at the *bimaristan*, it deemphasized the wall between theory and actual patient care. European medical students were only beginning to benefit from this hands-on teaching method—working with real patients—in the 18th century. To those preparing to practice, patients remained largely abstract entities little understood physiologically or psychologically. Aside from drawing patients' attention to such health factors as diet, exercise, and air quality or providing some useful pills or syrups to induce vomiting or stanch diarrhea, Western physicians had little that was effective to offer the suffering. Internal medicine, whether humoral or iatrochemical, was founded on misunderstandings of the human body and its functioning. Until the 17th century, experimentation was limited, though experienced physicians often noted which remedies or techniques worked and which did not. Although many important biological discoveries emerged from the Scientific Revolution, including the fact that the blood circulates through the vessels, being pumped by the muscular heart, they had little impact on medical education or practice. Though the microscope was in use for nearly two centuries, and scientists speculated about "animalcules" or other microscopic disease-causing agents, germs were identified, and germ theory became fruitful only midway through the 1800s. The learned explanation of epidemics such as bubonic plague—poisonous air (miasma)—did not change between Galen's time and the building of the first automobile despite centuries of direct experience with the disease. Some treatments, such as mercury for syphilis and bleeding for just about everything, were at least as bad as the ailment.

Some strides were made, however, though rarely by the medical world's heavy hitters. A diplomat's wife introduced inoculation for smallpox (with the virus) from Istanbul to Europe early in the 18th century, and country doctor Edward Jenner showed success with vaccinations of cowpox material at century's end (see Carrell 2003 and Jenner 1996). The vitamin-deficiency disease known as scurvy, which slaughtered long-distance sailors, was conquered in 1795 by introducing lime juice into shipboard diets, but only after nearly 50 years of recommendations by British naval surgeon James Lind (see Harvie 2002).

For the most part, however, early modern medical theory and education had little effect on people's general health and comfort. Physicians retained their high status, though prayer remained a powerful prophylactic and remedy among Christians and Muslims alike well into the modern era. Inexpensive and popular vernacular books of medical recipes and remedies circulated in Europe from the beginning of the 17th century, enabling common folk to have confidence in treating themselves and their own. Some of these were written by well-known practitioners, such as Nicholas Culpeper, who mischievously shared the profession's London pharmacopoeia, or official catalogue of medicinal plants and drugs, with the public at large (see Wooley 2004). Others came from literate women who sought to help others who needed it but could not afford a physician.

EARLY MODERN MEXICANS

In 1500, the Aztec people and state dominated the Central American region today known as Mexico. Theirs was a cumulative culture that benefited from earlier Olmec, Toltec, and other societies, and raised their own to a very high level. They had a well-ordered political organization ruled over by a king and clear traditions, held together by a fierce army of warriors. In 1519, Spanish conquistadors entered Mexico and began the disintegration of the Aztec state and the imposition of colonial government and the Christian religion that would characterize Mexico well past 1800. Aztec medical theory and practice was the norm until missionaries and royal bureaucrats introduced European medicine from the 1520s. While native medicine remained active in many places, where the Spanish held sway, their medical personnel, institutions, and practices dominated, though they were not averse to adopting elements of Aztec practice, especially the use of medicinal plants. (For further information on the Mexican tradition, see Alchon 2003; Cook 1998; Fields 2008; McCaa 1995; Kidwell 1997; and Ortiz de Montellano 1990.)

Aztec Theory and Practice

For the Aztec, the world was alive, and all things had impacts on all other things. Human life, including health and illness, was governed in part by the stars and sky deities, and those of the earth and its interior. In all things, there was a duality at work, which was best when balanced: hot/cold, male/female, up/down, order/chaos, creation/destruction. The gods were dualistic, in that they were both creators and destroyers, givers of health and of sickness and death. Health was the proper balance of the various dualities and forces of the body (*tonocayo*), and illness was imbalance. Aztecs imagined three bodily forces: *yolia*, located in the heart, was responsible for vitality, knowledge, and personality, and that spiritual force that survives death; *ihiyotl*, centered in the liver, was the power of respiration that could be polluted by immoral personal actions whose emanations needed to be cleansed with baths or sweat baths; and *tonalli*, located in the head, provided the body's correct (or incorrect) temperature, tending to wander away from the body during irrational states such as sex, sleep, extreme fear, drunkenness, or a haircut.

As in most societies, typical illnesses and accidents were treated by the sufferer or in the home, usually by women, along practical lines learned from experience. Diet, physical activities, accidents, and natural poisons were at the root of many maladies, but so were gods, spirits, witchcraft, and complex natural forces. When one's condition was serious, the *tíctl*, or healer, was called in. These apprentice-trained men and women were part priest and part doctor, recognizing the unity of the spiritual and physical worlds. They diagnosed conditions, at least in part by the body's temperature—indicating the condition of *tonalli*—and recommended courses of action. Diagnosis might also include divination and hallucinogen-induced trances to determine spiritual causes. They combined the skills of herbalists, surgeons, diviners, and magicians.

The few Spanish-mediated texts—original native works in the Nahuatl language were destroyed by the conquerors—discussing medicine also mention specialists. Further training in the Aztec temples in astrology and other arts enhanced one's supernatural abilities and reputations, earning him the title of priest-healer, *tepoxtlatl*. Other practitioners that served ailing Aztecs included their equivalents of surgeons, women midwives, bonesetters, specialists on the eyes and teeth, and blood letters (the last to be expected given the important place of human sacrifice in Aztec religion). Therapies ranged from such psychosomatic practices as appearing to pull an ailment-inducing object from the sufferer's body (by *techichinani* specialists), offering prayers and sacrifices to malicious gods such as Tlaloc (the gods who induce suffering can relieve it), bleeding to balance the body's temperature, and providing medicinal plants and their blends to be taken internally or used externally.

Colonial Mexican Medicine

European medicine and practitioners entered Mexico with the conquistadors, missionaries, and royal bureaucrats that oversaw Spanish colonization. The first physician to arrive was Diego Pedraza in 1525, the same year that Spanish Mexico City appointed Mexico's first civic barber-surgeon. Smallpox and other infectious diseases ravaged the native population, inflicting a crushing demographic and psychic blow. Spanish sources report a native willingness to adopt the newcomers' medicine, perhaps because they associated the murderous diseases with it (who hurts can also heal) or because they noted the failure of their own. In 1570, a Mexican press published the first medical book in the hemisphere, and by 1578, Spaniards had established the New World's first medical school in Mexico City.

Of course, transplanted Spanish medicine followed the Galenic model, and education in the New World paralleled that of the Old. There was a twist, however, in that Spain's kings Charles I and Philip II insisted that colonists seek out anything medically useful from the new conquests. This especially applied to plants used by the natives: one of the earliest colonial medical books included 60 native remedies. This openness ended in the 1570s, perhaps with the university's founding.

Placating the rain gods with human sacrifices necessarily came to an end, as did the native practice of male circumcision with amazingly sharp obsidian knives. The latter was associated by the Spanish Catholics with Judaism and fell afoul of the religious authorities. Bathing, which the Aztecs embraced, was denounced by orthodox Galenism as a means of opening pores and letting "corrupted" air into the body. Other "superstitious" practices such as divination were likewise rooted out. The Spanish licensed physicians through the *protomedicato*, the Mexican medical office. As important as qualifying skills was religious "purity of blood," which kept formal preparation and practice out of the hands of Jews, Muslims, blacks, or non-Christian natives.

The limited number of physicians opened the door to the *curandero*, an unlicensed practitioner who tended to blend native and European medicine with strains of African medical culture. Following the Aztec model, the *curandero* was often from a family of medical folk or apprenticed with a recognized healer. Most avoided any overt religious rituals or overtones to their practice, though Spanish authorities often found them objectionable. The early modern Church, colonial authorities, and patrons continued to impose European medicine on Mexico through the provision of hospitals, infirmaries, and other elements of the Western system, marginalizing but never eliminating the native healing traditions.

AFRICAN SLAVES IN THE CARIBBEAN

After imported infectious diseases savaged Native American populations during the early 1500s, Spanish and Portuguese slave traders began the transportation of millions of West Africans to the Caribbean islands and the Atlantic coasts of North and South America. They were expected to accept their new status and perform whatever labor was needed for the dominant agricultural or mining concerns among which their owners placed them. Over time, generations of enslaved blacks populated the Caribbean islands, but until the slave trade was finally abolished, fresh infusions of native Africans continually renewed the island populations. As in Mexico, Europeans in the Caribbean controlled productive land and its exploitation, having brought with them culture, technologies, and medicine. In a very uneven way across the West Indies—colonized by Spaniards, French, Dutch, and English planters and their African slaves—European and African medical traditions and practices either clashed or blended as slaves struggled to maintain their health in an unforgiving climate, performing physically draining tasks in the midst of indigenous and imported diseases and the psychic drain of their dehumanizing condition (Sheridan 1985; Voeks 1993).

African Traditions

Like the Aztecs, West Africans viewed the visible and invisible forces of nature, natural and divine, as simple aspects of the same unified world. An ultimate divinity oversaw all, but less powerful spiritual entities influenced or controlled the natural world inhabited by people. The spirits of dead ancestors also had powers to influence the natural order, perhaps using reward and punishment to enforce moral codes of the tribal societies. When a person fell ill, the first level of explanation was basic cause and effect: he fell from a tree and the fall broke his leg. When such a relationship was unclear, or the curious sought to know why he fell from the tree, spirits and ancestors filled in the blanks. Diseases and other painful conditions were readily attributed to spirits, and there was a fine line between the physical practitioner and the spiritual one. It seems that typically the physician was both priest and magician. Understanding the spiritual causes behind suffering, or divination, was the highest skill or gift, because the proper explanation led to proper remedies and success. Spirit possession—allowing a divinity or ancestor's spirit to enter one's consciousness—was one especially dramatic technique of divinatory diagnosis.

Medicine in early modern West Africa, then, was as much about pleasing angry ancestors or bribing mischievous gods as it was about setting a broken leg or curing stomach cramps. It was about ritual as much as herb lore, charms and amulets as much as cutting out bladder stones. Healing spirits needed to be invoked and the malevolent ones appeased. Human health was essentially part of a continuum of natural success, from earth's fertility to a child's birth, and the same societal specialists sought to understand the divine patterns. Of course, diviners could use their knowledge of the spiritual to harm as well as help, to expose people to malevolent powers as well as to protect them. Less potentially dangerous folks handled the less alarming medical emergencies, from childbirth to abscessed teeth and battle wounds. Some in each community had command of local plant lore, providing internal means of resolving many health issues.

Slave Medicine in the Caribbean

There was a wide range of white planter attitudes and behaviors toward black slaves and their health. Down to the 18th century, it was not unusual to work labor to death, literally, investing as little as possible in medical personnel, service, facilities, and supplies. Some owners relied on their own family members to tend sick or disabled slaves. Pressures from enlightened intellectuals and abolitionists had an impact on French and British plantations in particular, however, especially as the threat against the slave trade made the prospects of simply "buying more" less and less likely. Most planters had access to white physicians and surgeons who varied widely in training, experience, and competence. Humane planters

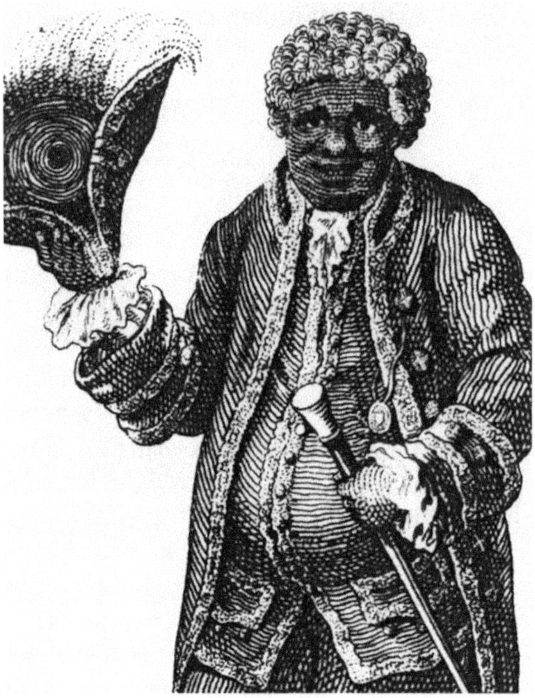

Illustration from 1796 depicting Graman Quacy, who was enslaved as a child in the area of present-day Ghana. Quacy became a freed man in Dutch-controlled Surinam and gained international renown as a healer and botanist. He created a bitter medicinal tea made from the plant *quassia*, which killed intestinal parasites. His European-style clothing and especially his feathered hat denote his high social status. (National Library of Medicine)

provided some type of infirmary facilities and both regular and emergency practitioner visits as needed. As the prospect of abolition loomed, midwifery and infant care took on a new importance. In the British West Indies, a medical manual for slaves (John Grainger's *An Essay on the More Common West Indian Diseases*, London, 1764) lagged behind the first for whites by 85 years. Grainger dealt with the universal conditions of worms, fevers, diarrhea, tetanus, dropsy, cholera, throat sores, and hepatitis, and the predominantly black conditions of leprosy, yaws, night blindness, Guinea worm, hernias, burns, and ulcers.

Slaves who had long been resident or had grown up in captivity understood the owner's medicine as a means of preserving or restoring their health. For new arrivals, however, the strange inattention to the gods and spirits made much white medicine a very alien thing, even when it proved successful. Language barriers aside, the white healers were far too reminiscent of the slave traders, inspectors, sailors, and brutal overseers to be trusted very far.

Both the shortage of competent white medical personnel and native distrust of white healers led to the employment of enslaved medical personnel in both French and British Caribbean colonies. Large French plantations featured crude slave hospitals overseen by enslaved black women known as *hospitalières*, who were aided by less respected *infirmières*. These women relied largely on European-style healing and the use of native plants as materia medica. They had high status among the slaves and were generally privileged by whites for their position and skills. Karol Weaver's study of 18th-century French Saint Domingue found that *hospitalières* could be domineering and insufferable or noted as excellent caregivers and administrators. There was little in the way of preparation for such a position, though it is likely that *hospitalières* tended to come from among the *infirmières* (Weaver 2006, 48–55).

Eighteenth-century English island colonies had similarly varied provisions for sick and injured slaves. Larger and wealthier plantations featured well-built infirmaries staffed with slave personnel, including a "doctor" or "doctors," assistants, nurses, an attendant for children, a cook, a midwife, and an attendant for those with yaws. A study of 10 plantations owned by John Tharpe in 1805 lists 51 black medical personnel for 3,000 slaves. Thirty-four were women, 23 were African-born, and only 6 of the 51 were declared "able" to do field work; the rest suffered from some disability, from missing a leg to being "insane." Those who could not work healed (Sheridan 1985, 89–94).

Among the slaves who worked in the fields, there were self-designated healers of the older African type. In French colonies, *kaperlatas* were practitioners of both spiritual and natural medicine who had high status among the slaves. They sold and traded familiar drugs, amulets, charms, and rituals, and were believed to be possessed of traditional powers to interact with the spirit world. As blacks empowered by their own people, they were naturally subversive leaders who represented the freedom of the Old World, and some helped foment rebellions that expressed the slaves' desire for self-determination (Weaver 2006, 3–5, 10, 113–119).

THE CHINESE

Practitioners

As in other early modern societies, China's late Mingand early Qing ("ching") dynasty leaders supported a wide range of healers. When a person suffered an illness, his or her choice of practitioner was dictated in part by availability and cost, by the sufferer's worldview, by the nature of the malady, and by the reputations of available and affordable healers (for further information see Furth 1999; Ping 1999; Unschuld 2010; and Yuan-Ling 2009).

China's religious traditions, especially Daoism and Buddhism, provided spiritual practitioners who specialized in protecting people from, and ridding people of, the onslaughts of angry ancestors, malicious ghosts, and demons. In both China and Japan, various anthropomorphic "disease gods" explained widespread epidemic outbreaks of measles, smallpox, and other infectious diseases. These entities inflicted ill health and disease on good people and bad alike, which explained why the good suffered. The stricken person wore amulets or talismans and had prayers, spells, rituals, and even exorcisms performed to placate or neutralize the troublesome spirits. This was no mere peasant superstition, as even well-educated medical professionals admitted the powers of spiritual forces, especially in adverse mental conditions. Other healers, perhaps the most common, relied on folklore and their own experience at using herbs and other common substances as remedies. The Chinese did not discriminate between men and women whose knowledge and techniques were rooted in long traditions. Where priests and monks learned their healing crafts in temples, these empirics usually came from families recognized for their practical medical skills, or had studied the craft as informal apprentices. Other popular, itinerant, or illiterate practitioners with special skills included midwives, bonesetters, magicians, acupuncturists, and specialists on body parts such as skin, teeth, and eyes.

China also had a long history of formal medical theory and practice. This was established in an expanding set of classic texts. The first was the *Yellow Emperor's Classic Canon of Internal Medicine* (Veith 2002), supposedly by the ruler and physician Huang Ti from the third millennium B.C.E. The heavily edited and commentated book is known from what was probably a second- or third-century-C.E. text. Ambitious men of the upper class studied these as a standard part of their preparation for careers as local or imperial government bureaucrats. Many who could not pass the rigorous examination for metropolitan civil service (the *jinshi* degree, for which an estimated 1 in 3,000 passed) established medical practices as scholar-gentleman physicians (*ruyi*). The Imperial Household in Beijing also sponsored a formal medical academy (Great Medical Office) educating 300 students at a time, whose curriculum shrank across our period as its integrity shriveled. These scholar-physicians, whether self-educated via the classics or formally at the academy, were solidly in the Confucian tradition of acquired expertise and social benevolence through public service. China's medical elite, they were generally unavailable to the common sufferer and made their fortunes and reputations by treating the wealthy. They formed a true profession based on their shared body of knowledge (the classics) and Confucian values (which underwent a revival in the 17th and 18th centuries), and status and privilege conferred by society (see Unschuld 1979, 56–106). Theirs was a growing profession fueled by economic prosperity, growing affluence, and competition for business. The profession was also formally supported by the Chinese state through its ritual temple worship of Huang Ti and two other early medical authors—the Three Emperors—as divinities, a move probably meant to undermine the status of Daoist and Buddhist religious healers.

The Dao, Yin and Yang, and the Five Elements

Formal or learned Chinese medicine was intimately linked to the place of human beings in the cosmos. As with Chinese religions and most philosophies, medical theory explained the universe as a living and moral entity. Humans were enveloped and interpenetrated by the natural forces of the cosmos. Human action and development were meant to be in synch with the flow of the universe: this defined good health. The Dao, or Way, was the Chinese expression of the proper conduct that kept one both physically healthy and morally good. The doctor, priest, and philosopher all sought to keep people on the Dao. The famed philosopher Confucius (551–479 B.C.E.) taught the application of balance and moderation as the foundation of the individual good life as of the good state. The health of each was at heart a matter of correct choices, of human action and self-discipline. Harm followed immorality.

In the human body, the principles or forces that needed to be maintained in balance were labeled "yin" and "yang." Yin was associated with earth, night, water, cold, damp, dark, contraction; female, wife, the earth being fertilized, the body's interior; constructive, conservative, positive action; lowliness, disease, evil, and death. Yang was essentially the opposite of each yin characteristic: sun, day, dryness, heat, light, expansion; male, husband, the heavens fertilizing the earth with rain and sunlight, the body's exterior; aggressive, destructive, negative action; nobility, health, good, and life. Winter and fall were yin, and spring, summer, and late summer were yang. Human organs were either yin or yang, and the two forces coursed through the body with blood and air through imagined ducts or conduits. Habits, food, and other factors could rob the body of yin or yang, or replenish it. Bad health resulted from an imbalance. The mind, body, and spirit were all interconnected through the force of qi ("chee"), which was directly affected by the yin/yang balance. Maintaining proper qi was the key to Chinese medicine.

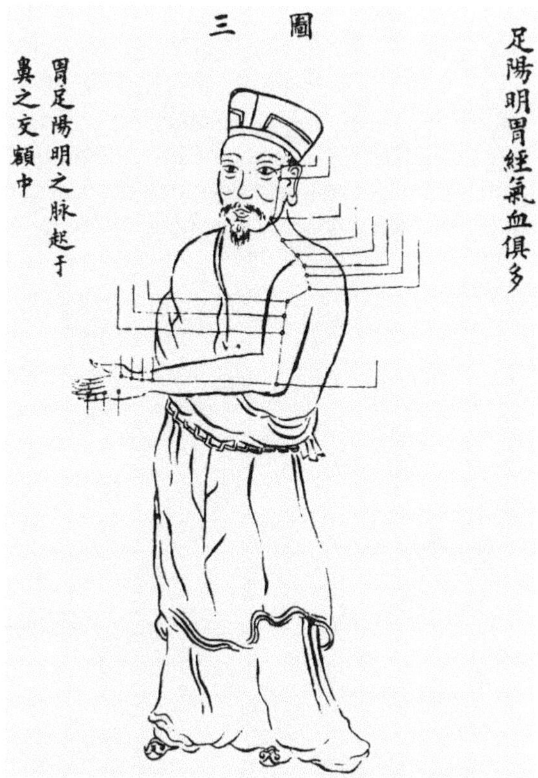

A visual guide to the points along the stomach meridian into which an acupuncturist would insert his needles, from Wen-chih Ch'en's *Yang K'o Hsuan sui*, 1628. In traditional Chinese medicine, the life force, qi, was channeled through meridians to organs. Hollow organs such as the stomach were associated with yang. (National Library of Medicine)

Further, the Five Phases or elements—earth, fire, water, metal, and wood—of which everything physical is constructed, including man, were connected to or associated with a long list of phenomena, including the seasons, planets, numbers, directions, flavors, odors, colors, emotions, the body's tissues and organs, and climate (wind, heat, humidity, cold, dryness). Spiritual "resources" as well as bodily fluids were associated with specific yin organs: liver with tears and soul; spleen with saliva and ideas; heart with sweat and spirit; kidneys with spittle and the will; and lungs with mucus and animal spirit. Of course, each organ is also associated with yin or yang. This whole system of yin/yang, seasons, elements, and concordances or correspondences was of ancient origin and found its first full articulation in the *Yellow Emperor's Classic Canon of Internal Medicine.*

Despite the dominance of Huang Ti's *Canon*, Chinese medical tradition and practice had long developed variations and schools that privileged one or another of the tradition's many complex variables. Treatments for the same disease might vary widely with the physician's understanding of the underlying cause of the ailment, be it the seasons, winds, diet, or demons. We have little evidence on how patients chose among physicians, other than the importance of reputation, but if a large swath of the educated Chinese had both studied medicine—as part of their general education—and provided the learned physicians with their clientele, it is likely that the physician's "school" often mattered.

3

Religion and Medicine

For most of human history, healing the human body was understood as being ultimately in the hands of God, gods, or other entities that transcended mere mortals. In many cultures, the shaman, witch doctor, or priest remained a major healing figure throughout the early modern period. Jesus and other religious figures healed miraculously when they walked the earth, and control over bodies and their sicknesses was considered a sign of power over life itself. Humans contacted these entities—spirits, jinn, ancestors, ghosts, gods, demons, saints, or the Almighty himself—through religious ritual, and did so because their faith and culture told them to do so. By 1500, many cultures had blended spiritual healing with remedies or rituals that were medicinal in nature. In the West, European cultures were in the process of segregating the body and spirit, the medical and religious: to the detriment of religion but the benefit of the sufferer. When European cultures took their medicine across the globe, they sometimes imposed Western religions and Western medicine on those they met.

The following short studies examine ways in which medicine and religion intersected within and between cultures across the globe between 1500 and 1800. They are meant to be indicative of certain patterns of human response and are by no means exhaustive of a rich and variegated topic.

THE EXPANDING CHRISTIAN WORLD

Roman Catholic Saints and Western Medicine

Healing bodily ills was long the stock-in-trade of Christian saints, or holy people, since Saint Peter's shadow was said to have cured the lame. Early stories of saints often featured miracles of healing—even resuscitating the dead—that were meant to be signs of God's favor with them. Christians did not believe the healing power was the holy person's but that God worked miracles through her as a benefit and a sign. Once deceased, the holy person properly came to be called saint and his or her ability to display God's favor through medical miracles remained.

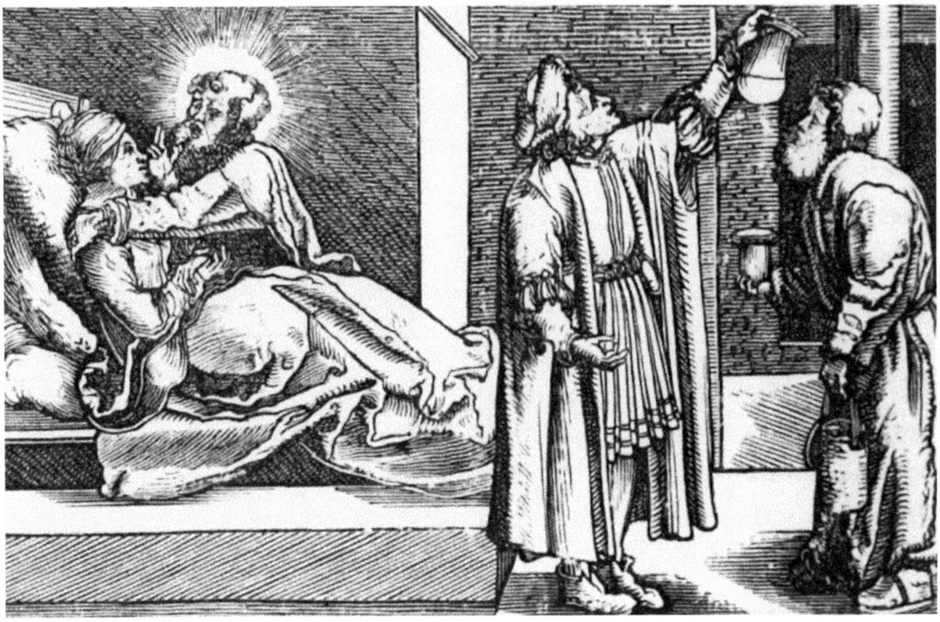

While a physician and his assistant examine a dying man's urine—a stereotypical medical activity—the patient is miraculously cured by the haloed saint who appears by his bedside. Copy of a woodcut attributed to Hans Holbein, from the German translation of Boethius' sixth-century *Consolation of Philosophy*, 1537. (Lacroix, Paul. *Science and Literature in the Middle Ages*, 1878)

From the early 1500s, the Christian Church experienced the split known as the Reformation. Factions that "broke away" from the Catholic Church—Lutherans and Radicals in Germany and Scandinavia; Calvinists in Switzerland, France, Scotland, and the Netherlands; Anglicans and others in England—discarded many traditional Christian beliefs and practices, including those associated with helpful saints. In response, the Catholic Church reemphasized the roles of the saints as sources of help from and advocacy before God. Certain saints had long been associated with specific diseases, such as Saints Job and Lazarus with leprosy, or more recently Sebastian and Roche with plague. Some were generalists, such as the ancient Roman physicians Saints Cosmas and Damian; others were believed to help with childbirth or broken bones or smallpox. Still other saints had local or regional reputations, such as plague saints Rosalia in Palermo, Sicily; Archbishop Carlo Borromeo in Milan and Vienna; and Saint Januarius (San Gennaro) in Naples. Jesus's mother Mary was a universal advocate on whom any faithful Christian could call for help. She was often depicted spreading her cloak around her devotees protecting them from disease or other threats.

The line between the saint as advocate asking for God's help and the saint as powerful in his or her own right was often very thin. When a Catholic prayed to a saint for help, he probably did not make a clear distinction in his own mind between the two. Either way, if the supplicant survived, he might thank the saint by depositing a thank-you gift of a small statuette or painting in a local church or shrine. These served as testimonials to the saint's aid, bidding others to depend upon it. Wealthy thankful individuals might decorate whole chapels with frescoes of the helpful saint's life, or large portraits to be placed above altars. When a community wanted to give thanks for salvation from an epidemic, they might build special churches such as Venice's Santa Maria della Salute or Vienna's Karlskirche. Epidemics tended to spawn these expressions, since the belief was that ultimately God sent pestilence (as in the Old Testament) and the saint had convinced Him to direct His wrath away from the person, family, or community.

Canonization and Medicine

In 1588, Pope Sixtus V in the bull *Immensa aeterni Dei*, as part of the Catholic Reformation, regularized the process of canonization by which the central church recognized the holiness of its heroes. To be declared a saint by the Catholic Church, one had to have been true to Church teaching, heroically practice Christian virtues, and have a number of miracles clearly attributed to him or her after death. A formal proceeding, which included the "devil's advocate" who did his best to disprove the supporting evidence, now carefully gathered and examined sworn testimony to miracles. Much of this material has survived and has been studied by Jacalyn Duffin (Duffin 2009).

Duffin found that between 1588 and 1800, 91 percent of the miracles attributed to candidates were healing miracles. This compares with 96 percent (486/506) during similar 20th-century proceedings. The people who were cured were not just members of religious orders (only about 9% were), nor were they all gullible peasants. Of those whose status is known, nobility rank first, from kings on down. The impoverished are also well represented, but so are members of physicians' families. Those who testified to the miracles were also often doctors, and by 1800, if a physician had not intervened in the medical case, then the claim would be tossed out.

The Church's demands grew stiffer over time. The purported miracle had to be completely unexpected, unnatural, not due to medical care or procedures, ideally spontaneous, permanent, and clearly the result of the person or those around him calling upon (invoking) the candidate for sainthood. Duffin found various manners of invocation surrounding the basic prayer, from pilgrimages to having holy relics placed on the sick person. Miraculous healings spanned the range of human illnesses, with fevers and malaria predominant, followed by orthopedic conditions, neurological problems (especially vision), cancers (tumors), and a long list of other conditions. There were even 20 cases of resurrections, most of infants or children.

The Catholic Church in 1588 was still reeling from the Protestant split and sought to rationalize one of its most mystical practices. The process, and its effect, was powerful in its day and remains of note today, as in the cases of Pope John Paul II and of Mother Teresa—herself a powerful caregiver in life.

These traditions and beliefs spread to Portuguese, Spanish, and French outposts and colonies around the world. Their professional missionaries—Franciscans, Dominicans, and Jesuits—saw to it that they were preached for the salvation of the souls of Indians, Africans, Native Americans, Pacific Islanders, Japanese, Chinese, and many others. Where the European newcomers laid down roots, as in South America, Catholic beliefs and practices sometimes replaced and sometimes blended with those of native cultures. In many of these, healing saints and healing deities often melded, residing beneath the Church's radar but emerging in times of need.

Witches and Sorcerers

If the early modern Catholic Church was willing to side with rationality and the growing medicalization of society regarding canonizations, it was equally willing to remain downright superstitious for two centuries regarding men and women suspected of consorting with demons or the devil himself. Often the diabolical effect was sickness, plague, or even death of innocent victims of demonic arts. But Catholics were far from alone in their opposition to the devil and his minions. One only need remember Salem, Massachusetts, and its Puritan judges in 1692. Christians had a particular fear of witches since the Bible clearly commanded "suffer not a witch to live." Their conception of evil and harm was embodied in the figure of Satan, an entity clearly opposed to God. The linkages of witches and Satan in the popular and even learned imaginations tarred even the most innocently accused woman or man.

Part of the problem was with the healing abilities of many of the people labeled by their communities as witches. Just as the midwife knew both how to birth a baby and how to kill it through abortion or infanticide, so a community healer could, it was commonly believed, injure, maim, or even kill. If prompted by the devil, then harm was as likely as health. This paranoia was fueled when the ministrations of the "old lady in the woods" backfired, in fact causing injury. In an age that believed God sent plague and saints could heal from beyond the grave, it was perfectly logical that old ladies would consort with demons and slaughter farm animals or sour all the community's milk.

By the 18th century, both Catholic and Protestant authorities came to recognize that much of the witch craze had been irrational and misdirected. Not that people did not consort with Satan or that certain individuals did not have the power to injure. Such cases came to be seen as very rare, however, and fear of witches was branded as the hysterical superstition it usually was. Both sacred and secular societies in the West were adopting the Enlightenment era's rationalism with its disdain for the unscientific. As contemporary medicine made great strides in explaining many ailments, the "old lady in the woods" as causative agent disappeared with celestial conjunctions and the evil eye.

Protestant Religiosity

The Reformation redirected popular Protestant religiosity away from what Reformers considered superstitious reliance on saints toward God and the Bible. Though denominations and individuals differed in specifics, it is safe to say that

Protestants believed that their health and welfare were ultimately in God's hands. The best way to preserve or improve both was through adherence to His will as found in the Bible. As prayer and fasting are both mentioned in Scripture, Protestant persons, congregations, and entire nations (England, Denmark, Brandenburg-Prussia) accepted these forms of individual and group penitence in the face of sickness, especially epidemics.

When plague broke out in 17th-century England, both Anglican and Puritan leaders urged prayer and fasting, even publishing prayers and directions for leading families in a godly direction. The practice was carried to the New World and informed colonial civic life in New England as well as the British West Indies.

Dutch Calvinists held the same beliefs, though they seem to have been less insistent in carrying these with them to their far-flung holdings. In rejecting Catholicism, all Protestants rejected its ordained and sacred clergy, especially its professional missionaries. The result was that where Catholic colonization directly reached out to evangelize the natives—whether Japanese shoguns or Mayan farmers—Protestant efforts were only as effective as their spirit-driven congregants. This began to change with the rise of Methodism in the 18th century and other English evangelizing movements in the 19th century, especially in Africa.

AFRICANS AT HOME AND ENSLAVED

West African Medicine: Body and Spirits

The peoples of early modern West Africa by no means constituted a single cultural unit. Their environments, languages, beliefs, practices, and shared experiences differed widely. They did, however, share certain fundamental beliefs about the natural world, the realm of spirits, and the intersections of the two. "Intersections" is probably an incorrect term, since for African societies, there was no distinction between one and the other. Spirits—whether gods or ancestors—operated as truly and significantly among living people as did any natural phenomena. Their impacts could be positive or negative, just as those of an animal, plant, or the weather could be either.

Sickness or other physical ailments were often conceived of as the result of spirits' anger, vengeance, whim, dissatisfaction, or service to a malevolent devotee. Conversely, gods or ancestors who imposed sickness could also protect one from it, cure it, or lead a healer to identify (diagnose) the problem and apply the proper remedy. Some gods were thought to control certain diseases. The powerful earth god Sakpata was believed to impose, cure, and protect people from smallpox. Others, like the largely destructive Legba, were associated with a wide range of maladies: "Legba has many *gbo* for headache, for colic, for dysentery, for leprosy, for eye trouble, for rheumatism, and for all other kinds of illness" (Sweet 2011, 125). *Gbo* were physical objects associated with avoiding sickness or healing, including talismans, amulets, and other ritual items. Keeping such entities satisfied meant good health or quick recovery, and West African healers were as much priests or shamans as practitioners of medicine in the European sense (see Voeks 1993).

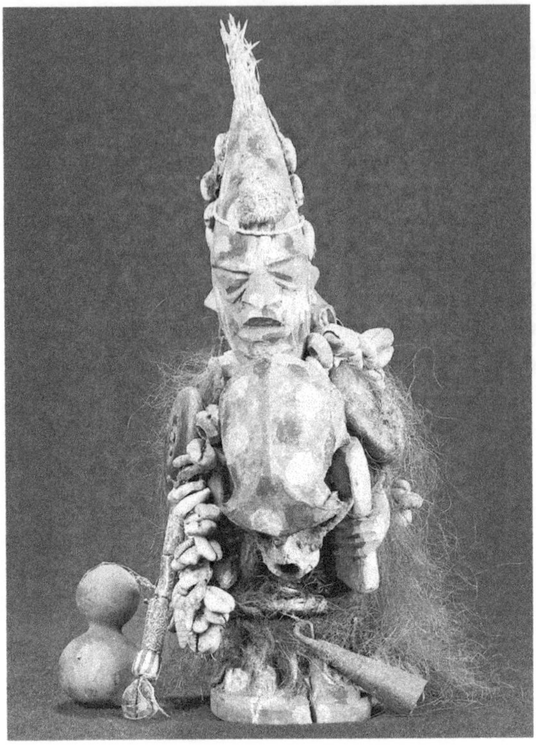

Modern rendition of a traditional West African figurine representing Sakpata, the Yoruba god of smallpox. Adorned with layers of meaningful organic objects (*gbo*), such as shells and monkey skulls, these types of carvings have traditionally been created for protection against maladies such as smallpox. The blotches represent the characteristic red marks on the skin. (Centers for Disease Control and Prevention)

Gods or ancestor spirits required acknowledgment and sacrifice, rewarding the cooperative and punishing the others. Prayers, songs, dances, and other rituals blended together into a spirit-pleasing display, while sacrifices might include food, alcohol, live animals, or blood. Human sacrifices were not unknown, though unlike among the Aztecs, they were apparently rare. Best known were those of powerful expansionist rulers, such as Agaja of Dahomey, who was said to have killed 200,000 as sacrifices to the war divinities (Sweet 2011, 137). Due attention to Sakpata, Legba, or other appropriate deities allowed healer-priests to work with them, diagnosing and appropriately prescribing treatments. Ancestors and gods might speak to healers, revealing the cause or course of a disease and its remedies. More dramatic was spirit possession. The spirit was drawn down into the healer or other devotee by dance or another ritual, often aided by hallucinogens or other mind-altering substances. Enveloped in a trance, the devotee provided a mouthpiece for the helpful divinity. This technique was also employed when an unsolved murder required divine help to identify the responsible party.

Enslaved Africans in the Caribbean

The millions of West Africans transplanted to the Western Hemisphere during the early modern period brought their cultures with them. Without the ability to record their beliefs, and under the assault of masters and resident black slaves to conform to the norms of their new home and employment, the recently enslaved appear to have lost at least some of the key elements of their belief systems. Specific entities associated with the homeland may have come to be understood as regional or local in their scope and power rather than universal. Mixing with slaves of various origins, recent arrivals would have been exposed to differing names of divinities, and perhaps new spiritual pantheons. Christianity, too, had an influence, depending on the attitudes of the slaveholders and their religious backgrounds (Spanish or French Catholic, English or Dutch Protestant). But even if the spiritual landscape had changed, the role of spirits in imposing, protecting from, and remedying illness could not have.

Studies have demonstrated that slave masters of European descent imposed European medicine on slaves who were injured or fell ill (a good example is Harrison 2010). More difficult to demonstrate is the hold spirit medicine continued to have on enslaved blacks. Of course, spiritual medicine required the special priest-healers, who had very high status in Africa. Such powerful figures and potential leaders of revolt were undesirable from the white slavers' viewpoint and would have been culled out if known. As Karol Weaver shows, however, such healers and leaders did emerge in some African slave communities. It was through the success of their healing practices that their reputations were made.

Afro-Caribbean slaves also adapted elements of Catholicism in their new homes, a process that remains rather dim to modern observers. Savvy priest-healers realized the power of syncretic religion, which blended Catholic beliefs and practices with those of West Africa. Healing or helpful saints retained their place among Catholics long after Protestant churches abandoned them, and for many slaves, they replaced African tribal entities. Catholic prayer and other rituals, often led by strangely dressed celebrants and illuminated by candles, had an appeal to people who had lost their own spiritual guides. Catholic sacramentals—objects associated with prayer or other rituals—such as scapulars, rosaries, holy water and oil, and statues of Jesus and saints came to be seen as *gbo* and were adopted as tools with healing power. When wielded by enslaved priest-healers, they were sources of power taken from those who had physical power over them.

RELIGION AND MEDICINE AMONG THE AZTECS

Precolonial Religion and Medicine

Like many premodern peoples, including those of West Africa, the Aztecs of what is today Mexico had powerful beliefs concerning the intervention of gods and lesser spirits in human affairs. This included health and illness; the veil between medicine and religion was very thin. Aztec deities had the same dualistic powers to help or hurt that the African gods possessed. For example, the major rain god Tláloc could enrich the earth and its peoples by providing abundant fresh water. Conversely, he could withhold his gift and cause drought or inundate the land, killing crops, animals, and people with his flood. Lesser divinities governed elements of nature including geographic and weather features, such as mountains and winds, and could use their powers to help or destroy the people. Still others controlled specific diseases, inflicting, protecting from, or remedying as they saw fit.

Most of the Aztec pantheon had some role to play in human health (see Schendel 1968, 16–31). The sun god Tonatiuh was necessary for life itself; too little or too much of his gift and famine struck the people. Tláloc governed the rains but was also associated with human, animal, and crop fertility, tuberculosis, and other respiratory illnesses. The famous Quetzalcóatl, for whom the Aztecs mistook the conqueror Cortés due to his fair skin and beard, was noted as a teacher of medicinal herbal lore, as were the goddesses Tzapotlatena and Tonantzin. Xiptótec was the patron of healers and held sway over abscesses, scabies, (later) smallpox, and some other skin diseases, while Nanáhuatl handled more severe ones such as elephantiasis and leprosy. The war god Huitzilopochtli could determine life and death on the battlefield, while the goddess Tlazoltéotl determined whether mothers in labor and their infants lived or died. Xoaltecuhtli was responsible for the mind, and Amímitl for one's bowels and dysentery.

Aztec religion discerned a very strict moral code that the gods and spirits expected humans to obey. While the deities could be whimsical in their infliction of sickness or other misfortunes, these were usually the result of human misbehavior and divine punishment. Sorcerers could also call upon gods to cause pain or suffering, and gods could punish wicked parents by making their children suffer. The key was to redress the moral imbalance through prayers and rituals. The most dramatic ritual was human sacrifice, during some of which the beating hearts were cut out of victims' bodies. The most famous of these took place in 1486 at the dedication of the new temple in the Aztec capital, in which 70,000 people were said to have been sacrificed. At times of military defeat, drought, famine, or disease, the world seemed clearly out of balance, and the cosmos itself, not merely some petulant divinity, needed to be reset.

The scholar Bernard Ortiz de Montellano sees the Aztec worldview as essentially fatalistic (Ortiz de Montellano 1990). The norm of life on Earth is suffering, and the gods are the agents of that suffering through the instruments of misfortune, accident, and sickness. There are no guarantees in life—even the good suffer—but people must strive to obey the laws of nature and acknowledge the gods. An apt metaphor was living on the razor's edge of a mountaintop, with a deep crevasse on either side. As with the Greeks, balance (survival) meant moderation in all things and a stoical outlook on life. When that failed, the sorcerers ("owl men"), shamans, and priests went to work divining the causes—especially which deity or deities bore responsibility—and prescribing or carrying out the appropriate remedies. Allowing oneself to be possessed by a spirit and reading the message in a handful of corn kernels tossed on a table were among the forms of diagnosis or prognosis by divination. If it was determined that a spirit had caused the disease, then healers oversaw spiritual remedies ranging from confession of sin to sacrifices or the eating of ritual cakes. Spirits might also inhabit medicinal plants, whose natural healing virtues were thus increased. In each case, the healer was the bridge between the patient and the divine disease, "the Lord of transformations" (Schendel 1968, 167).

Colonial Mexico

During most of the early modern period, the world of the Aztecs was dominated by the Roman Catholic Spaniards and their descendants. In villages and regions where the Spanish presence was light, the local people continued their beliefs and practices. Even so, spiritual healers were always subject to persecution by the religious authorities such as the Inquisition. Where the Catholic presence was stronger and the expectation that all subjects of the Spanish king would be Catholic, the natives found much that was familiar in the new rulers' medicine. The Catholic emphasis on saints, sacramentals, and religious rituals coupled with a rather fatalistic outlook, a Galenic medical emphasis on moderation and balance (of humors), and a positive interest in native healing practices and medicinal plants made acceptance of European religion and medicine rather easier than it might otherwise have been (for example, see McCaa 1995).

Positive, healing saints replaced the dualistic gods; a new set of prayers and rituals took the place of the old ones; and the Indians saw transformative power embedded in miraculous paintings, amulets, and the Catholic priesthood. The same missionaries who led the religious liturgies and processions often also baptized the newly born, cared for the sick, and blessed the dying. Spanish culture could not abide the continuation of human sacrifices, but the new and healthful religion emphasized the healing power of the sacrifice of Jesus Christ (so powerfully portrayed through the crucifix) and of many of the Christian martyrs to whom Catholics prayed. Even the Catholic belief in the literal presence of divine Jesus in the Eucharistic bread that was consumed by believers paralleled native beliefs of spirit possessions and cures effected by eating ritual cakes—"god cakes"—in which one of the healing deities was thought to be present.

The replacement or blending of spiritual healing traditions produced the *curanderos*, who often served the far-flung native villages and rural communities. These healers utilized native and imported medical techniques and remedies as well as both Aztec and Catholic spiritual practices. Mexican Catholic authorities distrusted these practitioners because they feared that the *curanderos* derived healing power from the devil, a fear reinforced by the healers' retention of Aztec practices and the Church's inability to oversee the Catholic elements in their practice, such as prayers and sacramental (see Fields 2008 and Cook and Lovell 1992).

MING AND QING CHINA

Chinese Medicine: Worshipping the Ancestor Physicians

In traditional China, physicians were considered social equals of artists and other craftsmen, despite their role as healers. This status, however, was augmented by the Chinese practice of ancestor worship. Before the early modern period temples dedicated to the Three Emperors (*sanhuang miao*), ancients considered by many to be the founders of medicine, drew worshippers to sacrifices of pigs and sheep overseen by physician-priests. Temples held images of the three, with their four assistants, and 28 famed physicians. The Yüan dynasty (1274–1368) emperors and their bureaucrats mandated and patronized these temples as a way of emphasizing their connection with the divine but also as a way of maintaining an authoritative presence among physicians and their patients. This was useful, since the Chinese state played no clear role in examining, licensing, or otherwise controlling doctors or medical practice (Yuan-Ling 2007).

Ming dynasty rulers (1368–1644) shifted this support, as they concentrated attention on themselves and their capital. By 1500, the craft of medicine was firmly associated with the Three Emperors, but state officials sought to have their worship concentrated in the capital and under their control. Three kneelings, nine bows, and three sacrifices (cow, sheep, pig) for each emperor constituted orthodox worship. Local temples, however, languished or disappeared without state support. The Qing dynastic rulers (1644–1912) continued the pattern of reduced support for provincial temples, while centralizing worship in the capital.

Local worship also shifted, as both urban and rural people developed and expanded the cults of local medical ancestors and of the Medicine King (*yaowang*). The identity of this figure changed with time and place, but by the 16th century it was usually Sun Simiao (581–682), a physician still worshipped today. Patronage from local social leaders replaced state support for medical cults, signaling a new level of popular acceptance of medicine as more than a mere craft. Chinese elites, whether the emperor or wealthy local merchants, built and funded these places of worship because they shared the core Confucian virtue of benevolence. Elite physicians, itinerant healers, herb peddlers, and others associated with medicine hung about these *yaowang miao* (temples) awaiting and seeing patients, further associating their work with divine aid of ancestor-gods. Secondary temples and shrines dedicated to healing and healers also popped up with local support due to people's demand for them. None of this was entirely new, and much reflected venerable local village and urban practice and belief.

Chinese Medicine: Demons and Spirits

Very early Chinese medicine also had a dominant role for malevolent spiritual forces as causes of all sorts of human illnesses. Despite the development of a rational system of medical theory and practice based upon it, spiritual forces of "evil" continued to play a significant role throughout the early modern (Ming-Qing) period. Among the people, concern for demonic influences and effects probably remained the norm long after 1800. As late as the 18th century, spell casting was a formal academic medical specialty (though it was removed), and exorcists in both cities and villages had plenty of business. Every classically trained or learned physician had to know the principles and procedures of defeating evil, if only to placate certain clients. Virtually every Ming-Qing Chinese medical text has a place for spiritual cures, even if, as physician Chang Chieh-pin wrote around 1624, "demons are created in one's mind" (Unschuld 2010, 329). An 18th-century edition of the works of physician Hsü Ling-t'ai approvingly includes his opinion:

> Whenever illnesses were caused by demons and spirits, the uneducated claim that demons and spirits truly possess the ability to bring misfortunes to man. Educated persons, however, maintain that although the specific characteristics of some illnesses may give the impression, demons and spirits in reality do not exist. Both of these views are false. (Unschuld 2010, 337)

Ancestors' ghosts, those of unjustly killed people, and nature spirits had potential to assault one in a lonely place, usually at night. Possession through the nose or mouth could result in unconsciousness; other ailments could be imposed through natural channels. Since the Chinese did not separate the spiritual and physical aspects of reality or medicine, there was no effective barrier against malevolent activity. Confucianism, however, did provide a prophylactic: one protected oneself from spiritual malevolence through virtuous living. Just as bad behavior could lead to naturally occurring disease, so it opened doors to demons.

Despite its ubiquity, there was no standardized theory or practice by which to deal with spiritually caused sickness. No doubt the itinerant or village healer or exorcist had local or familial traditions upon which to draw. Talismans and amulets might keep forces at bay, and noise, smoke, and potions using peach leaves and twigs might expel them when one was possessed. Learned authors recommended that their readers use both spiritual and natural treatments if there were any question . . . just in case.

4

Women's Health

Woman's health issues differed from those of men almost exclusively in the realm of reproduction. Despite male domination of learned medicine in China and the West in 1500, across cultures healing women in need and aiding in childbirth generally fell to other women. Aztec women practitioners, however, lost out to Spanish males, and by the 18th century, across Europe and China, the medical specialties we may loosely label gynecology and obstetrics (*obstetrix* refers to "midwife") were falling under the purview of educated professional males.

THE AZTECS

Women played powerful roles in maintaining the health of the Aztec population. Life came into the world through the instrumentation of their bodies, and their bodies nourished each new and young life. Bringing death, whether through warfare or bloody sacrifices to the gods, was a male occupation. Women healers (spiritual healers, herbalists, wound tenders, etc.), therefore, were considered to be on a par with males, sharing practical training and preparation in the temples for both spiritual and medical treatments.

Pregnancy and Birth before the Spanish

The midwife, or *tepalechuiani* (one who helps), was considered a specialized *tíctl* (healer), with the same social rank as a male healer. When doing her duty of overseeing a pregnancy and childbirth, she prayed to the healing goddess Yoaltíctl for protection as well as to the goddess of water, Chalchiuhtlicue, at the point of birth. The midwife knew which prayers, herbs, and sexual positions helped induce pregnancy as well as methods of contraception and, when desperate, abortion. Special care went to the first-time mother and her family, and the midwife taught all to see that the young mother, usually a teenager, ate properly and avoided strong emotions and strenuous work. Other, less obvious, activities were also to be

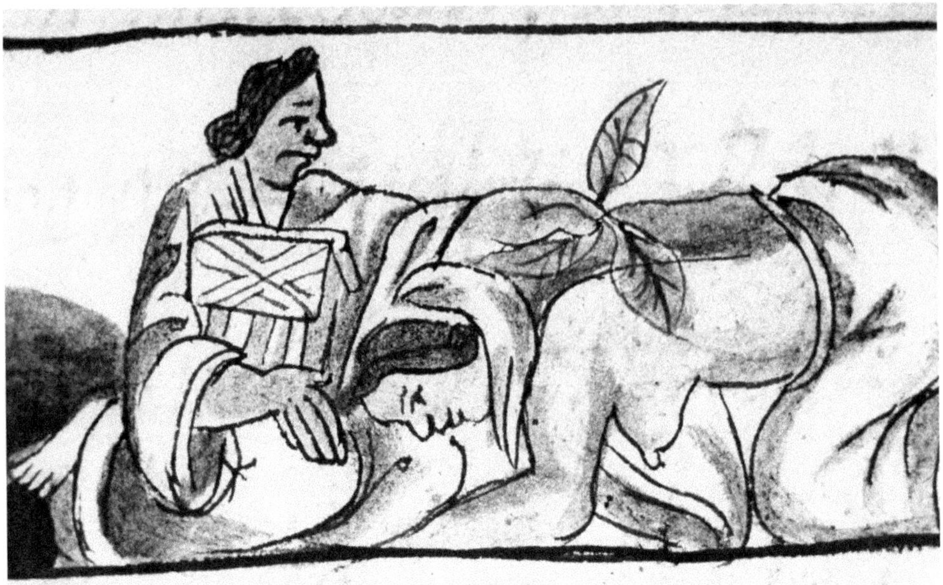

An Aztec midwife administers herbs to a woman after childbirth. One of the 2,000 native-produced illustrations from the 16th-century Florentine Codex by Bernardino de Sahagún, who died in 1590. (Biblioteca Medicea-Laurenziana, Florence, Italy/ Bridgeman Images)

avoided: viewing a lunar eclipse (believed to cause harelip in the child), chewing gum or tar (cleft palate), sleeping during the day (long eyelids), eating tamales from the bottom of the pot (could bring on a difficult labor), and viewing a hanging (could cause the umbilical cord to strangle the child) (Ortiz de Montellano 1990, 142).

During labor and birth, the Aztec midwife had full authority: the mother was "in your hands, in your lap, on your back" (Fields 2008, 47). The Aztecs respected cleanliness and kept the mother and birthing area relatively sanitary. The mother also received a steam bath to help induce labor and relieve stress. In his 1552 herbal, the native Martín de la Cruz provided the ingredients for washes to clean and lubricate the birth canal and a solution to be injected "into the womb" to reduce labor pains (Gates 1939/2000, 108–109). Cacao, which was considered good for inducing menstruation and conception, was also recommended for aiding labor, as was an extract of possum tails. Once the mother's water broke, the midwife positioned the baby from the outside as the mother squatted to give birth. In the case of a successful birth, the midwife cut the umbilical cord, washed the infant, and prayed "Goddess, be pleased that his [or her] life may be purified; that the water may carry away all stain, for the child puts him [or her]self in your hands, oh Chalchiuhtlicue, mother and sister of the gods." The midwife formally named the child (whether the parents had a say is uncertain). Herbs and poultices helped induce lactation, and further steam baths helped clean and relax the mother.

In the case of an unsuccessful birth, the midwife retained control and did all she could to save the mother's life. The midwife was equipped with a very sharp obsidian knife and tongs to dismember and remove a dead infant, and knew how to use them. If the mother died giving birth to her first child, she was hailed as a *mochihuaquetzqui*, a valiant woman, and she was carried by a procession of midwives to a special temple for burial. She was considered as if a soldier fallen in battle, and some parts of her body were considered relics and worn as amulets.

Colonial Mexico

With conquest by the Spanish in the mid-1500s, the roles and status of Aztec female *tícitl* declined. Male priests and physicians replaced female practitioners, and midwives fell in status to the subordinate place their sisters held in European society. As in Europe, pregnancy and childbirth only became medical issues when something went wrong, and the male surgeons and physicians stood by to handle any emergencies. From the spiritual side, priests and friars replaced the spiritual healers, both male and female, and prayers to the gods were replaced with those to the Trinity or saints, such as Anne, who oversaw childbirth. Midwives who retained their pre-Christian religious practices or who showed too much skill with herbs risked the label "witch" and investigation by the Inquisition. In general, Aztec women declined in status not only by virtue of their having been conquered but by their very sex (Kidwell 1997).

CARIBBEAN SLAVES

In many West African cultures, traditional healing lore and skills were passed from mother to daughter. Though male healers with special powers were necessary for serious medical cases, women healers tackled most common conditions of both men and women. Women were especially important for monitoring pregnancies, facilitating births, performing clitorectomies, and tracking children's growth and development, including the young woman's emergence into adulthood. Healing was far less an occupational specialty than a fundamental skill like cooking or making clothing (Sheridan 1985, 74–75).

In the world of the slave ship and plantation, the woman retained her role as healer and caregiver, though certain women rose to prominence for their skills. Some slave women tended the masters' children or other servants, and plantation mistresses sometimes chose to treat male and female slaves to the best of their abilities with European medicine. Of course, white male physicians and surgeons circulated through the slaves' world as needed, but women generally took on the full range of medical duties, as midwives, nurses, and herbalists and also as doctors, surgeons, and spiritual healers. Unfortunately, little is known of them or their service.

Early on, Caribbean planters of all nationalities imported primarily males, and the few female slaves were valuable for both their healing skills and their fertility. After a while, the low cost of importing slaves made keeping pregnant female slaves and supporting a nursery of slave children uneconomical, so "breeding" was discouraged. With the spread of abolitionism and restrictions on the slave trade in the 18th century, pronatalism returned, and female slaves were prized again for their fertility. In the British Sugar Islands, the Consolidated Slave Act of 1792 provided rewards for live births. When births were welcome, pregnant slaves were often protected by law or regulations from hard labor or brutal treatment, but even then miscarriages were common as were deaths from clumsy midwives and infection. Perennial problems of overwork, overheating, poor nutrition and living conditions, careless and inept health care, diseases, and sexual predation by both black and white males made pregnant or nursing young mothers terribly vulnerable (Harrison 2010 and Sheridan 1985).

THE CHINESE

Women Healers

By 1500, the Chinese had had a long and continuous tradition of learned medicine that recognized almost exclusively the well-read male physician as a legitimate healer. Writing was a carefully guarded and shared skill that few women healers possessed, so rather little is known about them from their own words. Of named Chinese medical practitioners only 1 in 200 (0.5%) is female. Of some 12,000 known premodern Chinese medical texts, women wrote only 3. The earliest was by the 16th-century physician's daughter Tan Yunxian, *Sayings of a Female Doctor*. Part biography and part case book, *Sayings* explains that Tan read the standard medical classics in her father's library and learned women's medicine from her grandmother. Most who sought her out were women, and she applied a variety of treatments, from diet recommendations to medicines, acupuncture, and moxibustion (Wu 2010, 21; also see Furth 1999).

Yet women healers always played a wide variety of very important roles in Chinese society. Like Tan, many were educated in healing by other female healers or their husbands or fathers, or they educated themselves informally. Their patients tended to be children and other women, but they also served as smallpox inoculators, pulse takers, herbalists and medicine sellers, religious healers, diviners, and caretakers for chronic sufferers. Wives of notables often tended the medical needs of servants, local peasants, and the poor. Midwives and "wise women" routinely advised and treated women for gynecological and obstetric problems, and Buddhist and Daoist nuns were noted for both their physical and spiritual healing treatments. Emperors of the Ming dynasty forbade male practitioners access to the women's rooms at court, relying on skilled women to tend to their wives and daughters. Yet the corps of learned physicians uniformly denigrated women healers for their lack of proper education and theoretical understanding, ignorance of proper practice, imitation of "genuine" physicians, and often lower-class origins.

Fuke, or Medicine for Women

Learned Chinese medicine had long treated the human body as male, with the female variations relegated to the knowledge and skills of women healers. In

651 C.E., the influential Sun Miao wrote that "illnesses of women are ten times harder to treat than those of men"; "they are unable to control their emotions by themselves, therefore the roots of their disorders are deep and it is difficult to cure them"; and "women's cravings and desires exceed their husbands' and they contract illnesses at twice the rate of men" (Wu 2010, 42–43). Four centuries later, the Imperial Medical Service formally recognized *chanke*—medicine for childbearing—and this was broadened into the medical field of medicine for women, or *fuke*. From the learned male's standpoint, however, basic biological principles (*li*) were more important than variations, so learned medicine in the 16th and 17th centuries downplayed the distinctiveness of *fuke* as a field of medicine (*yi*). At the same time, the later Ming dynasty witnessed the rise in demand for printed medical texts, including those on *fuke*.

A work such as Xue Ji's 16th-century *Revised Good Prescriptions for Women* collected much that was traditional from previous centuries but moved the theoretical emphasis away from blaming most women's medical problems on pulses and "cardinal channels" to the blood, its storage in the liver, and depletion through the menses and childbirth. In *To BenefitYin* (1620), Wu Zhiwang and his colleagues attacked the simplicity of Xue's work while preserving much traditional theory and practice dating back to the *Yellow Emperor's Canon* (Veith 2002). But *To Benefit Yin*'s popularity (34 known editions to 1911) was its acceptance of the complexity of *fuke*, given the structure of Chinese medical knowledge and genuine attempt to clarify its subject through organization and careful definition. As medical professionals sought to establish themselves on ever-firmer foundations of theory and book learning, more and more works on *fuke* appeared. These tended to reflect the greater emphasis on organic—as opposed to spiritual or even environmental—causes and appropriate treatments championed by Wu. Out went "baleful ghosts," sky spirits, unclear yin influences, and generic "wind" and "cold." Medicine sought to demystify the female body and to recommend treatments that fit the organic nature of both its structure and its illnesses. This accompanied a broader cultural shift toward emphasizing the reproductive nature and function of women. In 1757, Hsü Ta-ch'un could write in his *Forgotten Traditions of Ancient Chinese Medicine*, "There is no difference between illnesses affecting females and those affecting males except for illnesses related to the monthly period, to pregnancy, and delivery" (Unschuld 1998). Insofar as learned medicine could claim to understand and be able successfully to direct the care of pregnant or ailing women, it spread its professional control over the other half of China's population.

Midwives and *Fuke*, Pregnancy, and Birth

Through the 18th century, more treatises on *fuke* appeared—for example *Treatise on Easy Childbirth* by Ye Feng in 1715 (182 editions), *Childbirth Treasury* by Ni Zhiwei in 1728, Yan Chunxi's 1730 *Essential Teachings on Childbearing,* in 1742 the great compendium *The Golden Mirror*, and by the monks of the Bamboo Grove Buddhist monastery the *Secret Book for Female Tranquility* in 1786—as

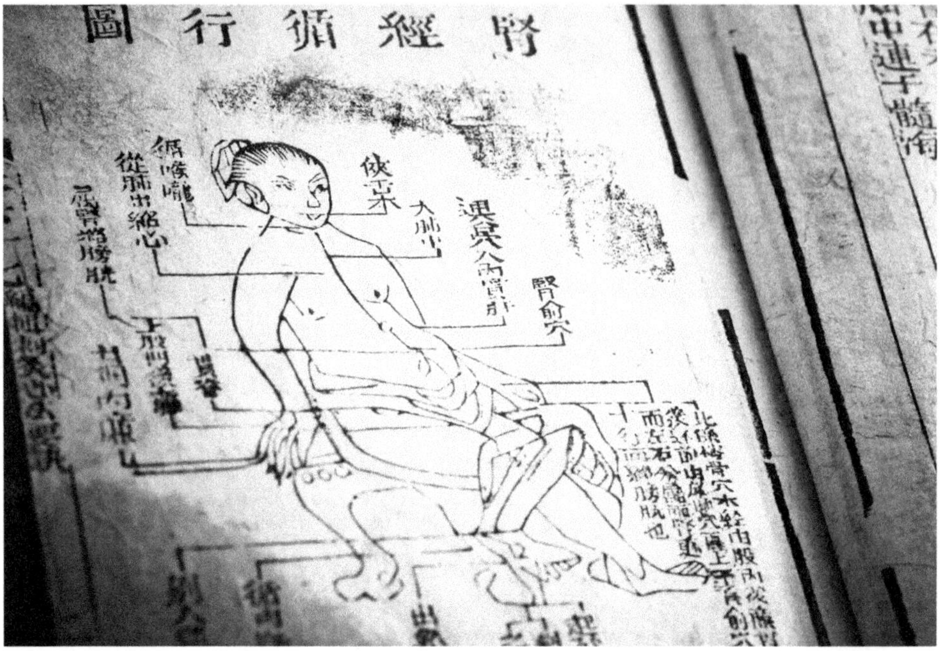

Page from the Qing dynasty's *Imperially Commissioned Golden Mirror of the Orthodox Lineage of Medicine* (1742). This specially produced collection of Chinese traditional and contemporary medical information included commentaries, clinical materials, and illustrations such as this in order to be useful to a wide audience. It was also notable for its inclusion of sections devoted to women's health, a field of increasing interest in the mid-18th century. (Photos.com)

male physicians continued to mark their new territory. But unlike the similar situation in contemporary Europe, Chinese physicians did not stoop to participate in child birthing. As before, they prescribed drugs and pronounced sage advice on prenatal care but left the birthing room to the women. Midwives remained despised even when vital, Ye Feng declaring them "frequently stupid and ignorant of the proper principles" (Wu 2010, 185). Their status fell as families invested in the new literature, which most midwives could not read, and physician-authors warned against employing "ignorant old women" to perform such an important function. In some ways, the new literature was meant to replace the midwives' prenatal direction and advice.

Yet advice on contraception, conception, and prenatal care remained traditional, as did the birthing procedures and options by most accounts. Blood was the yin manifestation of the life force qi ("chee") that joined with the male sperm to produce the fetus. Infertility might stem from insufficient quantity or quality of blood or interference in the womb by wind or cold (or demons or ghosts, though belief in these was waning). Careful inspection of the menses before an attempt at conception could alert one to future problems. Some blamed inappropriate temperatures inside or outside the womb or moistness/dryness inside, blocked blood vessels, insufficient penetration by the penis, weak sperm, or orgasms that were not simultaneous. To increase the likelihood of a male child, the male orgasm needed to be the stronger, the left or yang side of the womb had to host the fetus, and the day of conception needed to be a yang-dominant day, or the odd numbered days after the end of a menstrual period (Wu 2010, 94–120).

Prenatal care remained standard in principle from the seventh through the nineteenth centuries: a balance of rest, movement, and diet to regulate the qi of both mother and child; maintenance of emotional stability; and protection of the womb from physical trauma. The Chinese taught that failure in any area could mean a corrupted fetus, an overly long pregnancy (they believed the norm to be 10 months; more than that probably meant a stillbirth), and premature birth or miscarriage. Though the medical literature of the 18th century often ignored or taught against concern for ghosts, ancestors, demons, gods, or magic rituals, no doubt most families adhered to traditions with the acquiescence of the "ignorant old" midwife. Ye Feng swept aside the spiritual traditions, but he also embraced the idea that childbirth was an act of creation in harmony with the universe, and the norm should be relatively pain free and safe for mother and child. He objected to any interventions—painkillers, stimulants, forced labor, or manipulation of the child in the womb or in descent—that were supposed to ease or shorten labor. His disdain for midwives centered on their insistence on such unnatural interference.

Of course, the experienced midwife was invaluable if complications occurred during or after the baby presented. If the umbilical cord was strangling the child, if the child was dead and needed to be dismembered and extracted, if the afterbirth had not been ejected, or if the mother hemorrhaged, the midwife's expertise and demeanor could mean life or death. But just as the physician (if and when available) oversaw the prenatal mother, so he monitored the postpartum mother for damage to the genital area, for dangerous hormonal changes, for active lactation and the ability to feed the infant, for the replenishment of qi lost in labor, and for signs of infection or fever (see also Scheid 2007 and Yuan-Ling 2009).

THE EUROPEANS

Women as Medical Practitioners and Nurses

The existence of a small but learned and male-dominated medical profession in early modern Europe meant that the vast majority of medical problems were tended to by someone other than a physician. The tradition of the nurturing and caring woman anchored in the home ensured that mothers and grandmothers, sisters, wives, and daughters took care of ailing family members and servants, and neighbors watched sick neighbors. In rural areas, medical professionals were few; men and women relied largely on female healers from herbalists and wise-women to midwives, faith healers, and charitable aristocratic wives who learned medical recipes and procedures from a growing list of vernacular medical self-help books authored by men and women.

In cities, guilds of physicians, apothecaries, and surgeons, as well as male civic authorities, ensured that recognized or even licensed female practitioners were few and far between. Lack of access to education meant women were generally excluded from becoming physicians. Skilled wives or daughters of apothecaries or surgeons might be acceptable substitutes, especially during emergencies such as plague or war. But two societal trends worked against the ambitious female healer. One was the growing concern for the protection of the male professions from encroachment by each other, by nonprofessional empirics or quacks, and by women. The second was the fear of witches and witchcraft, claims of which often tainted female healers both rural and urban. If the patient lived, it was thanks to the healer's pact with Satan; if he died, it was murder at Satan's behest. Though rare before 1500, witch hunts had claimed perhaps 200,000 lives—men as well as women—across Europe by 1700.

The term "nursing" stems from the same root as "nourish" (as in wet nursing), and links the occupation of caregiving (as opposed to healing) to the woman's supposed place and function in the home. When hospitals, orphanages, pest houses, and other institutions required caregivers, the male administrators usually turned to women. Before the Reformation, most such facilities were Catholic and staffed by monks, friars, or nuns. The French began consolidating and secularizing their hospitals in the late 1400s, and Protestant states, including England, replaced religious with civic administrators and staff. Female nurses changed diapers and bandages, laundered and changed bed linens, fed and medicated the sick, comforted the dying, and laid out the dead for burial. Since male professionals visited weekly or as needed, the female staff had to handle all care in their absence. It was hard and dirty work, and in Protestant countries with low pay and status, turnover was common. In Catholic countries such as Italy, Spain, and Austria, nuns continued their service, providing spiritual as well as medical care and comfort. Some orders of nursing nuns predated 1500, but several were founded in the 16th and 17th centuries by pious and humane women, such as the Ursulines (1535) and Sisters of Saint Joseph (1650). The Sisters of Charity, founded by Saint Vincent de Paul, whose members served in madhouses, orphanages, hospitals, and even prisons, were not nuns but single and even married women who felt called to serve (see Whaley 2011).

Midwives

Though giving birth may not have been a "medical condition," it is and was often accompanied by hazards to both the mother and child. Both classical and Christian traditions considered women as humans who differed from the male anatomical and physiological norm, and formal medicine left much that was "gynecological" and almost all that was "obstetrical" to women healers, most often midwives. Women aiding other women in childbirth was traditionally a cross-cultural norm. In Europe, males were welcome in the birthing room only if an emergency occurred requiring a physician, surgeon, or priest. The local midwife was the expert on matters of reproduction from fertility to birth, and most physicians and surgeons were content to allow them to advise and practice both prenatally and during labor.

Most midwives had raised families of their own and had served neighbors and family during births. They learned much from older women, from their own experience assisting older midwives, and increasingly from vernacular manuals. For example, in Germany, Eucharius Roesselin published his *Rosegarden* (1513); it was translated into French in 1539 and English in 1540 as *The Birth of Mankind.* In Spain, Damián Carbón penned his *Book of the Midwives' Art* in1541; and in 1608, Frenchwoman Louise Bourgeois wrote her *Diverse Observations*, the first work by a midwife. Because giving birth was considered both an act of creation and a foul and polluting act, the Catholic Church began administering moral oaths to midwives, first in Regensburg in 1452. A midwife knew how to administer contraceptives and abortifacients, gave legal testimony on stillborn and abandoned infants and young women's virginity, and literally held the mother's and child's lives in her hand, and so had to be of high moral character as well as technically skilled. Yet even by the 18th century an errant German midwife could be denigrated by a court document as handling "a laboring woman with little skill and less concern, and instead of trying to raise her spirits with good words, prattles on with silly talk, smokes too much, and drinks brandy" (Lindemann 1996, 211). As early as 1512, England licensed midwives; in 1556, a French edict required that midwives be registered; and in 1560, statutes controlled Parisian midwives. The latter stipulated who could be a candidate, her examination by two midwives and two master surgeons, and her oath and moral requirements (baptize a dying infant, shun abortion, report illegitimate babies, help the poor without charge).

One trend across the early modern period was that midwives be registered, licensed, and, eventually, formally educated. The Anglican Church licensed midwives in England, and in France, medical practitioners, the Church, and the state all did so. In Venice, they were licensed by the state, but in most of Italy by local priests. In Germany and the Netherlands, municipal authorities licensed midwives, and in Spain, local physicians or the *protomedicato* (official medical office) did so. Another trend was toward a greater understanding of the female reproductive system, though this had minimal impact on the knowledge and practice of female midwives. This intellectual advance accompanied a trend toward professionalization among midwives. By the 18th century, this varied from place to place: increasing literacy meant a greater demand and greater supply of manuals and textbooks; some demanded (and some got) greater access to anatomical dissections and formal training, while others pushed for associations or guilds. At the same time, however, the male professions resisted the competition from women, and male midwives coming out of the surgeons' ranks began competing with the women. For many women (and their husbands), this was unacceptable, in part thanks to the thought of large male hands manipulating the emerging baby and its tender environment. For some, however, male midwives represented the cutting edge of proper science, combining theoretical knowledge as well as obstetrical training. They also used some new tools adapted to the purpose, such as forceps from about 1750.

Some women, such as Madame Angelique du Coudray in France, responded by providing across France formalized training of appropriate women, including the use of life-size models of the mother's birth canal. Du Coudray had been chosen by Louis XVI for the task, a reminder of the state's interest in healthy births. In Italy, Bologna opened one school in 1753, and between 1757 and 1779, another 13 midwifery schools appeared. Spain's first opened in Madrid in 1787. By 1751,

William Smellie of London had trained some 900 male midwives in two-week courses that tended to have practicing physicians and surgeons as students. Women's health care had to have improved somewhat by this embracing of obstetrics by the surgeon's profession, though this led to the further denigration of women midwives as ignorant and unskilled (Green 2008).

Contraception, Conception, and Abortion

Early modern European midwives, and many other women, knew how to avoid pregnancy or at least lessen its probability. This was possible by prolonging lactation by nursing, or by coitus interruptus (male's pulling out), by inserting a semen-absorbing sponge in the vagina, or by otherwise blocking the entrance with an impermeable membrane (as a female condom does today). Herbalists, apothecaries, and midwives knew of the supposed contraceptive properties of certain plants, but these, like black hellebore, were also powerful abortifacients and had to be used very carefully. Ignorant and rural Europeans often relied on talismans, chants, and rituals. Then as now, the Catholic Church condemned the intentional termination of any pregnancy, and civil laws often provided the death penalty for those involved in abortions. Nonetheless, woman empirics (guided by practical experience), wise women, and male charlatans peddled abortifacients, even advertising under the euphemism "restoratives."

When conceiving was the issue, the same range of practitioners suggested a vast variety of sexual positions, types of foreplay, control of orgasms, astrological timing, poultices, potions, rituals, prayers, diet and exercise regimens, and talismans. Galenic humoralism, astrology, pagan folk beliefs, Roman Catholicism, and family lore all contributed to the mix. To produce a "dry" male child, the French doctor Joubert recommended conceiving right after the mother's period before the menses collected and produced a "moist" uterine atmosphere. He further suggested the "dry" male would benefit from conception during dry weather and while the mother consumed a "dry and cold" diet. The Italian Dr. Michele Savonarola wrote that the boy-desiring mother should lie on her right side, since it was supposedly warmer. Ideas like these spread through vernacular editions and translations of manuals and from the literate to their friends and patients. Women were rarely dissected through the 16th century, so physicians had very little experience with women's reproductive anatomy—to the extent that many believed there were up to seven chambers in the uterus, with the central one that in which hermaphrodite babies were gestated.

Pregnant European women received what prenatal care they could. In cities, physicians, apothecaries, and midwives could provide advice and reliefs for discomforts and monitor the baby's development. To prevent miscarriages, practitioners prescribed all manner of prayers, amulets, jewels, ointments, and, more helpfully, strict regimens of healthful diets, soothing herbs, emotional stability, and plenty of rest. In rural areas, a male professional would have been rather rare and would have been useful only in the event of problems such as fainting or unexpected vaginal discharges of blood or other matter. The pregnant woman would have relied on family, friends, the local pastor, and the midwife (Gélis 1991).

Giving Birth, Nursing, and the Wet Nurse

The word "midwife" in English derives from the German phrase *mit weib*, "with the wife or woman." The most important task of both mother and midwife was to bring forth a healthy baby. In most European cultures, the midwife prepared the birthing room, bringing her tools and drugs, and ensuring warmth, water, towels, and some modicum of comfort. Other women may have been present to encourage the struggling mother or to pray if matters went awry. Men's presence was a matter of culture. As labor began, amulets and precious stones were laid on the mother's belly; her vaginal area was lubricated and massaged, and she was given an enema (often ipecacuanha) to clear out her intestines and stimulants such as coffee or cocoa or an opiate such as laudanum.

The position the mother took to give birth was also a matter of custom, though over time it seems mothers were given multiple options. During the 18th century, as males took greater roles in birthing, the German birthing chair with its restrictive stirrups became widely popular, as did a special "lucinary bed" complete with stirrups, a reclining back, and a seat at the foot for the midwife.

As the baby descended the birth canal, it was best if the mother's effort alone could give it help. Urgent cries of "push!" in every European language accompanied the infant as it rotated in the canal and eventually emerged. When the baby was ill-positioned, however, the midwife earned her pay. Before the invention of the forceps in mid-18th-century England (apparently), and for long after, the skilled hands of the midwife gently but firmly assessed the situation and did what they could. If she proved helpless, the surgeon was called in to do what he could. Assuming the baby was emerging intact, he still might have the umbilical cord wrapped around his throat, choking, and need further manipulation.

Through all of this ran the constant threat of serious wounding: the baby could be damaged or deprived of air; the mother could be badly bruised or slashed accidentally by one of the midwife's tools or left with hemorrhaging from a torn uterus. The constant threat was a vast variety of infections, from bacteria natural to the mother's interior, to those on the midwife's hands or tools, to those on bystanders or in the air or the dirt floor of the hut. In institutions where births were carried out, such as 18th-century lying-in hospitals, puerperal (from *puer*, "boy") fever—a type of blood poisoning—could run rampant among recuperating mothers, in a week or so killing from 10 to 100 percent. The problem, of course, was lack of cleanliness in everyone and at every stage of the birth-giving process. For the woman, each birth was a gamble with death. Lindsay Wilson states that 1 of every 10 babies was stillborn (or killed during birth) and that 1 of every 80 births resulted in the death of either mother or child. One of every 10 adult women died in childbirth in 18th-century France. Another study showed that in England around 1650, there were 160 maternal deaths for every 10,000 births, dropping to 105 during the early 18th century and 75 as 1800 approached (Wilson 1993, 140).

For most women between 1500 and 1800, there was no question whether the new mother would suckle her own child. Women of the middling and upper class, however, could forbear nursing and hire a wet nurse who had recently had a child of her own and was still lactating. The fathers were usually the ones who vetted and hired wet nurses and decided whether the child and nurse would live at her home—often in the cleaner country air—or in the urban family home. Like midwives, wet nurses needed reputations for morality and responsibility. This was especially important if the child were to be left with her but only little less so if she joined the infant's family for a couple of years. The practice of wet nursing had had critics among churchmen and others for centuries, and enlightened society began to turn against the practice in the later 18th century. This was spurred in part by the opening pages of Jean-Jacques Rousseau's *Émile* in which he decries the practice as unnatural (Read 2011).

Hysteria

Sixteenth- and seventeenth-century Galenic physicians accepted the Aristotelian notion that women were by nature humorally cold and moist. Being thus physically and intellectually weaker than males, they were subject to a wider range of both physical and emotional illnesses than males. The uterus or womb served not only to host the fetus during pregnancy but to collect menstrual fluid, considered a poison, and other corrupted humors and noxious bodily fluids. These swelled the sack-like structure, causing it to move about the abdomen. It also released "vapors" that somehow rose to a woman's head and triggered abnormal behaviors. The resulting mental or emotional sickness took the name "hysteria" from the Greek word *hystera*—uterus—and it could range from mild to very serious. Symptoms included swollen abdomen, tightness of the throat and breathing problems, paralysis, loss of sensation, and uncontrolled contortions of the body. Menstruation and female orgasms released the substances that built up, but chaste women were supposedly deprived of orgasms and many women suffered problems with their menstrual cycles, for example, due to poor diets or back-breaking work. Thus did early modern European medicine view what it labeled hysteria (see Martensen 2004, Scull 2009, and Peterson 2010).

Midwives, who often handled women's medical problems, had their personal remedies, including manipulating the uterus to stimulate menstruation or an orgasm, or tightly strapping or lacing the lower abdomen to keep the wandering womb in place. Male physicians sought the same basic goals, without the manual part: fumigation of the uterus with foul or fragrant odors, herbal douches, exercise, purging, drugs, and diets that avoided moist foods. Some modern herbalists still recommend the harsh purgative herb black hellebore for "hysteria," promoting menstruation, and as an abortifacient (Riddle 1997, 124). Of course, if a demon, witch, or curse were to have brought on the condition, other measures were necessary, from exorcism to burning the offending witch. "Hysterical" symptoms of apparent loss of control appeared as what many believed possession by a spiritual force might look like. Exactly this way of thinking fueled the witch craze of the 16th and 17th centuries.

In turn, just such superstitions and ignorance provoked many later-17th-century scientific revolutionaries, especially in England, to shine the light of reason on "women's problems." Prominent physicians felt that ailing women should no longer be left to "quacking jugglers and old women" but deserved the benefits of science. Dr. Nathaniel Highmore, admittedly using analogy rather than scientific observation, declared that hysteria stemmed not from the uterus but from the blockage and sudden release of blood into the lungs, which created the familiar suffocating effect and other hysterical symptoms. It was a problem of the blood's accumulation and "fermentation"—a trendy process—so he duly bled his hysterical patients. In the 1670s, Dr. Thomas Willis also retained traditional Galenic therapies for what he labeled the "so-called uterine disease": bleeding at the neck, purging, and a regimen of diet, rest, and exercise. As a scientist, though, Willis shifted attention away from the womb and blood vessels to supposed blockages in the nerves. Along with others, he understood nerves to be tiny tubes through which "animal spirits" circulated through the body and back to the brain. Since everyone had nerves and a brain, hysteria was not a female problem at all. It was a "convulsive disorder," and thus similar in his mind to scurvy, asthma, and epilepsy. He went so far as to autopsy a woman who died during a bout of hysteria and found no abnormalities in her uterus.

Willis's writings led to the demise of the exclusively female nature of hysteria during the 18th century. Spanish physician Martín Martínez disproved the roving uterus in 1728; the Italian Giovanni Battista Morgagni advanced the alternative theory of nerve blockage two decades later; and even Pope Benedict XIV, a science enthusiast, embraced the new model. But women had to remain both special and inferior to men, even enlightened men. In defining hysteria, science had begun replacing Galenic humoralism with a more mechanical model of the brain and conductive nerves, but the medium by which sense information was conducted to the brain and signals to the body's limbs and organs were conducted from the brain remained poorly understood and defined. Just as Isaac Newton labeled the famous force that attracted the apple to the earth "gravity"—heaviness—so Willis and others called the supposed medium "spirits": sometimes "animal" and sometimes "vital" spirits. Following John Locke's famous statement that we learn only by our sensory experiences, the theory was that through the flow of spirits, the brain accumulated information, and the person learned and became smarter. In males, the flow was stronger, and thus the male was both more intelligent and, by virtue of the greater flow to the limbs, had greater physical strength than the female. They believed women's less robust nervous system, smaller brains, and naturally weaker control over their emotions made them more susceptible to what were now labeled nervous disorders, though men were subject, too. Delicate women were associated with the aristocracy, and so were many types of nervous disorder; hence they became rather fashionable. Since no one had a clue as to how to treat weakened or blocked nerves and spirits, physicians retained Galenic guidelines of good living but added some of the many new patent drugs that claimed to strengthen female "vitals" (Vila 1998).

The Cutting Edge: Mesmerism

From about 1750, Europe, and especially France, experienced an epidemic of "nervous disorders," or so practitioners proclaimed. In 1782/83, the English Royal Society of Medicine sponsored an essay contest whose entries explained why "nervous disorders are very widespread, and have never been more common in the two sexes" (Wilson 1993, 127). The pressures of court or bourgeois life, childbearing and rearing, greater luxury and little exercise, repressed sexual urges, and other sexual anxieties topped the largely female-centric list. By the 1770s, "vitalism" was in decline, however, as research in electricity and magnetism fascinated the fickle philosophical crowd, especially in Paris. But it was in Vienna that Franz Mesmer first demonstrated that the nervous "spirits" were actually a magnetic *fluidum* that could be externally manipulated by magnets or even his own biological magnetism. His cure of Franzl Osterlin made him famous, but his botching of the treatment of Maria Theresa von Paradies's blindness drove him to Paris. Here he broadened the claimed value of his treatments—handholding, hugging "magnetic" trees, demagnetizing baths—to cure pains of all sorts. Mesmerism was officially debunked in 1784, but Mesmer retained many faithful supporters, especially among women (Dormandy 2006, 139–150).

5

Infant and Children's Health

Until recently, social historians and other scholars of early modern European family life often depicted parents as choosing to remain emotionally distant from their children. Their reasoning was that since childhood death rates were so high—for example, around 1700, 50 percent of London children died by age 12—parents did not want to get emotionally attached. Evidence included the practice of sending newborns out to nurse, frequency of abandonment and even infanticide, and the lack of a clear "culture of childhood" supported by families. More recent historians of childhood have redrawn the picture, portraying European culture as being truly invested in children, especially by the era of the Enlightenment. One view is that the nuclear family—as distinct from the extended family or clan—was invented during the 17th century by the urban middle class. Along with that was the invention or recognition of childhood as a distinct period of a person's life (Bell 1999, 135). The facts of early modern childhood have not changed, but they have been reinterpreted and added to. In this chapter, we survey the facts of childhood in various places rather than its interpretative history.

The emerging notion that children were not merely "little adults" but people in a unique phase of life had some important consequences. The early 18th century seems to have been a turning point. In Europe, the term "pediatrics" was coined to indicate the medical side of childhood and labeled a new framework for understanding and addressing the problems of childhood. New educational theories by John Locke and Jean-Jacques Rousseau emphasized the psychology of early learning and the importance of experience. From the states' point of view, children were valuable as the next generation and thus a resource to be nurtured and protected. At the same time, the industrialization taking place in Britain and elsewhere made claims on the small bodies, small hands, and nimble fingers that the young could bring to the new factories. With the assault on the vile practice of the slave trade plantation, owners prized Afro-Caribbean slave children as never before, since they alone would be the next generation of labor. The late 18th century even saw the emergence of maternity facilities and nurseries for slaves' children in the British West Indies (Sheridan 1985).

THEY ARE BORN: NEONATAL AND INFANT HEALTH

The Trauma of Birth

The child's entry into the world was natural but traumatic and hazardous. In many cultures, the experienced midwife handled most issues, but she was supported by the surgeon or healer who waited in the wings to rescue the child and/or mother in an emergency. The child in the womb could have had any of many weakening conditions stemming from genetic inheritance or the mother's behavior or accidents. The trip from the womb to the world had its threats. He might not be situated correctly for the voyage and have to be repositioned manually; she might be tangled in the umbilical cord; he might not rotate as needed during descent; and she might contract dangerous germs from the birth canal itself or the midwife's unsanitary hands. The midwife might poke or pull the small body with too much force, crippling him for life. Once emerged, the light blow or spank might not get the lungs breathing properly; the cutting and tying of the umbilical cord could introduce infection or accidentally puncture the infant. Bacteria could cause diarrhea and accompanying dehydration. Though usually treated carefully, one would imagine, the light, air, sounds and other unfamiliar sensations assaulted the newborn as she was held upside down to drain the throat and ear canals and then washed and wrapped tightly. For mother, child, and midwife, the successful live birth was a true triumph, however natural, for many passages into the world ended in tragedy (see Gélis 1991).

Infant Care and Nursing

Many early modern communities debated the rationale and wisdom of having newborn nurse with someone other than his or her birth mother. Poor families had no real options, and mothers breastfed their own if at all possible. Wealthier mothers, however, could become pregnant again sooner if they did not breastfeed, a choice often dictated by the male head of the household. Women who had been badly weakened or infected during labor or in its aftermath might choose not to nurse, and men who had fathered babies with unmarried servants or other women also often chose to send the baby away. Hiring a wet nurse, however, could mean either having her stay in the family's residence or sending the child to the wet nurse's home. Generally the fathers made the contracts, and generally with the nurse's husband. Reliable statistics are difficult to come by, and historians Rudolph Bell and Stephen Ozment warn against overestimating the practice in Italy and Germany respectively. On the other hand, Barbara Dunlap estimates that in later-18th-century Paris, of some 20,000 babies born each year, only around 3 percent were breastfed by their own mothers, and 92 percent were sent to the countryside to be fed by a stranger. In his *Èmile* (1762), French philosopher Jean-Jacques Rousseau, who fathered several children and sent them all to foundling homes, strongly advised breastfeeding by mothers as a healthier practice that bonded the two. In a modern study of British infants for the same period, deaths were shown to be 30 percent lower among those who were breastfed by their mothers (Bell 1999, 135–136; Dunlap 1997).

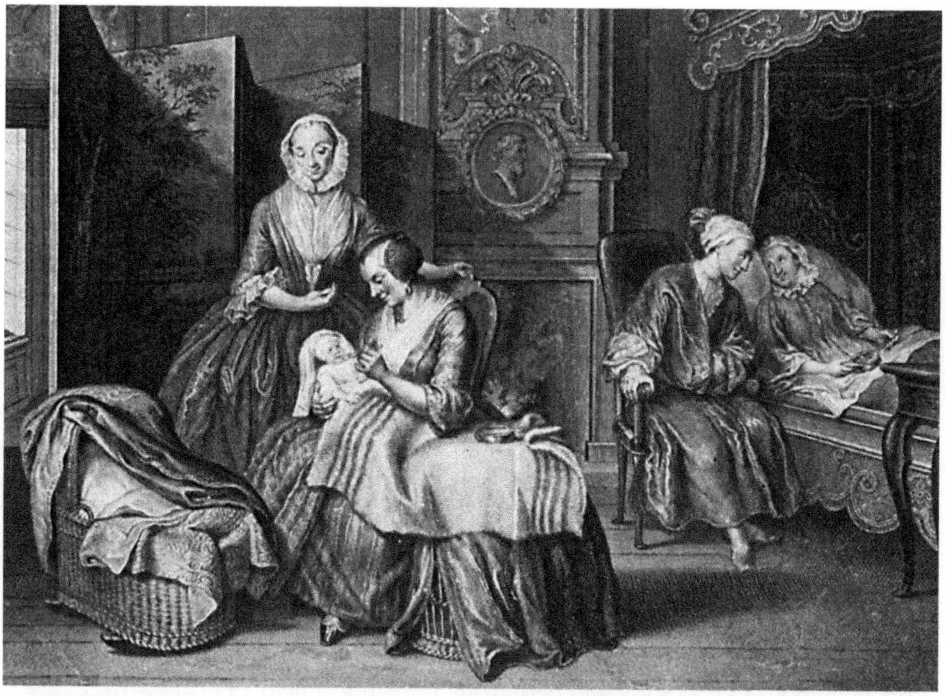

In this engraving of a work by Cornelis Troost (1697–1750), a wealthy Dutch woman rests in bed after childbirth, while the seated wet nurse prepares to feed the newborn infant. (National Library of Medicine)

Of course, the healthfulness of the milk was in many ways dependent on the diet of the mother. In situations of slavery, poverty, or social disruption, or where vitamin-rich diets were simply not available, a nursing child might suffer nutritional deprivation. Tuscan mothers generally nursed for two years, and West Indian slaves for three when allowed. Slave children often suffered from beriberi, scurvy, pellagra, rickets, and other diet deficiency conditions thanks to the poor diets generally afforded by their owners.

Threats to Infant Health

The Shadow World

The shadow world presented a hazard only slowly disposed of across our period. Demons, ghosts, elves, fairies, demigods, breath-sucking cats, gnomes, jinn, witches, and a host of other religious or folk entities were invoked to explain sudden deaths, emotional traumas, emergent skin deformities, and other abnormalities that very young minds or flesh suffered. Aztec families feared that "emanations" (*ihiyotl*, or "garbage air") from adults who broke sexual norms—homosexuals, adulterers, prostitutes—adversely affected the state of nearby infants' *tonalli*, or animating life force. Invading Spaniards brought the notion of the evil eye (*mal de ojo*), a parallel threat from unhealthy adults or witches, whose glance could cause a variety of maladies. In both cases, infants were protected by objects colored red, including coral necklaces, and cured with magical rituals involving eggs and herbs (Ortiz de Montellano 1990, 223–225). By the late 18th century, most cultures had eliminated these forces from medical considerations or at least reduced their perceived role.

Disease

Ming Chinese physicians considered smallpox to be the single greatest threat to a newborn's health. Smallpox was endemic in China and was linked directly to a notion called fetal poison. By the 17th century, many believed that the sex act creating the infant was polluting to both child and mother, and neonatal diseases, including smallpox, were the result. A paste of the child's roasted and dried umbilical cord and purgative pills of licorice and cinnabar became popular oral prophylactics against these diseases. Neonatal smallpox and other skin-manifesting conditions came to be seen as generated from within the baby's body as the poisons engendered in the sex act rose to the surface to escape. Rather than life threatening, they came to be seen as necessary to cleanse the body for a healthy childhood. These insights were collected by a new breed of physician who took interest in the ills of both women and children, a trend that later had important effects on both gynecology and pediatrics in China (Furth 1999, 178–182).

The infant also faced a wide range of other diseases. Infant syphilis was encountered and discussed in Europe as early as the 1490s. Mothers could pass this on in the womb, or it might be encountered in the birth canal. Doctors and laymen alike blamed it on the wet nurses when possible, and on the mother's own milk when used. Nine or ten days after birth, the infant might develop tetanus of the navel from exposure of the tender area to dirt and the germs. An estimated 25 percent who contracted this died. Measles, mumps, rubella, scarlet fever, flu, whooping cough, chicken pox, tuberculosis, various rashes, and other so-called childhood diseases plagued many in a given community, and any might turn deadly if the conditions were right and especially during an epidemic.

Those born in late-15th and early-16th-century Latin America were swept away in huge numbers by the many infectious diseases introduced by European and later African newcomers. When in some cases the germs destroyed adults more readily than children, the loss of their caretakers left infants helpless even when unaffected themselves.

Infanticide

Infanticide is the intentional killing of an infant. It might have been accomplished simply by leaving the child exposed to the elements and wild animals or by physical abuse of almost any kind. If it appeared that the murdered child was stolen or killed by accident, the murderer might even receive sympathy from the community. Sudden infant death that occurred in the parents' bed, whereby the infant died naturally or was crushed or smothered by one or both parents, could be a natural tragedy, an accident, or a tragic act of desperation. Both Jewish and

Church authorities often imposed spiritual penalties on parents regardless of its determined cause: even an accident was attributed to God's punishment for the parents' sins. Among Catholics, infanticide was usually punished with excommunication. Infanticide was most commonly associated with situations of rape or incest, adultery, or some clear physical disability or mental defect on the child's part (Shahar 1992, 126–139).

A related phenomenon was infant sacrifice, practiced, for example, among the pre-Christian Inca of Peru. According to Spanish observers, Incan culture apparently considered infants and children to be "natural resources" possessed more by the community than their families. These "commodities" were among the finest of sacrifices made to the gods at communal turning points such as coronations, wars, and, ironically, epidemics. Among the Aztecs, the young were annually sacrificed to the god of rain, Tlaloc. For some reason, the deity preferred those with hairlines sporting twin forelocks or widow's peaks (Dean 2002, 44; Ortiz de Montellano 1990, 195).

Accidents

Birth itself was fraught with harm from accidents, and after birth, the child faced a long list of threats from accidents. Tightly wrapping swaddling clothes were often applied immediately to the newborn to protect her from the elements but also as a way of immobilizing her. Yet cradles could be overturned; children roll off of high furniture; animals wound, kill, or carry off infants. They could be smothered or choked, wounded by knives or other sharp household objects, burned by household fires or lamps, scalded by hot water, drown in tubs or ponds, or be injured by larger animals such as horses or wild boars. Toddlers, of course, could get into all sorts of danger moving about within the house or beyond into streets, yards, or fields. Threats came from rabid or poisonous animals, and from smoke, dust, worms, and other parasites and environmental factors. Children have always been prone to put things in their mouths, and given the unsanitary conditions so many lived in, poisoning had to have occurred. They were also prone to choking on small objects and harm from oral experimentation with sharp or pointed objects.

In poorer families, children often tended those younger than themselves, and the results could be tragic. Neglect was far more likely where no servant or family member was dedicated to caring for the very young. Of course, caregivers were just as capable of being neglectful, and even a mother suffering from postpartum depression might give her little one little or no attention.

HAZARDS TO OLDER CHILDREN'S HEALTH AND LIVES

That infants were a special type of person and patient was obvious to all. Older children who could walk around and speak meaningfully, on the other hand, at some point became adults. At what point, however, was unclear and a matter of culture or debate. Very often children were treated medically as they were usually treated socially: as little adults. But their small bodies simply could not undergo purging or bleedings, and adult dosages of medicines seemed clearly inappropriate.

When ill, children often had a difficult time describing their pains or even articulating where on their bodies the unnatural feeling was occurring. Doctors could and did check pulse, urine, stool, and temperature (hot, cold, normal), but their diagnoses were necessarily limited.

Disease

Medical treatises on what came to be called pediatrics (child medicine) were not new to early modern Europe, whether for the professional or, increasingly, the layman. Mothers and female custodians of children were always their first line of defense when illness struck. In his 16th-century *The Godmother*, the Italian Brother Mercurio discussed 37 childhood diseases in 28 chapters. He divided them into "internal" and "external" problems, though his logic is not always clear. The internal were fevers, chicken pox, bodily swelling, suppurations, epilepsy, convulsions, paralysis and torpor, nightmares, sleeplessness, running nose, congested nose, coughs, breathing problems, earaches, strep throat, mouth sores, teething, hiccups, vomiting, bed-wetting, retained urine, stone, constipation, diarrhea, intestinal blockage, body aches, and worms. His external problems included cradle cap, lice, water on the brain, inflamed eyes, crossed eyes, cracked lips, scrofula, umbilical or navel problems, and distended colon. Importantly, he taught that none of these necessarily required a physician, and he provided practical and reasonable treatments for each. Near the end of the 17th century, English statistician John Graunt made the following list of diseases common to four- and five-year-olds: the fungal throat condition known as thrush; convulsions; the potentially bone deforming vitamin D deficiency known as rickets; worms; problems with one's teeth, and especially teething; chrysomes; and of course measles and smallpox (Knight 2006, 117–119; Bell 1999, 141–151).

Accidents

Older children were more capable of avoiding many of the hazards to the very young. Being much more mobile, however, they were capable of getting into far more trouble. Around the house, they were expected to work as if little adults, and this could lead to all sorts of accidents since their strength, coordination, and judgment were not as well developed as those of adolescents or adults. Falls from windows, stairs, or roofs, into wells or pits, down steep slopes, or from carts or horses could break bones or cause death. Scalding, burns, injuries from falling objects, cuts from knives, glass, or other household objects, kicks from horses or other farm animals, and bites from rabid dogs or other feral animals were also serious threats. The fear of being lost in a forest haunts many traditional stories and was no doubt a very real possibility.

Work-Related Hazards

In many urban settings, boys were expected to work outside of the family from an early age. The guild and apprentice system in Europe, for example, allowed boys as young as six or seven to be placed by their families with masters who would train them in an occupation over the next decade or more. Youngsters had value by performing certain simple but important tasks in almost any setting. Known as shop boys, they might be tasked with running errands, cleaning up, preparing materials, repairing machines, tending fires, fetching water, and a host of other jobs that differed by the occupation and as they grew older and more capable and experienced. They worked around men whose tolerance for childish misbehavior was probably typically low. They worked around dangerous machines such as printing presses and mill gears and by the 18th century in factories with steam-driven machines that were unforgiving of error. Children were used to clean chimneys from inside and squeeze into tight spaces to do the dangerous jobs grown men could not perform. Girls might help mothers who were laundresses, making themselves subject to the same problems the adults were and to the risk of falling into rivers and drowning. Even in the countryside, children were used to tend sheep or other animals and risked both the disease of anthrax and predator attacks—especially wolves. Girls who were sent out as servants ran the risk of sexual assault, and boys beatings or other abuse from employers, masters, or other members of their households.

Violence

Defenseless children in the early modern world were also threatened by violence from other corners. At home, naturally abusive, drunken, or mentally ill parents or other older family members preyed on children as they do today. Corporal punishment by parents was expected among all levels of society, and there could be a fine line between severe discipline and violence. In Aztec Mexico, physical discipline was considered appropriate from age 10 and could include beatings and forced inhalation of burning chili smoke, the equivalent of modern pepper spray (Lipsett-Rivera 2002, 66). Among older girls, there was always the threat of rape or molestation by older siblings or half-siblings or stepfathers; and stepmothers were stereotypically mean to and abusive of their stepdaughters. Bullying by older siblings or others could go too far and cause serious injuries. Because adult males tended to be given the benefit of the legal doubt in most early modern cultures, there was little recourse for those victimized in the household if the fathers did not intervene.

Outside the home, childnapping was known to most cultures, especially where domestic slavery was practiced. Of course, the very practice of chattel slavery was abusive, and children felt its sting as did their parents. In West Africa, native slavers seized athletic young boys to sell to the white slave traders, as in the famous case of Olaudah Equiano, who later gained his freedom and wrote of his enslavement and in favor of abolition (Equiano 1995). Among older children, pederast males preyed on boys, and girls could be stolen away or run away to lives of prostitution. Children also suffered from the ravages of war and other human-made disasters. Along with their parents or other caregivers, they were subject to being wounded, starved, stricken by disease, or physically abused. As violence swept through their world, they were often left orphaned and uncared for (see Brockliss and Montgomery 2010 and Martin 2009).

EUROPEAN INSTITUTIONS OF CHILDCARE

The Islamic Ottoman Empire had no orphanages or foundling hospitals. In fact, there was little provision for child patients in the *bimaristans* or other health facilities. The Muslim sense of family responsibility to its youngest members was very strong (Shefer-Mossensohn 2009, 132–134). Europe was different.

Children who lost or were abandoned by their families suffered a number of emotional and mental problems in addition to the possibility of being physically abused. All things equal, the younger one was, the less psychic damage was likely to be inflicted. Confusion, grief, sorrow, sadness, despair, and even guilt could accompany the change. These emotional states might be manifested in unacceptable behaviors including bedwetting, violent acting out, apathy and lack of affect, nightmares, disobedience, or eating disorders. In an age when children were to "be seen and not heard" and "spared not the rod," adult caregivers felt justified using corporal punishment to curb unacceptable behavior.

The Orphanage and Foundling Hospital

Christian charity had always pointed to the widow, the disabled, and the orphan as being worthy of support. Most children who lost both of their parents were taken in by other family members, neighbors, or, if old enough, guild masters who would raise them as apprentices. Both age and sex were important factors, since older children could earn their keep, and boys could be fostered or apprenticed out more readily than girls. On a farm, both girls and boys could be put to work as early as age five or six. Younger children or infants were a matter of pure expense, and even uncles would be reluctant to take them in. During times of famine, war, or epidemic, orphans proliferated, and support systems often disappeared altogether. Monks and especially nuns had traditionally cared for those otherwise left to their fate, and in Catholic countries, many still did.

In the later Middle Ages, and especially after the Black Death, wealthy Christians provided and staffed homes for orphans and abandoned infants in larger cities. Some of these were run by the Church, but increasingly civic authorities or secular boards managed them. One of the most famous was the Ospedale degli Innocenti in Florence. It was established in the last will (1410) of the local merchant Francesco Datini, himself orphaned in 1348 by the Black Death. He arranged to have one of Florence's chief guilds administer his gift, since he did not trust Florentine Church authorities. The Ospedale still stands: having been designed by the great Brunelleschi, it was one of the earliest masterpieces of Renaissance architecture. It operated beside the hospitals of San Gallo and La Scala, which also cared for children. In the 17th century, Amsterdam hosted 11 orphanages, providing shelter to some 3,400 children. One was specifically for the children of citizens and one for those of poor residents. Mennonites ran three, Catholics had two, and Lutherans, Huguenots, and members of the Dutch Reformed Church administered one each. City regulations required that each child brought in first be thoroughly washed and deloused (Gavitt 1991; Phillips 2008, 169–183). French cities had their *Charités* for orphans staffed by nuns and often attached to the

Maison Dieu charity hospital. In Paris, the Trouvés foundling hospital recorded having received 7,600 new charges in 1771 alone. Many of these died in the hospital, but city records also claimed that many Parisian newborns were simply left to die in the streets and fell prey to animals that roamed them (Barnes 2005, 142).

However well meaning the personnel that staffed these institutions, death rates, especially among infants, were horrific. In Renaissance Florence, upward of 7 in 10 died before their first birthday. In 17th- and 18th-century Paris and London, figures ranged from a third to 90 percent. Disease, neglect, accidents, sickness, and poor nutrition increased the death rolls, which were even greater during times of famine, epidemic, or war. Though practices differed, wet nurses were generally chosen to feed the youngest, and often this meant farming them out to the countryside with its hazards and uncertainties. Such wet nurses were probably paid little, resulting in many cases of children starving, being fed cows' milk, being neglected, or dying.

The poor, young mother leaving her infant in a basket at the door of a church or convent was not just a cliché; it was a reality for thousands. Unlike the orphan, the foundling was abandoned by his or her mother or by a father who lost his wife to the birth or other cause. Though of course the baby did not understand, society tended to blame the mother for her action. Often the mother was unmarried, and whether the infant was a love child, a side effect of a life of prostitution, or a product of rape, society viewed the mother as having been irresponsible. The children, too, tended to be tainted by social disdain, marked as having had immoral, uncaring, or even cursed parents. With perhaps 70,000 residents, Florence's women abandoned an average of 200 infants each year from 1450 to 1500. During the terrible years of the 1530s, the average more than doubled to 540 per annum. During this time, 22 percent of babies baptized in the city were abandoned (Gavitt 2011, 30–31).

Like those in orphanages, children in foundling homes lived in conditions varying from tender and loving to brutal. Mortality was high, and few lived to reach adulthood. Parents, mothers especially, could and did return to reclaim their infants. Some even gave birth, left the child with a facility, and then served as his wet nurse, gaining a small stipend for doing what she would have done for nothing. Such an arrangement served all parties involved, since the mother probably took much greater care of the child than if left to the staff and wet nurse.

Outside of cities, parish authorities often tended those left with them, arranging for appropriate care, feeding, and sometimes even education. In Catholic communities, some religious brotherhoods or confraternities and even formal orders of the Church, such as the Order of the Holy Spirit, were dedicated to infant care and placement. Where such organizations were lacking, desperate mothers or uncaring fathers resorted to infanticide or sale of the child into slavery or servitude (Shahar 1992, 122–125).

In European colonies, foundling homes were among the first institutions established by both religious and political authorities. Out-of-wedlock births among white men and women who were lower-class natives or slaves often resulted in the offspring's abandonment. As late as 1700, King Philip V of Spain received reports of newborns in Havana, Cuba, being tossed into the sea, smothered by parents, and left in streets to be eaten by dogs. In 1711, Casa Joseph opened to receive foundlings, the vast majority of whom were newborns. Yet this was no panacea, as in its early years, 75 percent of its charges died within six months of being admitted. Though conditions and survival rates improved (only 12% died in 1733), Casa Joseph had to close in 1755 due to misadministration (González 2002).

Lying-in Hospitals

The health of the mother was a major factor in the health of the child. When births took place under unsafe conditions, the infant often died, as did the mother. In Enlightenment Europe, patrons or communities began founding lying-in hospitals—often associated with foundling hospitals. These were facilities in which a pregnant woman—whether married or not was a community norm—lacking any other resources could give birth with relative safety. Pregnant prostitutes, servant girls, errant daughters, runaways, and poor but married women had the help of one or more midwives or midwives in training, as well as a surgeon or even physician on call. The child was thereby protected from abortion or infanticide, at least until the mother was released, and had the benefit of trained personnel if needed. If necessary, the hospital arranged for the infant to be left with a foundling home. In Paris's later-18th-century Hôtel Dieu charity hospital, 80 percent of pregnant women admitted were single and 90 percent of women who gave birth left their children behind to be cared for. Such facilities were not merely a matter of humanitarianism or Christian charity but of the state's concern for the survival of the next generation to bear babies, pay taxes, and fill the ranks of soldiers. Among the Aztecs before Cortés, newborn boys were given a small shield and a bow with four arrowheads as a symbol of their future profession as warriors. Infant mortality among the Aztecs was estimated at between 30 and 40 percent (Soustelle 1961/2002, 164).

Dispensaries

Poor urban mothers may have had their babies in lying-in hospitals, but if they kept their babies, they faced myriad health issues for which they had no preparation or resources. Religious houses in Catholic countries, civic physicians, poorhouses, and other charitable organizations helped when they could, but if a mother were single or of known low repute, the odds of help were slim. In 1769, physician George Armstrong created a new type of facility in London to help poor mothers and their sick infants. His dispensary was merely a point of distribution for advice and free medicines. There were no strings attached or questions asked. Of course, it is safe to say that the mothers who sought the help provided lived with their child or children in squalid conditions or filth, disease, and poverty. All too many of the children aided failed to live to pass it forward (Kilpatrick 1990, 254–255).

6

Diseases

Infectious diseases are those that are transmitted from someone or something that already has the disease's pathogens to someone who does not. No one "catches" a broken leg, a toothache, or diabetes from someone who already has the ailment, but one does "catch" a cold, plague, measles, typhus, malaria, or gonorrhea from an already infected source or carrier. Such diseases remained major causes of debilitation and death throughout the world and throughout the early modern period.

BACKGROUND

Pathogens and Epidemics

A carrier—which might be a fly, flea, louse, mosquito, tick, food, water source, or human—contacts a victim by sneezing or coughing, touching, biting, stinging, defecating on, injecting, or being consumed. The carrier thus passes the virus, bacterium, fungus, protozoon, or other pathogen into the new host's bloodstream, lymphatic system, lungs, digestive system, or other organs. If the victim is healthy, her immune system may isolate and destroy the invaders; she may already have immunity because of a previous infection by the same or related pathogen. If she is not healthy, and the pathogen is strong and numerous, it will overcome her body's defenses by outwitting or defeating them.

Some pathogens will do enough damage to kill their new host; others weaken her, leaving her unable to stave off subsequent, unrelated—opportunistic—pathogens. Still others, such as certain "childhood diseases," do minor damage and confer immunity by causing the body to create effective and long-lasting defenses.

Because these pathogens are passed through some sort of contact (even if only by breath), we call them contagious. In general, to thrive, these need large numbers of people living in close proximity so that the chain of contacts can be maintained and the organism can continue to survive and replicate. Where population densities are low, the pathogen runs out of victims and eventually changes or disappears. Where conditions are right, the carriers can contact many people. The chain begins and is sustained by new and susceptible victims. When many people are affected over a fairly short period of time, we speak of an epidemic; when a great many people are affected over a very broad geographic area and relatively long period of time, the outbreak is often labeled a pandemic. Prior to modern transportation, pandemics were rare because pathogens could be transported only at the speed of sail, river current, horse, or human legs (see also Gorbach, Bartlett, and Blacklow 2003).

Even so, during the early modern period contagious diseases probably killed more people than any other factor. This was especially true where pathogens landed in "virgin soil," among populations that had never experienced the disease before. This biological "naiveté" meant that there was no natural immunity in the population and no known defenses or healing processes. After contact with Europeans and Africans, natives of North and South America were slaughtered by such diseases, as were many native Pacific and most Caribbean islanders. In turn, European sailors, slavers, soldiers, missionaries, and colonists died by the thousands of unfamiliar tropical diseases in Africa, the Americas, and the Caribbean. The early modern period saw the world shrink through European "discovery," trade, conquest, and colonization. Huge numbers of Africans were transplanted as slaves into the Western Hemisphere, bringing their own pathogens that found new victims among natives and Europeans alike (see Byrne 2008 and Kiple 2003).

Limitations of Early Modern Medicine

Apart from gradual but inevitable mixing of populations and pathogen pools, the period was marked by a deadly ignorance of human physiology, microbiology, and medicine. No culture on Earth understood the medical model of the human body we take for granted today. Only fringe thinkers envisioned tiny "animalcules" causing horrific death tolls of plague or smallpox. Though inoculation as a means of protection against smallpox was known in Africa and other Islamic regions, and was adopted by Europeans in the 18th century, no one understood why and how it worked. And so it remained an isolated tool (see Carlin 2005).

The remainder of this chapter is a discussion of several among many major early modern infectious diseases, from plague to syphilis. They are organized by means and factors of transmission rather than by pathogen types or symptoms or another classification scheme that might be equally valid. People encountered these diseases in daily life or during epidemics through specific—if misunderstood—means.

THE CONTINUING SAGA: FLEAS, RATS, AND PLAGUE

The early modern period encompasses the second half of the Second Plague Pandemic (1347–1840s). Though sources are unclear about China, Europe and much of the Islamic world suffered recurring epidemics of bubonic and possibly pneumonic and septicemic plague. Though the medieval Black Death, the initial onslaught of the disease in the West from 1347 to 1352, killed perhaps 40 percent of the population and left few places unscathed, subsequent outbreaks were localized and usually much less deadly (see Aberth 2005 and Byrne 2006).

Plague and the Early Second Pandemic

Plague is an animal disease (zoonosis) caused by the bacterium *Yersinia pestis*. It lives in bloodstreams of a wide variety of rodents and other small mammals, and is transmitted when fleas suck infected blood from one host and then deposit bacteria when feeding on a second host. If the colony of rodents dies off, its fleas seek new hosts on which to feed. If the new hosts are human and fleas are many, an outbreak of plague can occur. Inside the human, the bacteria multiply rapidly, and many are collected in the lymphatic system. When accumulated in the lymph nodes of the groin and neck, the load of bacteria, pus, and other detritus causes nodes to swell into "buboes," a distinctive sign of bubonic plague. If collection is efficient and nodes handle the load, the patient lives; if not, bacteria spread through the bloodstream, affecting multiple organs. Malaise, fever, and delirium result, and the patient dies in about a week. If bacteria in the bloodstream are of a high enough quantity, death is swifter due to "poisoning" called septicemia. This deadly variation is septicemic plague, which kills so quickly that buboes have no time to form. Pneumonic plague results from *Y. pestis* bacteria being breathed into the respiratory system and acting quickly, and usually fatally, on the lungs. Though bubonic and septicemic plague forms require flea carriers for transmission, with pneumonic plague, simple coughing or sneezing can transmit *Y. pestis* to one or many others. Of course, at no point during the Second Plague Pandemic did anyone anywhere develop an understanding of the roles of bacteria, fleas, or rats. Medical practitioners and researchers, whether Christian, Muslim, or Enlightened, had much experience with plague but acquired little insight and no effective medical responses beyond isolation of the sick. Despite the Renaissance, Scientific Revolution, and Enlightenment, plague remained a matter of poisoned air (miasmas), and many continued to blame God and planets as the ultimate causal agents.

The Origins of Public Health Procedures

By 1500, plague was becoming an urban disease, though infected refugees or travelers might spread it to rural areas as well. At the same time, both Europeans and Muslims had learned to live with plague. Sixteenth-century European governments began adopting approaches pioneered by rulers of Italian city-states such as Venice, Milan, and Florence. Exercising a newfound willingness and ability to coerce their people, they imposed quarantines on suspect people, goods, and ships, and health cordons (no-go zones) around areas struck by plague. Closing city gates, erecting cordons, and quarantining merchant ships interrupted trade and interfered with profit, encouraging city officials to delay plague declarations until the outbreak was well established. Wealthier folks fled a city when plague was declared—usually determined by a certain number of confirmed plague cases

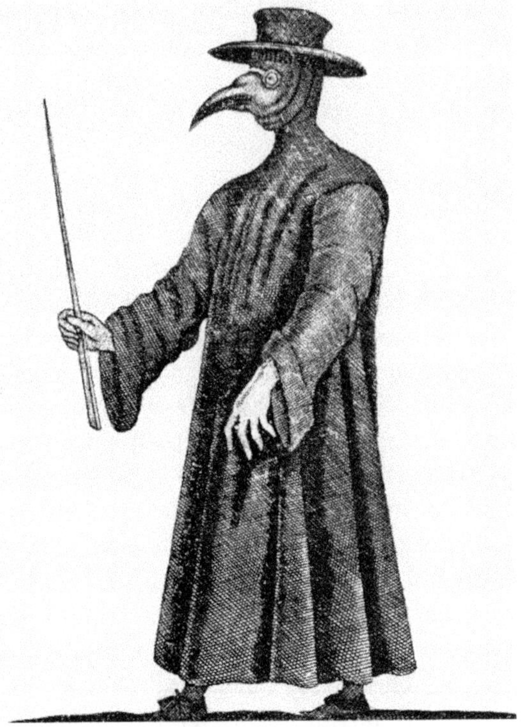

A physician sports the latest in plague-era protective clothing in this illustration from 1656. The wide-brimmed hat protects the head and face from poisonous precipitation, the oilcloth gown is impervious to the poisonous plague mists, the distinctive beak is filled with air-purifying herbs and flower petals, his hands are gloved, and he carries a wand to examine patients from a distance. (Wellcome Collection)

reported within a set time. Authorities then locked victims in their houses, built inadequate pest houses or lazarettos to house poorer victims, and had vagrants, beggars, prostitutes, and other undesirables expelled from their cities. London, Amsterdam, or Rome could become a ghost town in a week's time, leaving servants, apprentices, and the "lower sort" to fend for themselves. Shops closed, food became scarce, searchers patrolled streets for the dead, and corpses were tossed into rumbling carts and eventually mass graves. Bodies were also heaved into rivers that simply sluiced them downstream; they were also thrown into or dumped at sea, which in turn rejected them in horrible high tides of flesh and bone (see Byrne 2006 and Cipolla 1981).

In the Islamic World

People in Muslim countries, especially those around the Mediterranean Sea, experienced plague as often as Europeans did and for a longer period. Cities such as Istanbul, Alexandria, Cairo, and Damascus were drawn together more tightly after Ottoman Turks took control of Egypt in 1517. Increased contact, as among European port cities, meant increased opportunities for infection. But Muslims, even more than pious Christians, saw the hand of God in plague and adopted an acceptance of the disease that seems to have blunted attempts to prevent it. For the righteous, death by plague was martyrdom; for the wicked, it was just punishment. Therefore, as plague repeatedly swept through port cities, Turkish authorities did little to interfere. During the early modern era, they did rationalize the region's administration, paid more attention than previous rulers to sanitation and health care, and some sultans adopted elements of European medicine, but these advances did little to make life safer or more comfortable for the empire's peasants or workers. Islamic areas outside the Empire also continued to suffer: in the 1770s, a reported 2 million Persians died of plague, including 250,000 in Basra alone (see Borsch 2005 and Dols 1977).

The Second Pandemic's End Game

Between about 1650 and 1772, one major European city after another underwent one last major epidemic episode, followed by liberation from the pestilence. Civic responses were as sophisticated as they were going to get, as governments systematically engaged the tools they had acquired: civic bonfires to "fix" the corrupted air, quarantine, cordons, isolation, killing stray animals (even rats sometimes), burning the goods of victims, and executing those who bought or sold "infected" goods. Naples and Rome experienced their final plague epidemic in 1656 (together 173,000 died, though Rome suffered far less); Amsterdam in 1664 (35,000 dead) and London in 1665 and 1666 (70,000); Stockholm in 1711 (15,000) and Vienna during 1712–1714 (8,644 reported dead); Marseille and surrounding Provence during 1720–1722 (40,000 and 85,000 respectively); Messina, Sicily, in 1743 (50,000 of a population of 65,000); and Moscow during 1770–1772 (over 60,000): each in turn suffered and was seemingly immunized by the experience. Historians have long disputed why the disease retreated from Europe, but the dominant opinion is that human attempts succeeded in blocking recurrences due to importation of rats and fleas, especially by ship. Authorities bolstered efforts at cordons and quarantine, especially in the Mediterranean, as they saw Ottoman and other Muslim ports suffer repeatedly into the 1840s until they, too, successfully adopted these efforts (Byrne 2006, 281–297).

MOSQUITOES, MALARIA, AND YELLOW FEVER

Medieval and early modern people lived with rodents and fleas as common elements of their environments. This familiarity may have helped blind people to their roles in spreading plague. Malaria and yellow fever were Old World diseases spread by other ubiquitous pests, respectively the *anopheline* and *Aedes* mosquitoes. Early modern medical science was as ignorant of this connection as it was of the plague's bacterium-flea-rat-human chain, hence the name malaria, or "bad air" in Italian.

Malaria

Malaria is caused by parasitic protozoa of the *Plasmodium* family that are carried most effectively by mosquitoes of the *anopheline* family. The family is large, and 70 species can carry the protozoon. The mosquitoes prefer warm temperatures and still, stagnant water in which they lay eggs and that supports early stages of the insect's life cycle. Outside of humans, the protozoon reproduces sexually, but inside the human bloodstream, it does so asexually inside red blood cells, which are destroyed in the process. This happens over a two- or three-day cycle that accounts for the recurring "tertian," or third-day, fevers characteristic of malaria. Fever and anemia result, and the sufferer is weakened terribly by the combination. The protozoa can also hibernate in the liver for three-to five-year periods, emerging and causing the recurring fevers also associated with malaria.

Plasmodium has four types that can affect humans, and two—*P. vivax* and *P. falciparum*—that were common to Southern Europe and Africa, respectively. *Vivax* is the less virulent and plagued marshy areas as far north as England's Kent and East Anglian marshes. *Falciparum* is less discriminating about which red blood cells it invades, so far more cells are killed off within a victim, and many more victims succumb. *Falciparum* was far more common in Africa, and, despite its lethality, Central and Western Africans developed some natural defenses. Children who were bitten and survived gained a measure of immunity, and many developed and passed along the "sickle cell" trait that can lead to anemia but protects from *vivax* and, less so, *falciparum* (see Packard 2007 and Webb 2009).

Before the Age of Discovery, yellow fever was strictly an African disease, caused by an arbovirus (arthropod-borne virus) spread from victim to victim by the female *Aedes* mosquito. The virus requires the mosquito for reproduction, which it carries out in the insect's mid-gut. From there, it travels to the salivary glands from which it is deposited in the monkey or human bloodstream. Like other mosquitoes, *Aedes* reproduces in still water: pools, marshes, wheel ruts, or containers. For about a week after acquiring the virus, a victim suffers flu-like symptoms including chills, fever, and head and muscle aches. In a serious case, the kidneys shut down, and jaundice results from liver failure. The patient spews black vomit and hemorrhages. Within about a week, between 10 and 60 percent of patients die. Those who survive, however, do acquire immunity (see McNeill 2010, 32–52, 137–191; Kiple and Beck 1997; Pierce and Writer 2005).

Yellow Fever: The Tropical Scourge

Africans who lived with yellow fever and the more virulent *falciparum* form of malaria understood in their own terms the two diseases and had long developed ways of coping, both medicinal and cultural. When large numbers of these people were uprooted from their land and shipped as slaves to the Western Hemisphere, they and mosquitoes that lived and bred in ships' stagnant water supplies carried the pathogens with them. As the tragic cargoes spilled onto the wharves of colonial ports from Boston to Brazil, the diseases accompanied them. The mosquitoes fed indiscriminately on the immune and the uninfected alike, cross-infecting Europeans, natives, and blacks who had avoided infection or had been born in the colony.

The first major wave of yellow fever cases in the Caribbean began in the 1640s. As victims either died or were immunized, the epidemic cooled off for about 50 years. Spanish Havana, for example, suffered epidemics of yellow fever in 1649, 1651, 1652, and 1654, and again in 1709, 1715, 1730, 1731, 1733, 1738, and 1742. In 1762, during the Seven Years' War, an invading army of British troops was all but destroyed by the fever, while the largely immune Hispanic and slave population of Havana remained unscathed. After a 60-day siege and with the aid of North American militia, the British seized the city, which they had to return by treaty a year later. Though 696 British soldiers died of disease during the siege, during the two months following the surrender in mid-August, the hot season for yellow fever, over 4,000 British troops died of disease (McNeill 2010, 175–191).

Yellow fever, whether in the form of an urban epidemic or a military expedition-squashing outbreak among unseasoned troops, had a mortality rate that varied between 30 and 70 percent, depending on environment and season. *Vivax* malaria kills perhaps 1 percent of those infected, and the more lethal *falciparum* on the order of 10 percent. With *vivax*, the debilitation of the fever was the principal problem, one encountered in marshy European environments as well as colonial ports and plantations. Fever-weakened bodies were subject to a host of secondary diseases and conditions and of course needed medical care. While European population growth was accompanied by the mosquito-friendly expansion of cultivated land, with its irrigation and furrows, trenches, and other water-collecting features, by the 17th century Europe was in a climatic cooling period that tended to curb the insects' activity. At the same time, the discovery of malaria-inhibiting "Jesuit bark," or cinchona bark from the New World, made effective treatment a possibility, if an expensive one.

Despite their curative bark, the main ingredient in quinine, native Americans died of malaria at rates second only to the slaughter of smallpox, some scholars believe. Relatively benign *vivax* may have been present in low-lying coastal areas before European contact, but *falciparum* was clearly imported from Africa. Historically, yellow fever (largely a problem in settled areas) and malarial fevers killed or debilitated huge portions of the native populations, allowing much easier domination of the New World by the conquerors from the Old.

FILTH AND PARASITES: TYPHUS AND DYSENTERY

Early modern cultures differed widely in their understanding of what was an acceptable level of personal hygiene or cleanliness. Whether or how often a person bathed or changed clothes did, however, dictate whether and how parasites on the skin or lodged in dirty clothing next to it were eliminated. People living in hot climates tended to wear little in the way of clothing of any sort, and what they did wear tended to be very light and well ventilated. Northerners, however, had developed cultures that required coverage from head to toe, often with heavy woolens and furs. Cool temperatures and a medical prejudice against opening the pores during bathing made Europeans among the filthiest people on earth. And along with filth came parasites.

Typhus

Typhus (see Zinsser 1963; Sherman 2006; and Watts 2003) results from human body lice that live in clothing of dirty people. The louse feeds up to six times daily on human blood. If it is infected by *Rickettsia prowazekii* bacteria, it will transmit the pathogens to the human bloodstream or deposit them on human skin in its feces. Human scratching opens skin and rubs in the bacteria. Like a virus, these bacteria enter human cells and reproduce. Incubation takes 5 to 15 days, after which sudden fever, chills, nausea, and debilitation strike down the victim. A serious case will result in prostration, neurological damage to hearing and mental sharpness, collapse of the circulatory system, and death. Untreated victims tend to recover from epidemic typhus from 75 to 95 percent of the time, gaining a limited immunity from the experience. Though lice die from the bacteria, they can live long enough to invade other sets of clothing and spread the disease; uninfected lice consume human blood infected with bacteria, find new human hosts, and the cycle becomes an epidemic.

Typhus tended to be found where weather was cold at least part of the time, people wore layers of clothing without cleaning it or their bodies, and they lived closely together, which facilitated exchange of lice. Village families huddled together around the winter fire comes to mind, as do crowded prisons and campaigning soldiers with their filthy uniforms or stolen clothing. The list of early modern military campaigns that were cut short or protracted by typhus and attendant diseases is long indeed. Troop mobilizations were the largest population movements of the period, and they grew larger over time. When outbreaks erupted, they affected the troops, their camp followers, the enemy, and the populations through whom they moved and with whom they were billeted or with whom the wounded were left behind. Europeans' first notice was among Spanish troops in Cyprus around 1490. Redirected to Italy, they quickly spread the novel disease to Italy and thence it migrated to France, Germany, and the rest of Europe. Its symptoms were reported in Latin America, though heavy clothing was rare and bathing common, at least in healthy communities.

Dysentery

Dysentery is a disease of the lower digestive tract passed through the oral-fecal route. A person ingests infected food or water, and the pathogens exit the body through bloody diarrhea. Where control of human waste is lax, released pathogens taint food or water by direct contact (often by unhygienic infected food handlers) or by flies that alight on waste and then food; and the cycle continues. Inside the human colon, pathogens use and destroy the body's defensive cells, killing the organ's healthy cells and causing inflammation. A number of bacteria, including *Campylobacter*, *Escherichia coli* (*E. coli*), *Shigella*, and *Salmonella*, and the protozoon *Entamoeba histolytica* can cause the disease. *E. histolytica* become destructive only after they burrow into the colon's walls, causing bleeding, destruction of the walls, and possibly blood poisoning. Bacillary dysentery, caused by bacilli (bacteria), is clinically very similar to amebic dysentery, causing ulcers in the colon, bleeding, bloody diarrhea, and potentially acute dehydration.

Today, even though understood and treatable, dysentery kills tens of thousands each year. Usually dysentery becomes epidemic in large prison or refugee camps, third-world urban slums, or other environments where people are jammed together with little provision for cleanliness or waste disposal. In early modern times, dysentery regularly visited armies, both encamped and on campaign, and burgeoning cities of the 18th century with little public sanitation. Cortés's conquistadors spread (if they did not introduce) the disease to Mexico by campaigning and creating refugees. Among the natives in Portuguese Brazil, dysentery became epidemic in 1560, leading the colonists to begin importing Africans as slaves to do the work the sick natives could not. Dysentery may have helped Akbar the Great, Mughal ruler in India, expand his empire in 1601 by weakening and killing the defenders of the fortress at Asirgarh. Ironically, after reigning 50 years, he died of dysentery in October 1605 (Berinstain 2001, 71). Dysentery often accompanied other diseases, especially when customary sanitation and hygiene broke down, as in armies and besieged towns during the Thirty Years' War (1618–1648) in Europe, or London in 1623. Besiegers also suffered, as did the English during the siege of Jacobite Dundalk, Ireland, in the spring of 1689. A combination of deadly typhus, dysentery, and syphilis killed half of the English army, forcing its withdrawal, but not before striking the civil population as well. Until public sanitation and safe water, even Paris could suffer dysentery outbreaks, as in the winter of 1740, when it joined with influenza, tuberculosis, and typhus to slaughter thousands, especially among the poor. Epidemics accompanying filth often include several diseases since unhygienic and inadequate living conditions give rise to many related and unrelated conditions, from insect poisoning to digestive and respiratory illnesses.

WHEN THE AIR IS DEADLY: SMALLPOX, INFLUENZA, AND MEASLES

Many infectious diseases do not require insect vectors but are spread through the air by coughing or sneezing, as is pneumonic plague. Unlike plague bacteria, pathogens of smallpox, influenza, and measles are viruses that enter the human bloodstream rapidly through the respiratory system, invade human cells, and reproduce. Survivors of smallpox and measles gain immunity from the body's development of adequate defenses. Influenza, or flu, virus strains are extremely mutable, however, and the human immune system has to adjust to each new outbreak. Though smallpox has been eradicated from nature—thanks in part to its having only human hosts—and the flu and measles are either mild or easily controlled, each was a major epidemic killer during the early modern period.

Smallpox

Deadly smallpox was caused by a poxvirus, later named *Variola major*. It was passed in tiny aerosol droplets by coughing, sneezing, or even breathing, or by human contact with bedding or clothing on which the virus had been deposited. Around 12 days later, the victim suffered flu-like symptoms and malaise; within another few days, pustules erupted on the skin. If they dried, scabbed over, and the scab fell off, the crisis was passed, and he had immunity thereafter. In many cases, however, the pustules caused permanent pockmarks that permanently marred one's face, hands, and feet. The virus could also leave the survivor blind or, if male, infertile. But smallpox could also rapidly destroy the body, causing blood poisoning (septicemia), hemorrhaging, and death in 25–30 percent of its victims (Hopkins 2002).

By 1700, medical practitioners in Asia and Africa had long used various methods of introducing a powder of dried scabs into healthy people's skin to trigger a mild, immunity-conferring form of the disease. Known to the West as variolation or inoculation, the procedure came to Europe from Islamic Turkey in the early 1700s and even earlier to its colonies in the Americas with African slaves. The major problem was that the recipient underwent a form of the disease—from mild to deadly—and required rest and patient care. In 1798, English physician Edward Jenner did traditional medicine one better by replacing the smallpox material with biologically related cowpox material—vaccination—which immunized but did not debilitate recipients.

The Flu

Like all other diseases, influenza (from Italian for celestial "influence") was a mystery to early modern societies around the world. As we know from contemporary media reports, humans can catch the various forms of Orthomyxoviridae virus from animals as varied as birds and swine, and the strain of virus can mutate wildly. This makes modern vaccination programs problematical, since they tend to be effective against last year's version and not necessarily this year's. The famous "flu-like symptoms" of so many diseases make the disease difficult to pinpoint historically. Often called catarrh or grippe in early English sources, the disease was first clinically described in the mid-1650s by Thomas Willis. But influenza is an ancient disease, and its lethality was proven in the great pandemic of 1918 that swept the world and killed tens of millions (Patterson 1986; Quinn 2008).

Transmitted in the same manner as smallpox, the victim undergoes about five days of incubation before showing symptoms. During this time, he does not know that he is infected, but he is also infecting others unknowingly, since the virus can be passed along almost immediately after infection. This makes flu especially contagious and dangerous. The virus causes respiratory symptoms of coughing and sneezing—which help spread the virus—sore throat, fever, head and muscle aches, malaise, disorientation, vomiting, and diarrhea. Clearly, these symptoms weaken the victim, allowing other germs to invade and do further damage, often leading to death in the very young or elderly. The weakened respiratory system invites pneumonia, which can injure or even shut down the lungs. Unlike plague or smallpox, the flu opens the door to killer microbes that do the real damage.

Measles

Measles is caused by an airborne virus of the paramyxovirus family, which is related to several viruses that cause animal and other human diseases, including mumps. The fever and skin discoloration of measles created confusion with scarlet fever and rubella in doctors and even microbiologists until the 1880s. Though related to rinderpest, canine distemper, and other animal ailments, the virus that brings on measles is a strictly human pathogen, which has made measles a likely—though so far unsuccessful—candidate for eradication from nature through mass MMR (measles-mumps-rubella) vaccinations.

Early modern victims suffered a predictable and unvarying set of symptoms. After 10 days of incubation, respiratory inflammation, cough, and conjunctivitis develop, along with fever, a distinctive spotted rash on the inside of the cheeks, and the familiar raised, red itchy rash on the skin. The last tends to begin high on the body and move down, no doubt a frightening manifestation to cultures unaccustomed to measles. Complications included pneumonia, blindness, and encephalitis, and the disease was deadly to adults before modern medicine. Where it is endemic, as in early modern Europe, children tend to get the disease, which is generally mild and confers adult immunity. Among adult Native Americans, mortality rates may have been as high as 35 percent. Measles and smallpox appeared similar enough to confuse even medical practitioners. Though medieval Arabs seem to have distinguished the two, in Europe this had to await the efforts of Thomas Sydenham, the "English Hippocrates," who studied English epidemics of the disease in the 1670s. That measles was infectious was not proven until the 1750s, though no one understood how it spread.

Epidemics and Pandemics

An ancient disease, influenza was common in Europe, and it probably arrived in the Americas with Columbus's men. The period 1556–1560 saw a major European outbreak, which spread to North Africa and the New World. It appears often as an epidemic or even pandemic disease in the 18th century, beginning in Rome in 1708. Geographically isolated areas such as Spain, England, and Scandinavia were spared, but the disease struck across the rest of Europe. It returned with greater strength in 1712 and 1729, the latter outbreak affecting life from Central Asia to Iceland. This also spread by ship to the Americas. The years 1732–1733 saw another major outbreak, which swept even more widely, as it did again in 1742 and 1762. By 1762, European nations were fighting a world-encircling war (Seven Years' War) that probably served to reintroduce the virus to the Americas and India. In 1780, flu was reported in China, and it traveled widely in 1781 and 1782; and a Russian outbreak spread worldwide in 1788 and 1789.

Influenza may have been present in the Americas, but it would not have been the strain(s) brought over by Europeans during the 16th century. Historical sources often confuse flu, measles, and smallpox, or provide too little information for modern diagnosis of historical diseases. Nonetheless, it seems clear that the three tended to appear together with devastating results in the New World. They often arrived in a region long before the invaders, since carriers who were messengers, refugees, and travelers moved far in advance of European explorers. Unused to the frightening symptoms, natives responded to the fevers and rashes in ways, such as hot baths, that were dangerous rather than healing. Though infection conferred at least temporary immunity, which allowed the diseases to be endemic in Europe, they rapidly tore through the "virgin soil" of the Western Hemisphere, killing untold millions. As whole villages were stricken, there were few if any to tend the sick, providing them with vital food and water. Fever-ridden children quickly dehydrated and died. Frightened adults fled the horrors, spreading them further if they were carriers. Medicine proved fruitless, and rituals that ordered life and death disappeared as living conditions became intolerable and community leaders died off. Throughout the Americas, infectious disease eliminated entire cultures (see Alchon 2003; Cook and Lovell 1992).

By contrast, in Japan the result was vastly different. Though isolated by sea, Japanese people had long been in contact with many different peoples from the Indian and Pacific Oceans and Asia's mainland. The islands boasted many dense cities, including Edo/Tokyo, which had over a million residents in the 17th century. Smallpox and influenza were endemic, though smallpox outbreaks reached epidemic levels in 1523, 1531, 1550, 1619, 1654, 1679, 1682, 1702, 1708–1709, 1711–1712, 1720, 1723, 1746, 1748, and 1773. About the mid-18th century, the Japanese adopted smallpox inoculation from China, perhaps accounting for the fall-off in epidemics after 1748. Excellent Japanese records show that most deaths (in one study 95%) were of children 10 years of age or younger. Measles, popularly imagined as a large, bearded, black-robed man or speckled females, apparently never became endemic. Epidemics in 1506, 1513, 1523, 1535, 1578, 1587, 1607, 1616, 1649, 1690–91, 1708, 1730, 1753, and 1776 were sparked by importations of measles, at least some by Europeans, who were allowed access to Japan only from 1543 to 1639. Both younger adults and children suffered most of the deaths, probably due to the immunizing effect of the recurrent outbreaks. That none of these deadly diseases had deep effects on Japanese society may well have been because the Japanese understood the value of isolating the sick, or isolating the well from the sick (Jannetta 1987).

WATERBORNE DISEASES: CHOLERA AND TYPHOID FEVER

The human body requires water to live, but not any water will do. It will reject salt and sulfurous waters, but the really dangerous waters are those that appear to be clean to the sight, smell, and taste but are in fact home to various pathological microbes. When ingested, these could cause uncomfortable conditions such as "Montezuma's revenge," or even potentially deadly diseases, such as cholera and typhoid fever. Whereas ancient Rome drew its water from the surrounding hills through aqueducts and aerating fountains, burgeoning early modern cities around the world had water supply systems that presented the end user with a biological soup, however clear it might have appeared (see Hunter 1997).

Cholera

Cholera erupted onto the world stage in 1816, beginning a series of pandemics that circled the globe well into the 20th century. Before advances in travel such as steamships and trains, it tended to be confined to cities and narrow ribbons along polluted water routes. It had, however, long been endemic to China and the Ganges River Basin in India. After the Portuguese landed in India in 1498, they began chronicling cholera (*moryxi*) outbreaks, including one in 1503 that struck 20,000

Indian soldiers, killing many. In 1563, the Portuguese physician García de Orta first clinically described cholera. Colonial records from India between 1503 and 1817 contain 64 references to cholera outbreaks, which is no doubt the tip of the iceberg.

The pathogen is a rod-shaped bacterium called *Vibrio cholerae*. Being motile, it can move through water and needs no further vector. Transmission is a chicken-and-egg problem: A sufferer has it in her digestive system and passes it though her feces. When these pollute a water source, for example, a ground aquifer or surface stream, the bacterium is passed to one who drinks and digests the water. After a day or two in the body, *Vibrio* creates a toxin that induces cramps, as well as diarrhea and vomiting, which help spread infected waste even further. Up to 20 liters of fluid could flow out of a person in a single day, with 10,000,000 bacteria in a single milliliter. Other symptoms follow, but the acute expelling of bodily fluids dehydrates the sufferer, who may lose 10 percent of her body weight, including important electrolytes. Without rehydration, death is the likely outcome.

Typhoid Fever

Similar in many ways to typhus, typhoid is an enteric (intestinal) fever brought on by ingestion of a salmonella bacterium (*Salmonella typhi*) in infected food or water. Like *Vibrio*, it is transmitted within human groups through feces that may affect water supplies. Often, flies land on improperly treated infected waste and transmit it by their feet to human food. Unlike some other food-poisoning agents, typhoid pathogens enter the human bloodstream and various organs. Symptoms are slow to manifest, making identification of the source difficult to pinpoint. Fever, abdominal pains, headache, and diarrhea slowly reduce victims to a malaise that may last up to four weeks. Because typhoid affects the whole body, complications may occur in many organs from brain to spleen, and even bones may suffer from osteomyelitis. Death rates from such complications were about 15 percent before modern medicine.

Well-ordered communities that cared for the sick and maintained high levels of waste disposal had little to fear. Where people were crowded together and water supplies were subject to contamination, typhoid fever was always a threat. Armies in camp and on campaign were prime candidates, as were cities struck by war or disaster. As European cities grew, they often paid scant attention to water supplies and sewerage; in some cases, the two were barely distinguishable. In such cases, water, so necessary for human life, became a deadly poison.

WHEN SEX NEEDED DRUGS: SYPHILIS AND OTHER VENEREAL DISEASES

Transmission of a disease through sexual intercourse was labeled venereal in honor of Venus, the goddess of love but is now termed sexually transmitted disease. Low levels of hygiene can make sex a rather filthy act for a woman by allowing all sorts of bacteria to enter the vagina, whether from lingual, penile, or instrumental insertion. Males, too, may contract parasites or bacteria from contact with a woman's genitals, as early modern customers of prostitutes no doubt experienced. True venereal diseases are transmitted only through sexual contact, oral-genital, oral, or genital. Syphilis, or the pox, burst into the historical record in 1494 as a sidelight to the French attack on Naples, and gonorrhea was first described by a London physician a few decades later. In both cases the means of transmission was fairly clear, though no one understood the diseases' causes or how to treat them effectively and safely (see Arrizabalaga, Henderson, and French 1997).

Syphilis

Syphilis is transmitted by a carrier of the motile spirochete bacterium *Treponema pallidum.* During the three weeks after introduction through the mouth or genitalia, the pathogens enter the bloodstream and begin to affect the body's organs. A sore, or chancre, appears, probably at the site of infection. The lymphatic system sweeps many of the invaders and dead defenders to the groin's lymph nodes, which swell uncomfortably. After several weeks, a range of symptoms develop, depending on which organs are most affected. A red rash may develop; other lymph nodes swell with the bacteria and pus; skin spots, open sores, and large skin swellings filled with the active bacteria may appear in the groin and between the buttocks. Major organs swell up, anemia develops, and involvement of the nervous system can result in hearing and vision problems. About 60 percent of victims who survive slide into a long latent period during which the symptoms subside (though marks may well remain). The remainder move into a third stage, or tertiary syphilis, which badly weakens major organs, such as the heart, and the nervous system. A pregnant woman syphilis carrier may find that the disease has crossed the placenta and infected her baby.

Gonorrhea

During the early modern period, gonorrhea was considered a symptom of syphilis rather than a separate disease. In fact, it is a bacterial infection by the gonococcus, which is related to meningitis-producing meningococcus and several bacteria typically found in the human mouth. It affects both men and women, causing a distinctive cloudy discharge from the penis, urethral swelling, joint pains, and eye problems in men. Women develop arthritic joints, inflammation of the pelvis, and scarring in the reproductive organs.

Early Modern Spread and Treatment of Venereal Diseases

The armies that departed Naples in 1494 spread syphilis far and wide. Within only a couple of years, it was reported across Europe. Most observers regarded it as sexually transmitted—a penalty for illicit sex—though some reused the standard theory of miasma, or poisoned air, and others the conjunction of the planets

Saturn and Jupiter. Prostitutes and bathhouses were regulated or forbidden by civic authorities accustomed to stanching plague outbreaks. In 1497, the Scots isolated sufferers on the Isle of Inch until they recovered or died. The 16th-century Italian physician Girolamo Fracastoro gave the pox its Greek name, that of the main character in his poem "Syphilis." The Portuguese took it to India in 1498, the same year it appeared in Azerbaijan; then China (1502) and Japan (1512) began seeing cases. Whether it began in the New World or was imported from Europe remains an open question (the first reported date of 1494 is very suspicious), but it was soon found among American natives and colonists alike.

Arabs had long used mercury as a treatment for skin diseases, and around 1500, some European practitioners began using the potentially lethal substance on victims of syphilis. Symptoms of mercury poisoning were ascribed to the disease, and its use continued through the 18th century. In 1517, Spaniards discovered the value of guaiac bark, which was harvested in South America. Known to many as "Jesuit bark," it was expensive and only moderately effective when boiled in water and the liquid drunk. Pox wards in hospitals and entire facilities devoted to syphilitics appeared across Europe and in its colonies. Moral and hygienic imperatives, such as avoiding prostitutes, washing before sex, and inserting sponges into the vagina, may have had some effect in reducing the initial onslaught of syphilis (and gonorrhea as well), but it also appears that the disease lost some of its initial virulence. When disease pathogens are too deadly, they kill their hosts and cannot survive or reproduce in the long run.

Taken together, infectious diseases killed millions across the globe and damaged the lives of many millions more. Records of the premodern world allow for only a partial reconstruction of even the best-documented outbreak or epidemic, but those that survive paint a grim picture indeed.

7

Environmental and Occupational Hazards

Where and how one lives is sometimes a choice and sometimes dictated by genes, culture, technology, economics, or history. Some environments present regular, natural threats to human safety and life, and some suffer extraordinary and unexpected disasters. The following section scans some of the many endemic biological threats to human life in sub-Saharan Africa during the early modern period; and it focuses on two unforeseen ecological disasters in 18th-century Western Europe. The second half of the chapter outlines the hazards associated with certain early modern occupations.

ENVIRONMENTAL HAZARDS

The concept of environmental health is as ancient as Hippocrates and China's oldest medical texts. The climate, air, winds, water, seasonal changes, and other environmental factors played important roles in medical theory throughout history, as they still do. Endemic disease could be a major factor if it was potentially fatal and the society had no effective way of limiting it. Unusual conditions or events sometimes have complex or terrible effects on human populations. Hurricanes, tornadoes, volcanic eruptions, droughts, floods, deep freezes, and earthquakes are some of the environmental events that have marked the history of human health. Epidemic outbreaks of infectious diseases may also be considered environmental hazards, but these are specifically outlined in chapter 6.

The Sub-Saharan African Environment

Apart from a few major population centers, most early modern sub-Saharan Africans lived fairly close to nature in small settlements. Though some were influenced by Muslims from the east and north, and after 1500, by Europeans landing along the west coast, most lived tradition-circumscribed lives shaped by their physical environments. Africa is a huge continent possessing many types of landscape, and generalizations should be either avoided or highly qualified. One that is unavoidable is that the climate is hot and often very humid, though in certain regions prone to drought. Heat can cause many medical problems, even for those used to it, including dehydration and heat stroke. Another is that there is a very rich endemic disease environment in central and southern Africa. Both of these factors prevented the very mobile and aggressive Europeans from doing more than seizing much of the population of the central west coast between 1500 and 1800.

Every region of Africa did not host every major disease, but an overview of some of the major examples is instructive. Oliver Ransford divided them into the epidemic, the crippling or deadly, and the debilitating (Ransford 1983, 36). Of course, no one in the world understood how any of these diseases functioned or how they might be effectively battled. The epidemic diseases included typhus, bubonic plague, yellow fever, smallpox, relapsing fever, and meningitis (see chapter 6). Today, they all still plague the continent, but modern medicine reduces their carnage. Some deadly and crippling endemic diseases included the following:

Malaria has four forms, the most dangerous of which, caused by the *Plasmodium falciparum*, was very common throughout southern Africa. Some historians believe it was so devastating to local populations that it prevented the type of historical urban and civilizational development found in other areas of the world. The female *Anopheles* mosquito loves heat and standing water and transmitted the protozoa among the people off of whose blood she fed. The previously unexposed victims, especially pregnant women and children, died very rapidly, while others suffered recurring fever and chills that effectively crippled the individual. Africa's pattern of rural settlement was conducive to the *Anopheles*, and its tropical climate made malaria a year-round problem (Ransford 1983, 92–108).

Sleeping sickness affected both humans and animals and was caused by a protozoon (*Trypanosoma*) that was spread by the tsetse or Glossina fly. The protozoa in the victim's body created mild symptoms, including sluggishness and lack of balance, sores, inflammation and lung problems. When they attacked the central nervous system the brain swelled (encephalitis), often leading to coma or death. Animistic natives blamed witchcraft while Muslims pointed to God's punishment of apostates (Ransford 1983, 109–132).

River blindness, or onchocerciasis, was caused by the residence of pairs of male and female worm-like flukes, *Onchocercus volvulus*. These were carried about on flies known today as *Simulium damnosum*, which preferred life in proximity to fast moving fresh water. Growing up to 50 cm in length, the female fluke burrowed into human skin and rolled up into a ball with her much shorter mate. They produced up to a million offspring annually, and these moved about inside the human host, creating irritation that could even be maddening. The real problem occurred when these entered into the eyes and eventually caused blindness, which was far from unusual. Though the sightless were often given light agricultural tasks, many communities abandoned prime riverine areas to avoid the disease.

Filariasis was caused by round worms or nematodes of the family *Filariodea*. These were also carried by biting flies and mosquitoes that fed on infected human and animal—cattle, horses, dogs—blood. The parasites lived under the skin or within the lymphatic system, causing symptoms that differed with the parts of the body affected. These, too, could cause river blindness, swelling of the joints (arthritis), skin rashes, and the deformation of the skin known as elephantiasis.

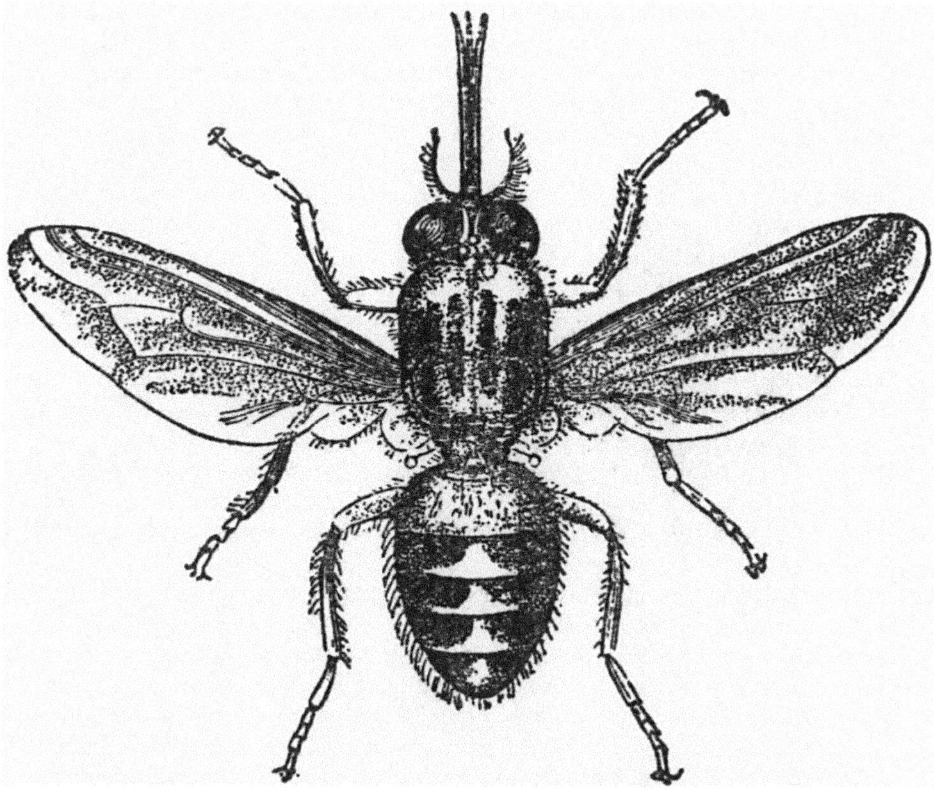

Engraving from 1880 of a tsetse fly. Found living between the Sahara and Kalahari deserts of Africa, the insect transmits the protozoan *trypanosoma*, which causes sleeping sickness in humans. (*Meyers Konversations-Lexikon*, 1888/1890)

Hookworms were roundworms (helminthes) that lived in warm, moist soil and as larvae could burrow into human skin. They traveled through the victim's circulatory system to the heart and lungs, and from there to the pharynx from which they were swallowed and eventually settled in the small intestine. Eggs were passed out in human feces and into the soil. They fed on the human host's blood, resulting in protein loss and anemia. This weakened the victims' resistance to other diseases and made them very weak and sluggish.

Ransford's debilitating and less severe diseases include the following:

Dysentery was a disease of the gastrointestinal system caused by *Shigella* and similar bacteria. The bacilli were carried on the legs of flies that had landed on contaminated human waste to feed and then landed on humans' food and contaminated it. In the body, the bacteria attacked the intestines, inflaming them, killing their cells, and shutting down their function. The victim suffered from bloody diarrhea and dehydration, but in modern cases many recover naturally as the body's defenses flush out the bacteria and repair the damage. While climate has nothing to do with the spread of *Shigella* and its equivalents, human waste management does. They often struck where normal ways of life were disrupted, as by natural disaster or war: to which early modern Africa was no stranger.

Leprosy was also a bacterial disease, one probably passed along by direct human contact—though modern research is questioning this. The bacteria prefer the cooler surface regions of the human body and thus caused skin and extremity deformities from scaly rashes to the falling off of toes or noses. The nerves were also susceptible to attack, resulting in symptoms from local numbness to blindness. Carriers were often asymptomatic and lived perfectly normal lives, but the symptoms could be disturbing and even revolting to those around one, resulting in a community's banishment of the sufferer, or worse.

Yaws was a condition of the skin caused by direct contact in the environment with the spirochete *Treponema pertenue*. Infection probably occurred when the germ entered the feet or legs through an open sore or wound, and in modern times, it especially affects children, who are more likely than adults to go barefoot. The deep open sores were limited to the lower leg but recurred repeatedly even after a single exposure. Over time the disease could attack the bones and so weaken them as to cripple the person. Among the African slaves in the Caribbean, yaws was so common that some plantations had special "houses" for treatment of the disease.

Worms and flukes entered the human body through the skin or orifices and lived as parasites inside the person. The Guinea worm lived under the skin consuming the body's fluids and could reach a meter in length. Lacking ways to kill the invader, African healers waited until the victim's skin opened to release the worm's larvae and tried to hook the worm itself, pulling it out by winding it around a spool. Schistosomiasis is also known as bilharzia, named for the European scientist who first discovered how the disease worked (Ransford 1983, 149–159). As larvae, the *Schistosoma* flukes penetrated the victim's skin within a few minutes of contact in fresh water. They traveled through the circulatory system and within a few days matured and mated. The female then anchored herself in such a way as to release her eggs into the host's urinary system or large intestine. From here, the eggs reentered the freshwater environment and the cycle continued. These flukes could live half a dozen years, and they evolved to have a rather minimal effect on their hosts. Nonetheless, urinary and enteric complications certainly arose as cycle followed cycle. (For more information on the diseases in this section, see Ransford 1983; Byrne 2008; and Osterfeld, Kessing, and Eviner 2008.)

European Disasters: The Great Winter in Lyon, 1709

Lyon, France, was a center of French finance and the silk industry at the confluence of the Rhône and Saone Rivers. Its 90,000 souls relied on imported foodstuffs for survival, and these arrived via both rivers and the several roads that met at the city's bridges. In May of 1708, unusually heavy rains struck the region, destroying or retarding much of the region's young wheat crop that would feed the city in the fall. Nervous citizens hoarded grain, and merchants gouged locals with high prices, as grain was shipped away to feed Louis XIV's military. Discontent rose until government interaction ensured that there would not be a winter of shortages.

Nature turned on the French, however, as temperatures plummeted in early January 1709. Rain-saturated land froze hard, killing or retarding all manner of trees and vines. Frozen rain destroyed winter crops; the rivers froze at Lyon, and ice blocked or impeded much of that lifeline for several months. Deep snows and icy winds joined the bone-chilling temperatures in February, killing herds of animals and taking a further toll on agricultural resources. Some people froze to death, and many more suffered frostbite from exposure. People stoked great fires trying to keep warm, which sometimes turned into conflagrations, laying waste to homes and warehouses. It was a legendarily brutal season.

In March, many peasants defied a royal edict and plowed under the ruined wheat crops, planting barley, oats, or buckwheat, which promised to grow more quickly. Faced with another greatly reduced crop, prices rose and people panicked, with serious rioting breaking out on March 25, usually around bakeries. As supplies dwindled and prospects soured further, mobs, soldiers, and royal officials seized grain shipments bound for Lyon even as increasingly desperate peasants began to swell the city's population. Economic disaster hit the city's elites as creditors called in accounts and debtors defaulted, ruining Lyonaise credit and cascading through the society. Imports dropped off, and even wine shipments fell by a third. State bread donations rose six times to 60,000 pounds in May, even after "foreign" poor had been herded out of the city in April. By May, the price of wheat had risen by 300 percent in the small village of Grenette, and royal troops had to guard the roads and waterways so grain could pass to Lyon unmolested. Surrounding regions were as desperate as Lyon's, and foreign wheat seemed the only answer. In late July, 15 barges loaded with wheat began the trip from Toulon to Lyon, but nature again intervened as red coral banks blocked the Rhône's mouth. On September 28, however, the barges arrived and the grain flowed into the granaries.

For many, this was too late. For numerous reasons, August was the year's deadliest month, the average death toll for August rising half again as high as the July average. In 1709, August saw nearly twice the average number of deaths (366 as opposed to 190), as the weakened population succumbed. As usual, during this crisis period, most deaths did not occur from starvation—few usually do starve—but malnutrition leads to anemia and gastrointestinal illnesses and weakens people's resistance to disease. The influx of rural folk introduced unusual pathogens; the lack of wine led to the drinking of tainted water (typhoid fever and dysentery); the cold winter led to unusually close living conditions and a lack of hygiene, which fostered lice-borne typhus and skin diseases. In the winter, endemic influenza and tuberculosis thrived, and children were stricken with smallpox and diarrhea. Though conditions never became epidemic, urban dependence, natural forces, and delayed human action combined to undermine or destroy the health of thousands during the crisis of 1708 and 1709 (see Monahan 1993).

European Disasters: The Lisbon Earthquake, 1755

> My right arm hung down before me motionless, like a great dead weight, the shoulder being out, and the bone broken; . . . my legs covered with wounds, the right ankle swelled to a prodigious size, with a fountain of blood spouting upwards from it: the knee was also much bruised, my left side felt as if beat in, so that I could hardly breathe: all the left side of my face was swelled, the skin beaten off, the blood streaming from it, with a great wound above and a small one below the eye, and several bruises on my back and head (Shrady 2008, 17).

The British merchant Thomas Chase was 26 years old when the great earthquake leveled the city of Lisbon, Portugal, at 9:30 a.m. on All Saints Day (November 1) in 1755. He was living in the same house in which he was born, and which collapsed atop him (he survived, recovered, and lived another 33 years). This was the 8.7 to 9.0 Richter scale earthquake that shattered the philosopher Voltaire's optimism in man's capabilities and led him to write his masterpiece, *Candide*. Like most of the 30,000 to 60,000 who died in the quake, Chase was struck and buried by falling debris. The well-built residences of the wealthy fared better than the ramshackle tenements of the poor, but even the best were damaged. Many who survived and were trapped were incinerated by conflagrations started by disrupted kitchen fires, shop lights, and the thousands of candles in the well-lit churches on that religious feast day.

But the earthquake also spawned three tidal waves whose backwash swept into Europe's third-busiest harbor, engulfing debris, ships, docks, warehouses, and people and washing them out to sea. Barbados and Martinique in the far-distant Caribbean felt the tsunamis. When the major tremors and tidal events subsided, both the desperate and the criminal took what they wanted in the ensuing anarchy. With the city's food supplies gone or spoiled, and the infrastructure for resupplying it in tatters, the survivors made for the countryside or rioted until order was restored. Dysentery and other diseases of the disrupted human environment swept the survivors. To this was joined the fear of miasma and plague from the rotting corpses, many being washed up from the ocean. For all of their wealth and culture, before the fury of nature and nature's God, the Portuguese stood humbled (Shrady 2008, 3–49 and see Paice 2010).

OCCUPATIONAL HAZARDS

Many early physicians recognized that people in certain occupations tended to suffer from the same ailments. Hippocrates discussed the problems of tailors, horse wranglers, fishermen, dyers, metalworkers, and farm laborers. Galen noted patterns of sickness in wet nurses, students, farmers, and wrestlers. Sixteenth-and seventeenth-century physicians wrote about soldiers, miners, metalworkers, melancholic scholars, mothers, and other specific groups and the risks they faced. The real founder of what we can call occupational health, however, was the Italian physician Bernardino Ramazzini.

Bernardino Ramazzini, Father of Industrial Medicine

Ramazzini spent most of his productive life in and around the city of Modena, at whose university he held a chair of medicine. Rather than being a medical theorist, he spent much of his time as a healer and observer of the sick and well. He visited and interviewed workers in many occupations but also read widely among the ancient and modern medical authors. His writings are liberally sprinkled with references to Hippocrates, "the Divine Teacher." He discussed his interest in the medical problems common to people in various trades with other physicians. He was a keen observer and a man of the early Enlightenment who wanted to see the improvement of working conditions and medical care for the men and women of his day.

To this end, he penned *The Diseases of Workers,* which was published in 1700 (Ramazzini 1940; see also Franco, Franco and Paita 1999). This first edition contained descriptions of the health risks for workers in 43 occupations. A second appeared in 1713, which included an additional 12 trades. In this case, he published it in a size that was easy for the practicing physician to carry with him, firmly believing that one of the first questions a patient is asked should be "What is your occupation?" Two common themes that came out of his research were that a person should be physically and temperamentally suited to his or her occupation and that most "diseases" stemmed from environmental causes, such as noxious vapors from materials or from the "violent and irregular motions of the body" required by the job. Though he was perhaps the first medical writer to rely solely on statistics for a study, in *Diseases* he used little in the way of quantification.

Women Workers in Ramazzini

Of the 55 chapters in the 1713 edition of *The Diseases of Workers*, only 3 dealt specifically with women. Midwives were susceptible to any diseases the child might have, but he was less clear about the mother's passing along any illnesses. The nature of contagion was still an open question, and as close as he came is to note that if the mother had syphilis, the infected lochia could cause the midwife's hands to become inflamed. Even uninfected but "corrosive, acrid" lochia could damage the skin, as could the "poisonous" menstrual fluid that was released as part of the afterbirth. He did cite several authorities who dismissed the ancient fiction of poisonous menses but concluded that the fluid did have "a certain latent malignant quality." Even breathing the vapors could sicken one. He recommended often washing the hands with water and wine or vinegar during labor. Oddly, it was to protect the midwife and not the mother. Ramazzini also noted that Italian midwives used the birthing chair unlike women elsewhere. This required the midwife to lean out over the mother's legs with her arms outstretched to receive the baby. In the short run, fatigue set in, but over time, this posture could cause real skeletal damage, he noted (Ramazzini 1940, 157–167).

In his lengthy chapter on wet nurses and nursing women in general, Ramazzini summarized that they were subject to "gradual wasting, hysteria, pustules and scabies, headache, vertigo, respiratory trouble, and weak eyesight." The very act of holding or carrying the nursing infant could cause "itching irruptions," and a mother could suffer from curdling milk, cracked nipples, and abscesses. Since lactating suppressed the menses, Ramazzini could blame many of the side effects on the accumulation of the "poisonous" stuff. He recommended the typically Galenic remedy of letting blood. A wet nurse who lived in a rich man's house, away from her husband, had two other problems. One was that she consumed rich foods to which her body was not accustomed. The other was the absence of sexual intercourse. These combined with the menstrual suppression to cause hysteria in many women, Ramazzini believed. The fathers would do well, he wrote, to allow the nurse to have sex with her husband from time to time to prevent this condition.

Finally, the nurse could suffer "wasting" from feeding the infant too often. On the other hand, women who nursed often tended to have even fewer breast tumors than nuns who never did, Ramazzini wrote (Ramazzini 1940, 167–201).

Laundresses worked in a constantly damp environment, which damaged the lungs and skin. Having their feet and lower legs immersed supposedly suppressed their menses, as did the clogging of their skin pores with moisture. He cited lung problems resulting from breathing the boiling lye soap and inhaling of the remains of "a thousand kinds of filth" that saturated bedding, underclothes, and other laundry. Like the midwives, laundresses' hands suffered, becoming inflamed by the lye, which could also cause fever, he averred. He noted the value of their service to the community and wrote that he always urged them to avoid all fumes as much as possible, to use butter to soften their hands, and to change their wet clothing after work. Women workers also appear in the chapter on textile workers and on Jews (seamstresses). In the latter, he mentioned the eyestrain caused by the close work their craft entailed (Ramazzini 1940, 253–255; 257–261, 287).

Anthrax: The Woolsorters' Disease

In his chapter on textiles, Ramazzini discussed flax, hemp, and silk but not the far more common wool. This was because Frenchman Nicholas Fournier had yet to articulate the connection of wool and anthrax (1750s), a disease typically associated with wool workers, especially female woolsorters. It is a disease of animals (zoonosis) that humans catch from contact with infected animals or their products. The bacterium traveled inside spores and could live in the soil or animal hides, meat, hair, or wool. In1758, there was a report from Finland of a bear that died from having eaten an infected animal. The man who skinned the bear caught the disease and died, as did four other men who prepared the skin. It produced toxins similar to cholera or tetanus and was quite deadly depending on where on the body the initial infection occurred. The French blamed "cursed fields" whose vegetation fed and contaminated the animals that butchers then slaughtered and marketed. By this means, what was an occupational hazard became an epidemic disease. Major outbreaks occurred in Southern Europe in 1613, when some 60,000 died, and in Guadeloupe and Saint Domingue in the Caribbean in the 1770s, when 15,000 people and thousands of animals perished. With no understanding of bacteria, Fournier and his followers located the cause of the disease in tainted animals. How the animals became diseased was another question: miasma, nonspecific contagion "germes," and spontaneous generation were all suggested. Modern science indicates that periodic floods disturbed the spores in the fields, grazing animals inhaled them, and an outbreak was set off (Jones 2010).

Bookkeepers and Scholars

While Ramazzini does not specifically address the plight of scholars, he does have a chapter on "scribes and notaries." Such workers, he says, suffer from three qualities of their profession: constant sitting, continual movement of the hand and in the same direction, and the mental strain of striving to copy the material correctly. Our culture is well aware of the problems of a "sedentary lifestyle" and carpal tunnel syndrome, and Ramazzini seems like something of a prophet. He cites medical problems such as "obstructions of the viscera . . . indigestion . . . numbness of the legs, a considerable hindrance of the circulation of the blood, and an unhealthy habit. In a word, they lack the benefit of moderate exercise." His take on repetitive-motion problems is equally modern, and he mentions a notary whose right hand had become paralyzed by his profession. Worst, he thought, was the mental strain from concentration that resulted in "headaches, heavy colds, sore throats, and fluxes" (Ramazzini 1940, 421–425).

Eighty years before Ramazzini, the English physician Robert Burton penned his lengthy *Anatomy of Melancholy* (1621). Melancholy was a recognized medical condition and not just an emotional state. It was caused by an excess of black bile ("melan" means "black"; "choler" means "bile"), associated astrologically with the planet Saturn, and a curse of the depressive and introspective scholar and artist. Early in the 1500s, German artist Albrecht Dürer created a remarkable woodcut entitled *Melancolia I* in which an angelic figure representing genius sits frustrated and impotent though surrounded by intellectual tools and symbols. This creative blockage was the result of the buildup of black bile due to a sedentary lifestyle. The Galenic explanation was that excessive contemplation or study had a drying effect on the mind and ultimately the whole body. The student's natural poverty meant that the stomach and liver were not properly fed, and the body became "desiccated." Burton wrote that this led to a bevy of symptoms: "gouts, catarrhs, rheums, wasting, indigestion, bad eyes, stone and colic, crudities, oppilations, vertigo, winds, consumptions and all such diseases as come by oversitting." Emotionally, of course, the melancholic person, whether a scholar or not, is still associated with depression and deep, unshakeable sadness. Burton's is a complex work with layers of moral teaching and not merely a medical manual, but the condition he described was taken very seriously.

Even before Burton, William Shakespeare gave his audiences Hamlet, the "melancholy Dane." The young man is a student at Wittenberg University. Home for break, he has to confront the death of his father and sketchy remarriage of his mother. Like the textbook melancholic, he is very smart but confused, unsure of himself, and frustrated from acting to avenge his father. He even contemplates suicide. Those around him are uncertain of and fearful for his sanity. In his brilliant monologues, Hamlet explores the anatomy of his own melancholy, a study that ultimately takes him down a path of death and destruction (Burton 1621/2008; see also Radden 2000).

European and Colonial Metal Mineworkers

In the early modern world, deep-shaft mining was common in many regions. In his treatment of miner's diseases, Ramazzini mentions mines for gold, silver, and copper and also mercury, vitriol, niter, and arsenic. The dangers of work in the deep-shaft metal ore mines were legendary. In the classical world, only slaves,

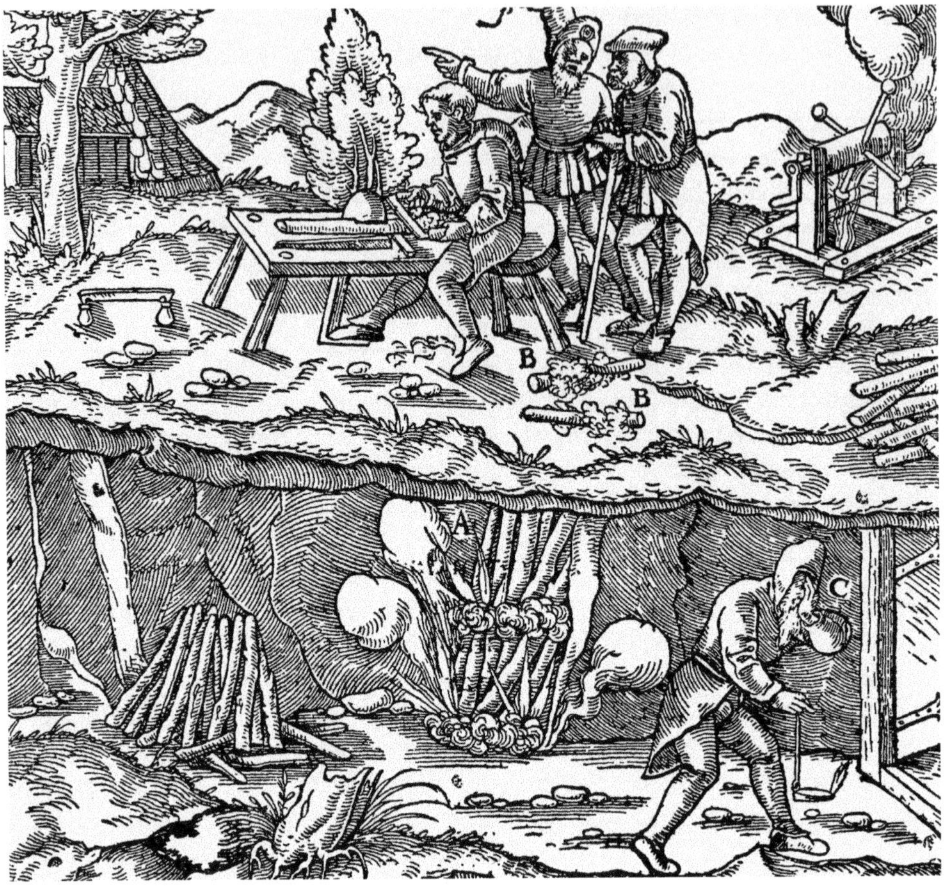

Tin mining methods as depicted in Georgius Agricola's *De Re Metallica* (1556). The author noted that the method of heating sealed tunnels unleashed a "foetid vapour," exposure to which was one of the many hazards of early mining practices. (Eon Images)

criminals, or prisoners of war were cast into the earth to reap its shiny bounty. In early modern Europe, miners were respected laborers—Martin Luther's Saxon father was one—and their problems and issues were noticed. Sixteenth-century German medical reformer Paracelsus wrote a three-volume work on the diseases of miners, and in 1551, German scholar and physician Georgius Agricola discussed a range of illnesses related to mining in his *De re metallica.* At Joachimsthal, small contributions from miners supported the "brother houses" in which disabled miners lived.

Spain had long had its own mines, and in gaining the New World imposed the industry on hapless natives. Critics at court decried exploitation of Indians as early as 1511. The royal Burgos Statutes of 1512 and regulations articulated the following year sought to limit the exposure of women and children under 14 to the rigors and hazards of the mines. At the Guadalcanal mines near Seville in Spain itself, the monarchs provided a physician with a nice house and high salary to treat the victims of fumes, "smoke and noxious vapors." Eventually the Spaniards imported German miners, whom they thought naturally better suited to the work.

At Almadén, Spain, the miners extracted mercury, a deadly toxin that was used in treating syphilis and in purifying silver from ore. This was shipped to South America until mercury was discovered and mined by natives and slaves at Huancavélica in Peru. For Spaniards, Indians, and African slaves alike, the exposure to and use of mercury were crippling. Nerve damage, palsy, and extreme debilitation; tooth loss and mouth sores; and outright madness were not atypical results. Later in our period, the use of mercury in making headgear gave rise to the phrase "as mad as a hatter."

High in the Andes, Indian workers chewed coca leaves, the high from which dulled some of the pain they had to endure. Colonial authorities did try to humanize working conditions by insisting on changes of clothing after shifts, reasonable working hours, and no forced labor. At the Potosì mines, officials imposed standards for shoring up the mineshafts and employment of a single daylight shift each day. Eventually a hospital with a physician, surgeon, and apothecary was mandated and established for the workers, which was funded from a 1 percent tax on the mine operators.

In Germany, Agricola emphasized the lung diseases, headaches, vertigo, and podagra from which miners suffered, and his contemporary the physician Paracelsus also concentrated on the vapors and fumes that led to pneumonia and what he believed to be a mix of tuberculosis, lung cancer, and silicosis. Andean mummies show clear signs of this last disease, with their lungs coated with the dust of silver, iron, copper, and silica. This condition was at least as deadly as black lung disease in coal mining. One of the main problems, of course, was poor ventilation in the shafts and the lack of respiration-protecting masks.

Ramazzini chose to open his work with miners' diseases, and his text reminds us that there were many early modern authors who either discussed the occupation and its dangers or mentioned miners when discussing diseases of lungs and brain. Early on, Ramazzini lists miners' problems as "dyspnoea, phthisis [tuberculosis], apoplexy, paralysis, cachexy, swollen feet [from the damp], loss of teeth, ulcerated gums, pains in the joints, and palsy." In the course of his discussion, he added asthma, ophthalmia, suffocation, and the threat of "certain small creatures that look like spiders," and "little demons and phantoms" that were "no fable as I used to think." True to his reformer's program, he wrote, "We ought study carefully the diseases of those workers with a view to their safety and suggest precautions and remedies." For the demons, he recommended exorcisms; for the others, his program was scanty: ventilation pumps, gloves and leggings, masks, milk and butter in the diet, and various medicines for specific complaints. What he does not address is what a general audience might regard as the most dangerous hazards: flooding and cave-ins that either trapped or buried miners. Nor does he treat the strains on the human body of mining, including hernias and repetitive-stress injuries, injuries from mishandled tools or falling objects, heat exhaustion, and eyestrain, just to name a few (Ramazzini 1940, 15–33; Pretel and Bremón 1999; Piekarski 1999).

It was a dangerous world out there.

8

Surgery and Medical Procedures

The learned traditions of China and the West clearly defined medical practitioners. Physicians were experts on intricate theories of human physiology and the food, drink, and medicines necessary to maintain health and cure illness. This was the high road to health and healing in both cultures. They distinguished other medical practitioners who, essentially, worked with their hands as inferior. For theirs was an art or craft, not a profession: it lacked the theoretical or "philosophical" underpinnings that marked the physician and his training. Yet the human body often needed the physical manipulation that physicians shunned. Wounds needed bandaging; broken bones needed to be set; babies needed to be delivered; cataracts and urinary stones needed to be cut away; teeth needed to be pulled, blood drawn, hernias removed, boils lanced, dislocations repositioned, and the list goes on. In some cultures, such as the Aztec, the African, and the Afro-Caribbean, these tasks simply fell to the healer's skills, with some known for what we might call specialization. In China, such needs literally fell to lower-class healers, often itinerant, who had no relationship to the learned profession. In the West, the situation was complex. Some specialized healers—lithotomists, wound doctors, bonesetters, oculists—operated under the radar of the physicians and most civic authorities. Others, with broader skill sets gained through formal apprenticeships, were given the name surgeon and organized into self-regulating guilds—like physicians, but of inferior education and status. During the early modern period, the roles and status of European surgeons underwent some major changes that reflected larger trends in society and culture.

THE AZTECS

Truly effective healing requires a fairly sophisticated understanding of human anatomy and physiology, but there is little evidence of this among the Aztecs. They were empirics in the true sense of relying upon their own experience, often guided by others. The Nahuatl *texoxtl* was the equivalent of "surgeon" and indicated a wide range of skills. More specialized was the "bloodletter," or *tecoani*. Medicinally, letting blood flow was simply a means of reducing certain types of swelling. The *tecoani* used flaked obsidian knives or maguey tree thorns to open veins. He had another important societal use, too. He carried out the human sacrifices required by the Aztec religion. He knew how to use certain narcotic plants—jimson weed, marijuana—to drug the victims, ensuring their cooperation.

The *texoxtl* learned his skills from others and worked in cooperation with herbalists, spirit healers, and other practitioners. Unlike Europeans, Aztec surgeons valued cleanliness, though having no conception of germs. This was especially useful in treating wounds, which could so easily become infected. According to one instruction, the wound was to be washed clean with water; further cleansed with fresh, warm urine (which is aseptic); slathered in agave sap, salt, and lampblack; then wrapped airtight. In his Nahuatl herbal of 1552, the native physician Martín de la Cruz recommended the following: "An inflicted wound will heal if the juice from the bark of the *ylin* tree, the root of the *tlal-ahuehuetl* bush [a low-lying cypress], wax salve and yolk of egg be injected" (Gates 1939/2000, 84). They had numerous poultices and knew how to suture a wound or incision, using a long human hair cleansed with honey and salt. If not bled, a swollen wound would be cleansed with papaya juice.

Maintaining dental health was important, and tooth powders (dentifrices) included combinations of salt and charcoal or white ashes in white honey. Caries, or cavities, resulted, they believed, from the rapid succession of hot and cold fluids in the mouth. If decay and toothache should occur, the tooth was to be punctured with an incisor and the damage cleared away. De la Cruz offered a compress to dull the pain (Ortiz de Montellano 1990, 155; Gates 1939/2000: 27–28). They also knew how to drill away and fill caries. For some reason, the eyes were often treated with powdered human excrement, yet Aztec surgeons could successfully treat cataracts. They also carried out trepanation, the drilling of holes in the skull, though whether it was to release fluid pressure on the brain from traumas or let spirits escape is unclear. Fractures received splints to immobilize the bone until it knitted itself back together. Bleeding or plasters were used to reduce swelling. If the bone failed to heal, they used a tool not seen again in the West until the 20th century: the intramedullar nail. A "resinous stick" was inserted into the halves of the bone to hold them together (see also Schendel 1968).

The first European surgeon arrived in Mexico City in 1525, and more soon followed. Other colonists valued these men and their ways, leaving the healing of natives, especially outside the major towns, to the old ways. In cities, though, the Spanish reproduced the pattern of surgical practice and its oversight that they knew in Old Spain (see Fields 2008).

THE CHINESE

China's ancient Confucian heritage revered the human body and shunned deliberate violations of it. This included not only invasive forms of medical treatment but even the study of anatomy and dissection of corpses. True medicine was learned medicine, and this involved balancing the yin and yang, strengthening the qi, and keeping channels of their flow open through daily regimen and largely herbal medicinal drugs (Veith 2000, 3). Kidney or bladder stones were treated with tea; no one cut for cataracts but instead there were medicinal herbs; and amputations were out of the question as far as formal medicine was concerned. Not surprisingly, the earliest Chinese work on surgery or external medicine, *Remedies Left over by Ghosts,* was rather late (c. 500 C.E.) and largely military in its concerns (wounds) (Wang 1999, 141–142).

Yet popular medicine had long run its parallel track, developing what we might call surgical specialties. By the early modern period, many physicians (*ruyi*) accepted the need for skilled mechanics of the human body and accepted them the way architects accept plumbers. The early modern period did see the appearance of numerous works on wounds, boils, burns, fractures, and other typical surgical concerns. But the period was one of neo-Confucianism, and critics such as late-17th-century physician Wang Weidei resented their interference and undermined the role of invasive medicine and surgeons in society. He represented one of three recognized early modern schools of external medicine (survival school). Chen Shigong and his school (the "orthodox") stressed a balance of internal medication and external approaches, and even the sterilization of instruments (*True Lineages of External Medicine*, 1617). The surgeon and *ruyi* Gao Binjun leaned toward internal approaches, noting that even skin diseases and carbuncles originate within the body. His followers were sometimes called the "study school," and he expressed his ideas in his *Collection of Heart-Felt Experiences in Sore Specialty* (1805) (Wang 1999, 233–237).

They learned their trades from predecessors, much as Western empirics did. Many were itinerant, quickly identifying where in a community the healers gathered to meet or treat their patients (often a religious shrine or garden). Wounds were tended, abscesses drained, and eyes treated with something other than drugs; some specialized in teeth, others cupping and phlebotomy; some practiced massage, setting fractured bones, and tending dislocated ones (Barnes 2005, 118).

Acupuncture and moxibustion are two therapies associated with classical Chinese medicine and popular practitioners. Acupuncture dated back to at least the second century B.C.E., and the standard Nine Needles to the Han Dynasty. Each type of needle has a particular form and function: for example, a two-edged one is for releasing pus and a round, sharp one is used in the treatment of acute maladies (Wang 1999, 24). Usually the needles were heated and carefully rotated or hammered into a very specific spot or spots on the body. The theory was that the needle was placed to open a closed conduit for blood or qi, whose blockage was causing the illness. The acupuncturist had to know the network of conduits that ran through the body, the best spots on the skin through which to contact the appropriate position on the conduit, and the most effective way to place the needle in the body. Many were Daoist priests (see Eckman 2007, 81–86). Moxibustion, used by both Indians and Chinese, consisted of the burning of a small cone of dried mugwort on a very specific spot on the body with hopes of the same essential effect (Barnes 2005, 110–115, 181–185). Throughout our period, both practices, which could be quite painful for the patient, were losing popularity as people preferred to take medicines (and the *ruyi* preferred to prescribe them). In 1757, Hsü Ta-ch'un wrote, "[Recently the use of] prescriptions and drugs flourished widely while no one spoke of the method of needling anymore. . . . Today's physicians insert their needles at liberty and do not care about any schema" (Unschuld 1998, 244, 247).

THE ISLAMIC WORLD

The Tradition by 1500

The Arabs, and by extension Islam, inherited the medicine of ancient Greece and Rome. Galenic humoralism emphasized the role of the humors and of regimens of lifestyle and, when necessary, pharmaceuticals. But Galen himself had tended gladiators, and most of their problems were not treated with "moist" or "dry" foods or herbs. The line between surgeon (*jarrah*) and physician (*tabib*) appears not to have been too broadly drawn, at least from the 10th century. Later medieval and early modern Persian and Arabic physicians seem to have performed certain surgical procedures themselves, leaving others to trained assistants, though no clear pattern of practice emerges. As in China, numerous manuals of surgical procedures circulated, and these display a truly sophisticated understanding of instruments and their use. This was true of even very meticulous tasks, such as work on the eye.

As for a working knowledge of human anatomy and physiology, however, despite some evidence to the contrary, it seems that Muslim doctors had little beyond Galen's problematic legacy. Anatomical illustrations remain crude, and there is no evidence of dissection for the sake of education. In the 13th century, the physician and critic of traditional medicine Ibn al-Nafis wrote:

> The veto of the religious law and the sentiment of charity innate in ourselves alike prevent us from the practice of dissection. That is why we are willing to be limited to basing our knowledge of the internal organs on the sayings of those who had gone before us.

Little had changed by the 18th century. In working with living patients, Islamic laws of personal modesty limited the amount of the body that one could expose to a doctor without scandal: off limits were navel to knees for a man and neck to ankles for a woman. Ignorance was so deep that physicians argued over the number of bones in the human body (which in fact changes with age as bones fuse). In Persia, it was said that a Jew had boiled a woman's body and found 248. This was confirmed by the ancient saying that one's number of bones was the same as the numerological value of the name of one's "original home." The value of the word *rahm*, or womb, was 248 (Elgood 1970, 131–139).

When operating, Muslim practitioners insisted on cleanliness, in part because blood was a ritual pollutant, but they had no notion of germs or the need for asepsis. In addition, anesthesia was limited to a few opiates, which would have made many procedures excruciating. Amputation of the hands, however, was a well-understood procedure since it was a judicial punishment. Certain routine concerns, such as bloodletting, dentistry, bonesetting, and suturing wounds, apparently fell to specialist craftspeople on whom the physicians relied. Some of these were women, especially in areas related to reproduction, but their wider participation was a matter of local culture (Pormann and Savage-Smith 2007, 121–135).

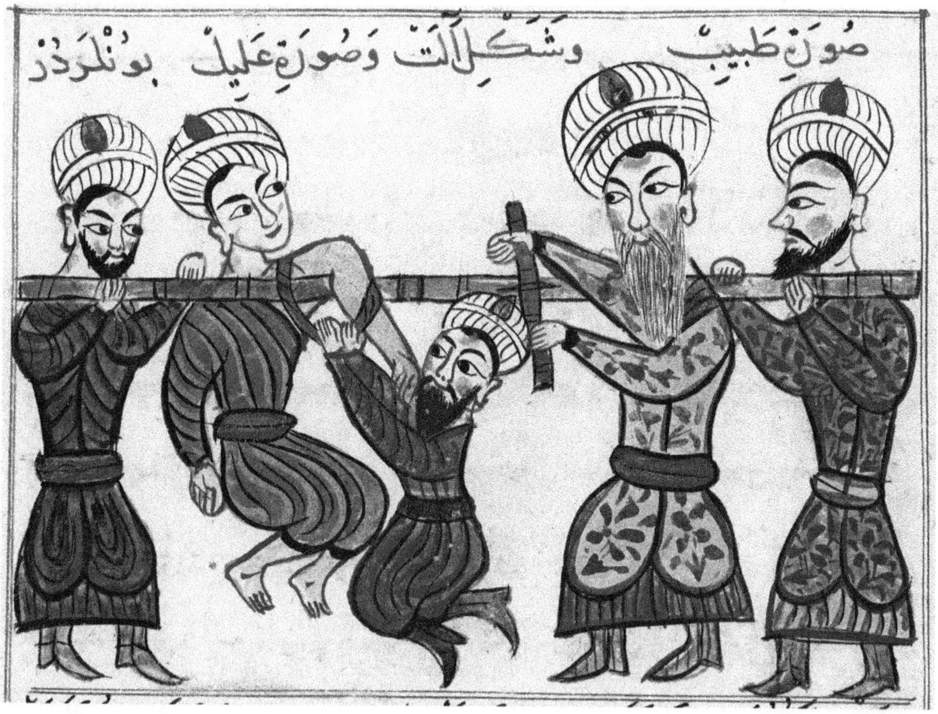

Illustration of bonesetters setting a fracture, from an Ottoman medical manuscript. (Leemage/UIG via Getty Images)

Ottoman Turks and Safavid Persians

The Muslim Turks who conquered Constantinople in 1453 and seized the Levant and Egypt in the 1510s inherited the Arabo-Persian medical system. Galen and Avicenna retained their pride of place, as did the surgical writings of the 11th-century Spanish Muslim al-Zahrawi. Nothing of medical knowledge seems to have been lost due to the conquest, but the Turks had little to add (with the possible exception of inoculation for smallpox). The surgeon (*cerrah*) and other specialists in external medicine worked in the urban hospitals alongside the physicians. They also served in the Turkish fleets and army, both to maintain the men's health and to do what they could in the wake of battle (Shefer-Mossensohn 2009. 45–56).

The Safavid Empire that centered on Iran suffered from the same antiquity of theory and practice, and yet their practitioners could be quite effective. They had barbers who cut, shaved, and dyed men's hair, bled, performed dentistry, cleaned ears, massaged, cauterized, cupped, and circumcised males (near puberty in Muslim Persia). They had bonesetters who had expertise in all of the bones and tools such as retractors, pulleys, ropes, and wheels. They knew how to set splints, what ointments to help bones heal, and which anesthetics were most effective. These included opium, marijuana, and drugs that were said to "induce unconsciousness" and "put the patient to sleep." They knew how to recognize cancers and cut many out successfully. They operated with a range of knives and other instruments whose edges were kept razor sharp by preservation in olive oil. Their suturing needles were made of steel or copper and were probably the same as those used by tailors and shoemakers. To stitch wounds, they used silk or cotton thread, horse or human hairs, harp strings, and even the heads of biting ants as tiny clamps, snapping the bodies off after setting them (Elgood 1970, 141–170).

One last disagreeable area of Safavid surgical performance was in using surgical removals to punish wrongdoers. Eyes were cut up and removed, gouged out, or skewered with a red-hot needle that penetrated the lens and optic nerve. Red-hot pokers and corrosive materials that ate away the eye were also used. When a new shah took the throne, it was customary to blind anyone who might threaten the throne, so even the oldest prince generally lost his sight as a matter of course: a man who could not see could not rule. Spoken insults or blasphemy easily resulted in one's tongue being cut off; a few teeth might be pulled out; ears, hands, and feet were amputated. Hands were not sawn off but hammered off with a mallet at the wrist, and the stump shoved into flaming tar to cauterize the wound. It may not be fair to end this discussion of Islamic surgery with this list of horrors, but it remains a reminder that under an autocratic regime, even healers could be used as instruments of torture and death.

THE EUROPEANS

Later medieval Europeans derived a great deal from Muslim sources. Some included medical manuals from antiquity and subsequent Muslim commentators and practitioners (in translation), knowledge of and access to pharmaceuticals, and certain surgical skills and practices gained from direct contact with Islamic medicine in the Near East, Sicily, or southern Spain. Of course, Christian healers had long used a wide array of their own traditional techniques for handling wounds, fractures, rotten teeth, and dislocated shoulders. Skilled and unskilled technicians could be found at noble courts, monasteries, and pilgrim hospices, and with armies in the field. Since its inception at Salerno in the 12th century, formal European medical education was based on Galen, balancing humors, and the use of dietary regimens and pharmaceuticals. Medical schools, at least outside Italy, had little to teach about treating the body for nonhumoral problems. Physicians, then, recommended, diagnosed, and prescribed. Virtually, everything physical—from bloodletting to setting a broken leg—was left to the trained but not "educated," surgeon or other specialist.

Organization

By 1500, however, a recognized craft of surgeon had emerged across Europe to the point that in towns and cities they had organized into guilds. Guilds regulated the education of young apprentices as well as the practices of their masters and limited access to those they deemed fit. They kept themselves busy by restricting the number of surgeons who could practice and often regulated scales of charges for typical procedures. One of the most typical was bloodletting, understood as important for regulating humors in the body. This was often linked to the cutting

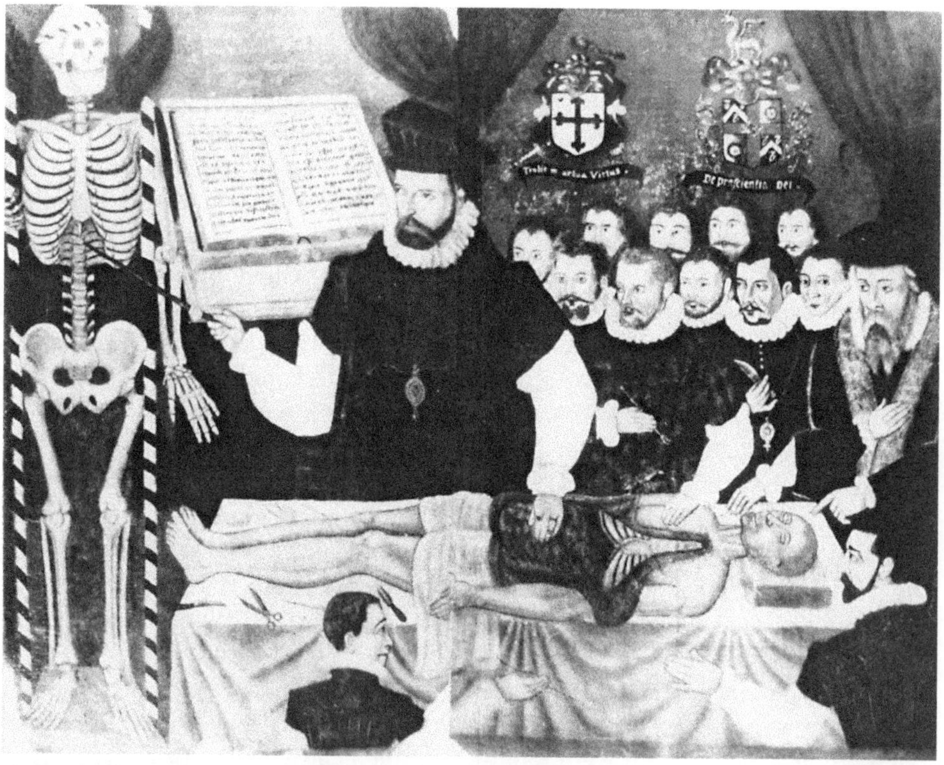

Oxford-educated John Banister—surgeon, medical author, and teacher—lectures at the Barber-Surgeons Hall, London, 1581. He conducts the lesson using a corpse, a text, and a display skeleton. Note that the onlookers are well-dressed men who are probably practicing surgeons. (National Library of Medicine)

and shaving of hair, which of course also required the use of extremely sharp cutting tools. Barbers and surgeons were often joined in the same guild, and were often the same people, as in Paris from the 14th century. Scotland's James IV required combining when he created the Incorporation of Barber-Surgeons in Edinburgh in 1505. In 1540, England's Henry VIII raised the status of barbers by linking their Guild of Surgeons with the Company of Barber-Surgeons (the largest of London's 39 guilds with 185 members in 1537). The result was the United Company of Barbers and Surgeons. Oddly, perhaps, only barbers could cut hair or pull teeth, and the regulations required seven years of apprenticeship. This arrangement lasted until 1745, during a period when surgeons across Europe were trying desperately to raise their status. In 1800, London achieved this with the foundation of the Royal College of Surgeons (a society, not a school). Spain's Philip II imposed the Barber-Surgeon's Guild in Amsterdam in 1556. By the later 17th century, Dutch tastes were craving French-style hair salons and stylists—no surprise that so many hair-preparation terms are French: coiffure, barrette, stylist, pomade, even salon—and by the 18th century, high-status barbers sought separation from the bleeders and wound stitchers (Ellis 2009, 37–39, 61; see also Pelling 1998, 203–229).

Anatomical Dissections and Medical Education

No one today has to argue that any medical training should require a strong background in anatomy and physiology. Yet Galenic medicine, that of the physician, required a bare minimum. The oldest anatomical handbook, Mondino de' Liuzzi's *Anathomie*, dated to the early 14th century, and its many misunderstandings and fallacies remained unchallenged for almost two centuries. Dissections were not unknown—even the pope called for autopsying some of the local plague victims in 1348—but they were conducted rarely before the 17th century. Students sat at a distance while a surgeon opened the body up and the physician/ professor droned on from an error-filled Latin text. This began to change in the 16th century with the new teaching and illustrating techniques of Andreas Vesalius. The Netherlander studied in Italy and here established his new model: the professor needed to perform the actual dissection, as Vesalius did, and anatomical texts needed to be rewritten to reflect reality. He also insisted that text illustrations had to rise to the same level of realism as contemporary painting and sculpture. Though the last of nine new anatomy works published between 1490 and 1543, his *Construction of the Human Body*, illustrated by a partner of the artist Titian, rose to a new level of verbal and visual accuracy. Vesalius alone corrected over 200 of Galen's verbal anatomical errors (Vesalius 1543/2003–2009).

The value of anatomical education was such that dissection/lectures were usually open to surgeons as well as well as medical students. They were offered more regularly and increasingly were required for medical licensing or degrees. Over the following 250 years, three trends unfolded: first, Galenism underwent a slow decline; second, the line between physician and surgeon began to blur; and third, the surgeon's status rose in recognition that his expertise in the mechanical—as opposed to the humoral—body was directly related to the major advances in medicine of the 17th and 18th centuries.

Empiricism and Medical Advances

Rooted in experience rather than theory and models, practicing surgeons in the 16th century began publishing manuals and studies that reflected their findings in real cases. Pierre Franco published his *Treatise on Hernias* in 1561 and other works on urinary tract stones and cataracts based on his own experiences and experiments. In 1597, Gaspare Tagliacozzi of Bologna first described a successful skin graft: arm skin to make a new nose. The Scotsman Peter Lowe helped organize the Guild of Surgeons in Glasgow (1599) but only after writing Britain's first full surgical manual, *Chirurgerie*, in 1597. Most famously, the French barber-surgeon and army surgeon Ambroise Paré published many works in which he shared his widely ranging new and successful surgical techniques. Like other surgeons, he wrote in his vernacular to make his works accessible. He very consciously sought to reform surgical practice, perhaps in a way like contemporary Protestants were reforming Christianity. Some of his advances came from the battlefield, such as employing ligatures to stop blood flow to a limb before amputation (instead of merely cauterizing afterward) or the prosthetic mechanical hand he invented for those who had undergone a successful amputation. Others ranged from improved methods of treating cataracts to an infant feeding bottle (Paré 1968). He and others experimented with and made advances in the treatment of urinary stones, gunshot wounds, tumors, and fractures, among many other ailments. Theirs was the spirit of the Scientific Revolution, which questioned authorities (Galen, Aristotle), trusted their own empirical evidence, shared their successes and failures, and sought to improve people's lives though their efforts.

Formal Education for Surgeons

Seventeenth-century discoveries about human anatomy and physiology joined with the practical and successful application of new surgical techniques to raise the social status of the surgeon close to that of the physician by the mid-18th century. Their tools were being made with greater skill and to standardized designs and quality by gold-and pewter-smiths rather than armorers and blacksmiths. Surgeons sought to raise their status, and they were enabled by separating themselves from barbers and their guilds. They did this by supporting the repression of empiric practitioners and even moving in on the practice of female midwives. Monarchs prized the surgeons that saved the lives of their precious soldiers and sailors, and increased their presence among the field ranks and shipboard. Few 18th-century British surgeons had not served in the military or navy. In 1752, Parliament's unpopular Murder Act guaranteed that the corpses of executed criminals would go to the Company of Barber-Surgeons for dissection. The British Royal Navy valued the advice of Scots naval surgeon James Lind to use citrus fruits to prevent scurvy aboard ship, testing it in the 1750s but refusing to adopt their use until the century's end (Harvie 2002). The Italian medical schools had long combined surgical education with Galenic humoralism, but Padua, Bologna, and other once renowned centers fell into a slump. In 1742, the overlord of Bologna, Pope Benedict XIV, set up a local "short-course" school of surgery: over 20 days students would study cadavers from two hospitals.

France was in the forefront of establishing surgical education, with the foundation in Paris of the royal School of Surgery in 1724. Barbers and surgeons in Paris were divorced in 1743, and the Royal Academy of Surgery was established in 1748. In Paris, widows were barred from continuing their husbands' practice in 1755, and after 1768, formal surgical education was required in place of outdated apprenticeships. In 1775, the school became the Collège de Chirurgie with a curriculum including anatomy, chemistry, and physiology (Gelfand 1980). Several German states followed Paris's lead by instituting state surgical schools, often as a way of ensuring a supply of trained surgeons and undermining powerful local guilds.

Perhaps following the Italian model, Spanish medical schools sponsored chairs of surgery at Salamanca (1561) and Alacalá de Henares (1590). In 1617, a royal decree mandated all universities have chairs of anatomy and surgery. Filling these positions remained difficult, and many professors were second-rate practitioners and teachers. Because the law required either two years' apprenticeship plus two of school, or four as an apprentice (after 1603 a total of five years), most Spanish surgeons had apprenticed and received little or no anatomical education. Since university-educated surgeons knew Latin and most apprenticed did not, society made the distinction between "Latin surgeons" and "romance surgeons" who knew only Spanish or Catalan. From 1583, Madrid's *Confradía*, or Brotherhood of Saints Cosmas and Damian, two early Christian physicians, included all the city's surgeons. Consisting mostly of romance surgeons, the group existed almost exclusively to protect its members and reduce competition from outside. It did virtually nothing to advance surgical practice and by its conservatism probably retarded innovation and change. In 1701, the Hospital General in Madrid received its first chair of anatomy, and four years later its anatomy theater for dissections.

Like many 18th-century Scots, enlightened Spaniards tended toward useful knowledge and practical projects for improving life in their country. The Benedictine monk and royal adviser Benito Feijóo helped found Madrid's Academy of Medicine and Surgery in 1734, and in 1748, a group of naval surgeons successfully lobbied to found the Royal School of Surgery, Spain's first, in the busy port city of Cadiz, and a second in Barcelona in 1760. The same year, Madrid's General Hospital began teaching a regular three-year anatomy course, but it was limited to physicians. The capital finally received its first surgical school, the Royal College of San Carlos, in 1787. San Carlos was built adjacent to Madrid's General Hospital and by 1790 had a 40-bed clinical ward for its students' use. The curriculum was based on those of the naval surgery's schools and was both practical and up-to-date (Burke 1977).

The training of surgeons took a different tack in Enlightenment London. The island's premier medical school was in Edinburgh, and it followed many of the reforms pioneered at Leiden in the Netherlands. One of these was having the professor and medical students "doing rounds," or making regular visits to patients in hospital beds. Young Scotsman John Hunter (d. 1793) avoided what he considered the nonsense of medical school and went to London to learn the surgeon's craft from his brother. He also apprenticed with William Cheselden, noted for his success in removing urinary stones with a mortality rate of 10 percent or less (despite advances the norm was closer to 40%). Hunter practiced surgery at St. George's and St. Bartholomew's hospitals and became the premier teacher of apprentice surgeons from England, Scotland, and even North America. He is believed to have trained 449 apprentices in 40 years of practice. He was an empiricist in the spirit of John Locke and the English and Scots Enlightenment: "Do the experiment," he taught his students. Hunter tried new methods, observed carefully, and recorded his findings. He studied the lymphatic system, the reproductive systems of pigs and dogs, and bone regrowth after fracturing, and worked with running tubes down the trachea (intubation). The age of the professional surgeon had arrived (Friedenberg 2009, 193).

A Range of Practitioners

As in China and the Islamic world, the European medical landscape was populated with more or less skilled craftspeople practicing surgical specialties. The poor and rural folk usually had to make do in silence with what they knew. Some household medical books from the 17th and 18th centuries contain recipes for rough casts to immobilize a fractured bone and oral solutions to unroot rotted teeth. The local blacksmith could usually pull teeth and reposition dislocated joints. In Germany, bathhouses made a comeback by the 18th century, and bathmasters were allowed to shave, cut hair, and let blood, as long as it was done in the bathhouse. Germany also had "wound doctors" who dealt with open sores, wounds, and bad bruising (Lindemann 1996). Other specialists either set up shop and were tolerated or moved itinerantly plying their craft(s). Lithotomists extracted urinary stones; oculists treated cataracts and a variety of eye diseases; hernia cutters removed these and other growths, often caused by the strain of hard work; and phlebotomists let blood. In general, medical guilds and colleges fought against these unlicensed empirics, though in times of need, especially during wartime or plague, authorities were happy to bend the rules. Another trend was to license skilled practitioners. In 1699, Paris licensed *bandigistes,* a category that included hernia cutters, lithotomists, bonesetters, occulists, and dentists, and Bourbon Spain followed some years later with the same list of special licenses (Burke 1977, 29–35).

But was the public in 1800 better served by all the licensing, educating, and organizing? Paré's insistence on applying a tourniquet above the wound before amputating no doubt saved some lives, but the horrible pain from the four minutes of bone sawing, the shock, and the nearly inevitable infection that followed no doubt killed as many as before. Anesthesia remained a major problem, and surgeons had their own concoctions, including alcohol and/or opiates, and made few real advances. Stone cutting, even by an expert and lasting only 30 seconds, often meant not only pain but hemorrhaging, shock, and infection. Complicated fractures or poorly set bones could knit together badly and result in loss of the limb or gangrene and death. Most surgeons, even formally educated ones, had limited knowledge of anatomy, even less of physiology, and no respect for cleanliness. Even the finest surgeons avoided invasive surgery beyond cutting for stones, hernias, or some tumors, knowing that deep, especially thoracic penetration simply invited hemorrhage, shock, and infection. Despite medical academies and manuals that spread news of discoveries, these often had little impact on the practicing surgeon and less on the unlicensed practitioner. Perhaps the widest range of practical surgical advances came from men who had served as army or naval surgeons, which, following a major conflict such as the Seven Years' War, might include a large percentage of practicing surgeons.

Dentistry

Maintenance of good teeth and removal of troublesome teeth was a major concern of early modern Europeans. Many factors had always threatened dental health, such as poor diet, trauma, or cavities, but new ones appeared between 1500 and 1800. Scurvy from months at sea damaged the mouth, gums, and teeth; the increased use of cheap sugar helped rot teeth away; and the increased use of mercury as an ingredient in cosmetics and as treatment for syphilis introduced a poison that undermined the teeth and gums. Poor dental and oral health more generally led to halitosis, ugliness, and disruption of speech, all of which were especially unwelcome in polite European society. Home recipe books almost always included tooth painkillers and toothpowders—including such abrasives as ground amber or coral—to cleanse the teeth, and many had herbal mouthwashes, heavy on the alcohol and mint. Across the period, a few professional works appeared, including sections of Paré's books in France and the German *Teeth Doctoring* (*Zene Artzney*), which was published around 1530 and saw 15 editions by 1576. England's first was Charles Allen's *Curious Observations in That Difficult Part of Chirurgery, Relating to the Teeth* of 1685–1687 (Hargreaves 1998; see also King 1998).

Barbers, surgeons, and tooth pullers handled most of society's needs. All could clean and pull, but only the talented, or skilled jewelers, could make artificial dental work. Artificial teeth date from the 16th century, when carved animal bone, agates, or tusks did the job. Human teeth, too, often pulled from dead soldiers on the battlefield, were fitted into new owners and secured by gold wires. Teeth specialists could drain abscesses, use a hand drill to remove decay, reroot teeth that had fallen out, and whiten teeth with acids or bleaching compounds. By the mid-17th century, tooth pullers had morphed into "operators for the teeth." One such, London's "High German Operator," John Schultim, advertised his abilities: "He also draweth broken teeth, and sets in artificial ones in their room, as firm as if they were natural, so that you may eat and bite with them: he helps loose teeth, restoreth decayed gums, and cureth the scurvy in the mouth" (Hargreaves 1998, 78).

The dentist, properly labeled and considered a professional, had emerged by about 1760. With license in hand, at least in Paris and Spain, the dentist emphasized his "painless" methods, and by the end of the 18th century, artificial teeth of porcelain and metal began to appear. In that often gullible Age of Enlightenment, many charlatans and outright frauds peddled dentifrices, painkillers, cures for halitosis, and other oral remedies, but tooth pulling remained the standard procedure for professional and itinerant alike (Jones 2000).

9

Mental Health

When a person fractures a bone, suffers from a high fever, or hemorrhages after giving birth, there is little doubt that some treatment is needed. Practitioners may argue over the cause of the fever or what damage is causing the hemorrhage but not over the need for setting the bone or stanching the flow of blood. When a person is uncharacteristically sluggish or excited, suddenly passes out, or begins talking to himself, both the need for intervention and what remedy is needed are far less obvious. Today's psychology and psychiatry may have answers about the underlying conditions that cause this series of symptoms. These may be serious and require medical treatment, or they may be simply situational: low blood sugar resulting from poor diet or preoccupation due to anger. We look to doctors to sort these out.

In premodern societies, the interactions among the brain, nerves, and outward behavior were understood only very tentatively if at all. People, including physicians, accepted and thought they understood divine or demonic actions, magic and curses, vapors released by bad humors into the brain, poisons, and negative astrological influences as causes for aberrant behaviors. Depression, panic attacks, epileptic fits, multiple personalities, rage, idiocy, senility, paranoia, and madness were often considered spiritual rather than medical conditions, or spiritually caused medical conditions. Different cultures approached those afflicted with mental problems in different ways, depending in part on the level of disruption their behaviors caused. Across the early modern period, most mentally or emotionally ill people whose symptoms were tolerable were probably treated by the appropriate priest, shaman, cunning woman, or "mad doctor" and then hidden away by the family. A much greater problem was posed by those unfortunates whose behaviors were extreme and threatened themselves and others around them.

THE AZTECS

Much of what is known of Aztec medicine was transferred through the Spanish, though some writers were themselves of Aztec origin. Aztecs believed the heart and not the brain was the seat of mental activity. Thus the root of behaviors such as epilepsy, idiocy, and mania was to be found in the heart. They did not have as wide a set of labels for mental illness as the Europeans did, and most behaviors were categorized as either passive or active insanity. It seems that passive indicated those symptoms that made the person quiet and easily manageable, such as depression, lack of affect, dementia, or catatonia. Active insanity would have made the person unpredictable and difficult to manage, such as epilepsy or frenzy. Aztecs blamed both behavior patterns on what the Europeans called phlegm collecting in the area of the heart (Schendel 1968, 49–50).

This could occur naturally but could also be the result of self-poisoning with certain drugs used for their psychotropic or other effects. In this case, detoxification by purging and withdrawal of the person from the offending substance was supposed to return him or her to normal. In the 1552 Aztec herbal, written in Nahuatl by native Martín de la Cruz, appear several entries dealing with what we would call mental problems. The first is for epilepsy "recently aroused." First, the patient drinks the juice of a purgative root, then a wicked mixture of hot water with stones found in specific bird stomachs, the root of a highly odiferous plant (*quetzalatzonyatl*), deer's horn, white incense, human corpse hair, and the ashes of an incinerated mole. This should cause him to vomit profusely. Right before a fit begins, he is to undergo a second treatment including the consumption of boiled wolf and weasel brains, and incensing with the "odor of a mouse's nest." The very macho Aztecs treated "fear or timidity" with a potion made of several plants and a poultice made of "the blood of a wolf and a fox, a worm, the blood and excrement of the *acuecueyalotl*, laurel, [and] swallow's excrement." Temporary "stupidity of mind" was treated first with a vomit-inducing purge; days later a drink including the "heart plant" should drive out "the evil humor in the chest." Then a cocktail of powdered bird stomach stones and precious stones was to be drunk and poured over his head. After this, if he takes to carrying around yet another bird stomach stone, "his sanity of mind [will] be restored." Just in case, his head should be anointed with ravens' brains, and he should wear an amulet of a swallow's stomach stone around his neck (Gates 1939/2000, 94, 97, 98).

As with other maladies, however, a cause other than nature or self was also possible: evil spirits. Some of the elements of each of the remedies above probably contain elements that were meant to propitiate or drive away malevolent entities. But priest-practitioners, at least in pre-Christian Mexico, had their exorcisms and other rites for restoring the mentally troubled to their communities. The Catholic Church did what it could to eliminate the Aztec priesthood, replacing native with Catholic exorcisms, but the low state of 16th-century mental health practice meant that the Spaniards had little to teach the Indians. The first mental hospital in the Western Hemisphere was San Hipólito in Mexico City, used exclusively for the insane from 1589 (Kidwell 1997; Leiby 1992).

CARIBBEAN SLAVES

Over the 300 years covered by this book, several million Africans were forcibly taken from their homes, held as captives in dank, prison-like conditions, and then shipped under utterly inhumane conditions to a strange land where they were to serve in baking, disease-ridden landscapes as field slaves for the rest of their lives. Perhaps the surprising thing is that any preserved even a shred of their mental health. Because slaves were gathered, sold, bought, and used as property, records on their mental health and illness are hard to come by. Slaveholders and their agents simply did not tolerate the kinds of manic, depressive, demented, or otherwise disruptive behavior that are often associated with mental illness. While a physician might have been called to treat a fever, a surgeon to mend a broken limb, or a midwife to help with a woman's labor, only the whip and other instruments of discipline waited on the bodies of the mentally or emotionally troubled.

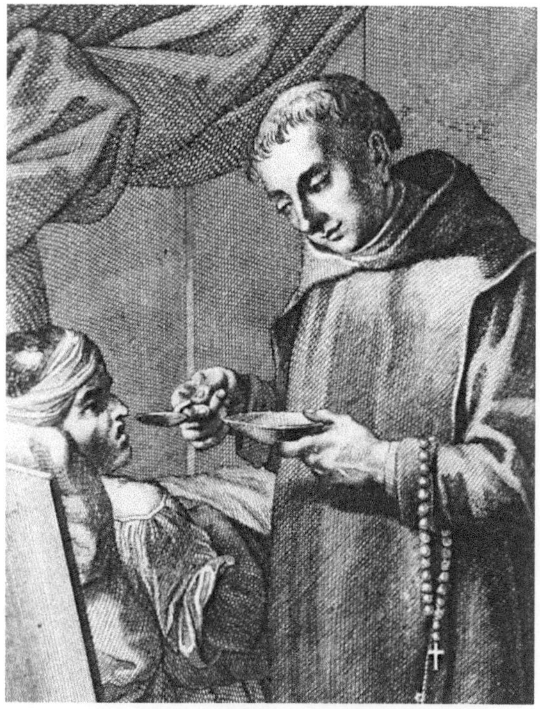

Sixteenth-century religious brother Bernardino Álvarez, founder of the earliest mental hospitals in the Americas. He came to New Spain as a soldier and became a wealthy businessman who used his wealth to build health facilities. He founded a religious order named for his asylum of San Hipólito in Mexico City. (National Library of Medicine)

While certain congenital conditions may have been sifted out of many African populations by the harsh and demanding realities of daily life in the tropics, the trauma of the descent into slavery would have left many in a miserable emotional state. From later slave narratives, we know the terror imposed simply by the white-skinned slavers, by the unfamiliarity of the pounding surf and endless ocean, the rocking of the fetid ship. The new slave's sense of self was stripped not only by the shackles and chains but by the babble of strange voices, the loss of identity and freedom of action, and the utter uncertainty of the future. Anthropologists have pointed out that typically Africans built their senses of self through identification with their natural and social environments in Africa. Modern—or even postmodern—people define themselves at least in part by their independence to define themselves by their economic liberty and their choices. Africans defined themselves as individuals who were a part of a larger whole, a kin group and tribe that provided for all of the individual's needs and whose circle was the source of personal fulfillment and happiness. Outside the circle was social death. The African was a person only in relation to his family, ancestors, and divinities. The living landscape, of which he was an integral part, not only provided food and shelter but was the matrix that gave meaning to life.

Capture, captivity, and enslavement ripped all of that away. Life became a matter of confusion, weariness, pain, disease, fear, and death. Many chose suicide, either at their own hands or at those of their armed captors. All had suffered a social death and had few resources with which to build a new self. Those whose bodies survived the Middle Passage intact found new homes as the property of Spanish, French, Dutch, or English masters. Their new communities were formed of people whose languages differed and whose customs and manners sometimes clashed. Foods, gods, and medicines were a mixture of the familiar and the strange. The hostile climate, numbing labor, and endless hours invited illness of mind and body, and weakness made the body susceptible to greater ravishment still. Slaves were brutalized by overseers and rented out to neighbors who had little incentive to treat them humanely. While slave owners would have recognized certain behaviors as medical illness among their own social group, the weariness of depression, epileptic fits, or unpredictable outbreaks of mania were simply intolerable breaches of discipline, no matter how involuntary. Those whose mental capacities dropped considerably were given tasks suited to their new conditions, while those whose behaviors became chronically disruptive often simply disappeared and were written off, as there was neither madhouse nor market for an insane slave.

THE CHINESE

Early modern Chinese medicine revered its ancient roots and the literature in which it was expressed. Like Aztec and African traditions, Chinese medical traditions held that the human body, mind, and spirit were all organically interconnected and that proper treatment accounted for all three aspects of the unwell person. Mental or emotional illness could be the result of physical or spiritual causes, and the two could appear very similar. For example, madness could be caused by an excess of "mucus" around the heart, requiring the administration of drugs that would break up and remove the troublesome substance. But spiritual forces including demons, angry ancestors, or the spirits of victims of injustice could also induce madness. Comprehensive treatment thus required a spiritual specialist's methods, such as exorcisms and sacrifices, as well as organic or physical remedies. The same held for emotional problems: for example, anger was directly related to the liver, and if a person's proper liver functioning were disrupted, then uncontrolled verbal or physical manifestations of anger could result. Of course, spirits might also cause such displays (Unschuld 2010, 216).

As early as the *Yellow Emperor's Canon*, Chinese physicians recognized the two types of causation. One was physical: imbalances in or among the body's yin and yang, Five Phases, emotional centers in the organs, or the seasons. The second included a wide range of spiritual conditions both particular to the individual, such as a "loss of soul," or external assaults such as spirit possession or disfavor by the gods. Alternative medical practitioners, the highly spiritual Chinese Daoist masters emphasized the role of religious ritual, such as sacrifices, and spiritually powerful objects such as amulets. When Catholic priests arrived, the masters recognized and welcomed the power of the foreigners' healing rituals (the Mass, prayers, hymns, exorcisms) and variety of sacramentals (religious objects including rosaries, holy water and oil, communion wafers, icons, relics, crucifixes, and candles) (Ng 1990).

The *Canon* also distinguished two main types of illness. *Dian* was an overabundance of yin that led to behaviors as different as depression or catatonia and unwarranted euphoria or giddiness. Too much yang resulted in *kuan*, which manifested in many ways, including aversion to heat, loss of appetite and inability to eat, irrational anger, and uncontrollable urges to sing, undress, curse, climb things, or lord it over others. In the seventh century, Sun Miao added "wind" as a cause: it entered the conduits of the body's yin or yang resulting in the disruptive imbalance. Twelfth-century Liu Wansu emphasized the importance of the "climatic influences" heat and fire in bringing on *kuan* behaviors. This immediately recommended physical therapies that reduced the body's heat and fire and sleep that naturally cooled it.

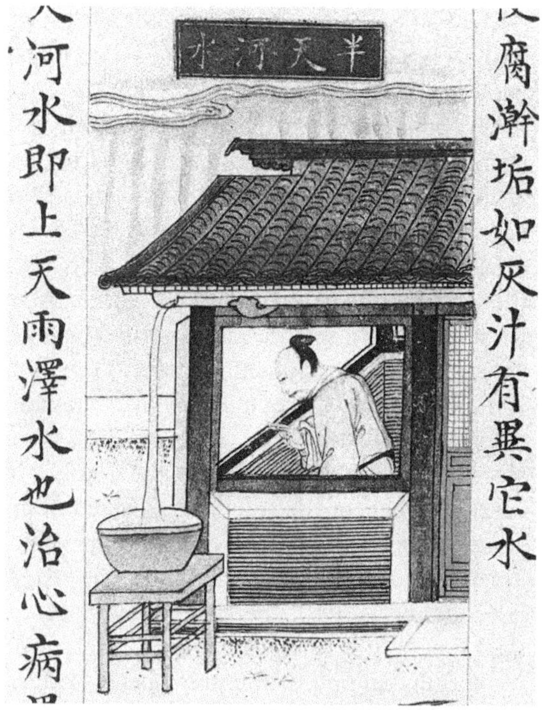

Illustration of a man collecting "mid-air river water," from the anonymous Ming-era dietetic herbal, *Shiwu bencao*. The accompanying text refers to rainwater as being pure and clean and as such a useful tool to fight heart disease, madness from demonic infestation, malign qi, and noxious poisons. (Wellcome Collection)

As part of their campaign to increase their status in Chinese society, physicians increasingly emphasized the "medical" causes of and remedies for mental illness and emotional distress. If a sufferer or her family consulted a physician, he would seek the organic cause and recommend herbs, potions, acupuncture, and/or moxibustion as means of addressing it. From the 13th century, there was also a move toward what we would call psychological treatments. The physician might seek to provoke laughter from a person with no outward emotion or induce a person who refuses to eat with his favorite foods' sights and smells. Reverse psychology suggested countering exaggerated emotional states with their opposites: trying to anger or depress the giddy, for example. With the decline in physicians' emphasis on spiritual causes for mental or emotional illness, which often had moral guilt associated with its onset (what had the patient done to anger the gods or ancestors?), personal stigma tended to fall away. At least it happened among those urban Chinese who accepted the official medical community's conclusions.

Even in cities, however, there were thriving communities of alternative healers with whom even the most sophisticated might consult. In rural areas, the range of choices was smaller, but the local healer was far more likely to be an empiric herbalist or religious master than a literate physician. As might be expected, older folk traditions held sway, and mental or emotional problems did imply moral failings, at least once home remedies failed. For Buddhists, sins took many forms, from killing animals for food to homosexuality. Given their concept of karma, Buddhists insisted that such actions had consequences—including mental illness in this or future lives—and offered sufferers small certificates after proper prayers for release from retribution. Buddhist and other alternative healers seem to have especially credited sexual sins with the onset of mental or emotional troubles.

Early modern China had no governmental asylums until the 1730s. Those with debilitating illness found shelter in their homes or Buddhist care facilities. Others simply wandered the streets and roads—at least until officials across China cracked down on the mentally and emotionally ill. In 1731, an asylum for the insane was proposed for Sichuan Province; this was provided, and the order extended to the country in 1740. The same law required all mentally ill to be housed, and in 1757, the government attempted to get the rural clans to register their mentally ill. Across China, clans refused to comply: a matter of clan solidarity and the stigma of mental illness. A decade later, the Board of Punishments declared the insane to be incapable of forming the necessary intention to commit criminal acts apart from murder or treason. From 1762, a mad murderer warranted imprisonment for life rather than execution. Also in 1766, the government insisted that the ill kept in homes or religious refuges had to be secure against escape, or they would be forcibly confined. Governmental facilities were for men only; women had to be maintained securely at home, a bow to the culture's traditional gender distinction. Officially, at least, the Late Imperial Chinese had come to regard the mentally ill not as victims—whether of demons or organic failures—but rather as deviants who needed to be confined and controlled (Ng 1990, 63–83).

THE TURKS AND PERSIANS

Early modern Islamic authorities considered madness to be an imbalance of both a spiritual and physical nature. As such, there were recognized degrees of madness, from those that caused mild behavioral problems to those that presented a real threat to the person or those around him or her. The first were generally accepted as colorful characters in society, often providing what we would consider unacceptable amusement by their babbling, dancing, or harmless emotional outbursts. Both medical and civic authorities allowed the harmlessly insane to wander as they would, living on what they could find, steal, or receive as charity. Public lunacy was often associated with substance abuse, and the line between intoxication and true mental illness could be easily ignored.

When symptoms became acute, however, the *bimaristans* took in the disruptively mentally ill person. In the Turkish world, they were controlled in special wards, being chained when needed. For those who were believed to benefit from therapy, there were soothing fountains and even a form of music therapy. Baths played a role in the attempt to rebalance the superfluity of overly "dry" humors. Lest this create an image of paradise, however, visitors also described vile living conditions of filth and disorder among the incarcerated insane. In Persia, physician recommendations apparently included severe beatings "about the head." In at least one case, staff were told that a patient "be shut up and so terrified that he dare not open his mouth" (Elgood 1970, 27–28). "Therapy" for the acutely insane included shaving of the head, branding of the temples, pulling of all the teeth, and beating with a leather strap or on the soles of the feet with a cane. However barbaric, such treatment was disciplinary and not punitive in meaning. Maintaining social order was of prime importance to the Ottomans and perhaps even more so to the Safavids and their officials. When lunatics seemed to threaten this order, even by their mere presence, the state was more than willing to act (Dols 1992; Shefer-Mossensohn 2009, 135–140).

THE EUROPEANS

In several famous books, the French intellectual and historian Michel Foucault laid out an influential model of European (especially French) reaction to mental illness. As he saw it, up to the 17th century, societies not only tolerated the presence of the mad in society but even celebrated their freedom from convention and alternatives to social norms. Renaissance works such as Erasmus of Rotterdam's *Praise of Folly*, Sebastian Brandt's *Ship of Fools*, Rabelais's *Gargantua and Pantagruel*, Cervantes's *Don Quixote*, and any number of Shakespeare plays featured disordered minds that often formed deeper truths than the day's philosophy (see Chakravarti 2011). Foucault described this acceptance withering beneath the burgeoning 17th-century state, which understood any deviance as a threat to its authority and power. The growth of the insane asylum paralleled those of the prison for the criminal and pest house for the plague sickened. Religious bigotry accompanied the targeting of "witches," and intolerance trumped diversity. Foucault's vision of our period has been refined and undermined, but it remains an important model for considering how a society defines and constructs a disease (Foucault 1965; Foucault 1977; see also Finzsch and Jütte 1996).

Early Theories of Madness

Early modern Western philosophy no less than medicine was uncomfortable with the problem of the connection and relationship among the mind, soul, and body. That the corporeal body and the nonmaterial mind and—eternal—soul interacted was accepted as obvious, but neither religion nor philosophy nor medicine could clarify how this worked. It became an issue when a person's behavior—fits, inappropriate babbling, catatonia—seemed to indicate a problem that was not merely physical.

Christian Europe accepted the power and interference of the spiritual world no less than did the Aztecs or Chinese. Biblical accounts of demonic possession and popular tales of curses by devil-worshipping witches or wizards seemed to confirm the role of the unholy in causing at least some cases of insanity or emotional imbalance. On the other hand were the saints, whose irrational acts and meditative states indicated God's favor and possession by the Holy Spirit. The French girl Joan of Arc heard voices she identified as those of saints: was she deluded by Satan, mentally ill, or truly blessed? In her day, her supporters considered her a prophet and her enemies considered her a witch, capturing and burning her as punishment. Today, she would probably be given medication and be shunned even by her own church. In 1562, the prescient Dutch physician Johann Weyer published an entire book on how demons indeed deceive people, especially women, into serving Satan, but he insisted that self-confessed "witches" were really poor wretches who merely suffered from melancholy, an overabundance of the humor black bile, or bad dreams, drug abuse, or hallucinations (see Radden 2000, 97–105).

From the ancient Greeks, and to a lesser extent the medieval Arabs, Europeans inherited a natural model of mental and emotional illness. Most problems were a matter not of spiritual interference, whether possession or curse, but of a physical imbalance in the body itself. That this affected the body's behavior—hallucinating, passing out, uncontrollably cursing—was not an issue, but how this was caused by the mind, or itself affected the mind, was not at all clear. The Greek medical paradigm of Galen posited the body's four humors—blood, phlegm, black bile, and yellow bile—as the determiners of most forms of illness, including mental or behavioral illness. Each humor and its associated organ needed to function properly and in balance with the others for good health.

For at least the early part of our period, many physicians also accepted that each person was influenced by the planet under which he or she was born, each of which was associated with a specific humor. This astrological effect was dominant in the 16th century, being heavily supported by the writings of Marsilio Ficino, a physician and head of the Medici Academy in Florence. The planet imprinted itself as a kind of genetic predisposition to a dominant mood. It did this by stimulating the production of its particular humor. For example, those born under Saturn's influence were subject to overabundance of black bile, and this buildup would stimulate a number of responses including creativity and emotional depression, or melancholia (literally "black bile").

In his *Three Books of Life* (1482), Ficino further explained that human behavior could be an important causal factor as well. The kind of intense mental work and concentration that was required of the artist or scholar had the physiological effect of drying up the brain. This eliminated the important moisture that retained important heat, making the brain cold and dry, which were the characteristics of the melancholic. Still further, the sedentary artist or scholar did not move about (exercise) in such a way as to "exhale" the "thick, dense, clinging, dusky vapors" that "overcome the soul with sadness and terrifies it" (Radden 2000, 90; see also Ficino 1998). How physical vapors could terrify the immaterial soul remains unexplained. For other practitioners, melancholy was brought on by "vapors" that rose from one or more of the body's organs and dried out the brain. Warm and moist substances such as cinnamon, saffron, sandal, and "milky" foods could help prevent melancholia, while it could be treated with moist foods and baths or a warming ointment of lavender. Wearing a talisman with the properties of Jupiter could also ward off the effects of Saturn. Handling melancholy successfully was important because many believed that if unattended it developed into the more serious mania. But in 1549, the Montpellier physician Denys Fontanon wrote that mania resulted rather from yellow bile or too much blood around the brain (Porter 2006, 243). Four decades later, in England's first treatise on *melancholia*, Timothy Bright distinguished melancholy caused by black bile, which could be treated successfully with typical dietary remedies and purging, from melancholy rooted in spiritual anguish or guilt, which called for repentance and religious healing.

In a broader sense, exercise, one of the six classic "non-naturals," along with rest, diet, evacuation (helped by purging), and healthy climate were believed to help maintain humoral balance, while ignoring a healthy regimen courted imbalance and illness. Galen taught that epilepsy, usually associated with divine disfavor, resulted from the rising to the brain of vapors of phlegm or black bile. Of course physical trauma to the head could result in diminished mental capacity or disrupted emotions, and emotional traumas such as losing a loved one or witnessing a shocking horror could also bring on a disordered mental or emotional state. Some believed trauma could unbalance the humors in the head, while others understood that "corrupted air" found its way into the head. Popular English 16th-century remedies for illnesses of the head included herbal plasters for headaches, a plaster of vinegar and mustard for a migraine, lily of the valley or rosemary for memory loss, primrose, sage, and powdered human skull for inability to speak, and for insomnia alcohol, poppy syrup (an opiate), or a mixture of valerian, hops, and passiflora (Knight 2006, 128–143).

The Early Asylum

As the chapter on early modern medical institutions makes clear, many types of confinement or isolation facilities for special patients sprang up across Europe between 1500 and 1800. Yet family members, villagers, and townspeople either tolerated eccentricities or locked the more dangerous folk in sturdy rooms, attics, or cellars. This was in part to protect the dangerously ill from hurting themselves or others, but it was also to shield from the public the family shame. Throughout the period—across the globe—most insane people were cared for and isolated by their own families. Some hospitals and other semimonastic facilities had special wards or rooms for the seriously mentally ill—including those suffering from the madness brought on by late-stage syphilis—but many more excluded the disruptive and dangerous.

Housing the mad seems to have begun in the 15th century, with the Casa de los Inocentes (House of the Innocents, 1436) in the Spanish port city of Seville as an early example. Perhaps based on Muslim models in Granada, others soon appeared in Valencia, Zaragoza, Valladolid, Toledo, and Barcelona. The beliefs that lunatics were insensitive to most sources of discomfort and that maniacs were possessed of extraordinary strength meant that madhouses needed few luxuries but strong doors, window bars, and at least some shackles and chains. The infamous Bedlam

Hospital in London began life in 1247 as the Priory (religious residence) of St. Mary of Bethlehem (Bethlem). In 1403, it housed at least six insane men. During the Reformation, the city took it from the exiled Catholic Church, stripped its incomes and chapels, and appointed the board of governors of Bridewell Prison to run it as an asylum from 1547 (to1948). Inmates could be discharged to known friends, but they were not allowed to beg. A 1598 report listed 20 inmates: 11 women and 9 men, 6 sent from Bridewell and 14 committed by courts or families (both poor and wealthy). Overseers treated physical wounds or sicknesses, but governors provided nothing in the way of mental therapy. Located between two open sewers, the place naturally stank, all the more so since it was never cleaned out. In 1618, King James I ordered conditions raised to the level of those at the city's hospitals. In 1643, the Puritan government enlarged Bedlam and doubled the population but banned curious sightseers and insisted on more sanitary conditions (Arnold 2008; Smith 2007; Andrews and Scull 2001).

New Bethlem (1674) was the first purpose-built hospital in London since 1519. Located in Moorfields on the City's old moat and funded by loans and private donations, it was designed by Robert Hooke (of microscope fame) as a long neoclassical block 720 feet by 80 feet deep. Its 120 rooms were surrounded by walls 14 feet high, and for half a century, it was London's biggest postfire (1666) building project after only the Exchange Building and St. Paul's Cathedral. Additional space for noninsane paupers was added in 1725 and 1733, allowing for a total population of some 220 (Andrews and Scull 2002, 8).

From at least 1610, Bedlam became a place to visit to watch the residents' antics, like a zoo. Some moralists considered this a good thing, insofar as they viewed the inmates as morally fallen humans who were suffering for their sins. By the 18th century this practice was seen as degrading and disruptive to residents, but it provided some £400 annually of very necessary income, and visitations reached a peak in the 1760s. Nevertheless, gawking visitors were first limited in number and then banned altogether in 1770.

In France in 1657, Louis XIV established in Paris the *hôpitaux généraux* named Bicêtre (for men) and Salpêtrière (for women). They included the insane, increasingly specialized in holding them, and gained reputations for their horrible conditions and inhumane treatment of the sick. At their height early on, they housed some 6,000 residents. In 1788, 245 of the males in Bicêtre were mentally ill (the rest were beggars and decrepit old men) (Shorter 1998, 6).

Central Europe lacked the metropolises of London and Paris and relied on churches and local governments to provide secure quarters for the mad when a family could not. From the later Middle Ages, many Catholic-run German hospitals housed "raving lunatics" in specially furnished rooms, but by the 16th century, they resided together with the blind, elderly, and crippled in urban hospitals. In Protestant areas, some old monasteries were converted for confining the insane, where strict discipline—even beatings and the use of cages—might be used to maintain order. Unlike hospitals in Catholic Europe, where friars, monks, or nuns often provided spiritual as well as physical care, Protestant hospitals in Central Europe were run as strictly secular institutions (Vanja 1996). Given the Russian love for their mad holy men, it should not surprise that when a Russian family

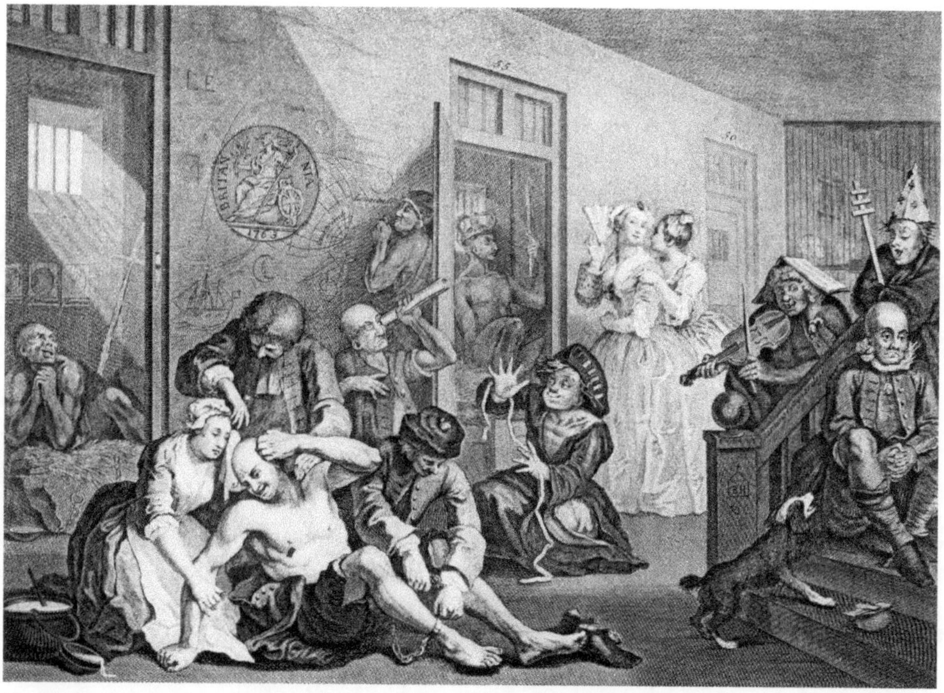

Engraving by William Hogarth depicting the interior of Bedlam Hospital in 1763. Based on Hogarth's earlier paintings for the series *A Rake's Progress*, the engraving shows the character of Tom Rakewell in the madhouse of Bethlem Royal Hospital in London. As in the real asylum of the time, in Hogarth's Bedlam, fashionable ladies have come to observe the lunatics as a form of entertainment. (National Library of Medicine)

could or would not care for a mentally sick member, he or she would be sent to a monastery.

Asylums were transplanted rather late to the New World, with the first in Mexico City in 1589: the Hospital of San Hipólito, which was hived off the facility La Caridad y San Hipólito. In colonial Boston, the Almshouse, which cared for the destitute, set aside a special ward for the insane in 1729, and the first public insane asylum appeared in Williamsburg, Virginia, in 1773. Ireland's first madhouse was St. Patrick's Asylum in Dublin, funded in part by reformer, cleric, and author Jonathan Swift.

Emerging Theories and Therapies

In early modern Europe, more than any other part of the world, traditional medical models of mental illness were challenged by the discoveries and theories of scientists and physicians. In turn these suggested new treatments. For example, the nerves, envisioned as tiny tubes that connected the brain to the rest of the body, were believed by some to circulate "vital spirits" that somehow provided sense data to the brain and directed the brain's commands to the body. Blockages in the nerve-tubes or other types of damage to them explained many types of illness and gave rise to the notion of "nervous disorders" and "neurosis" (coined by Dr. William Cullen in 1785). This mechanical model replaced "rising vapors," humoral imbalances, and the wandering uterus. It also opened the door to hydrotherapies that utilized baths of mineral waters, such as those found naturally at Bath, England; Spa, Belgium; Wiesbaden, Germany; and Plombieres, France. These and other "watering holes" drew Europe's elite and became seasonally fashionable to aristocrats and hangers-on. This fad grew with the notion that being a bit "nervous" was a sign of a "sensible" person of high breeding. By the century's end, though, the elites had discovered the sea as a natural source of dissolved minerals and salts, and they abandoned the spas for the seaside resorts that canny entrepreneurs established along the Atlantic and Mediterranean shorelines.

The fad for bathing joined with the fascination for magnetism and early electrical experiments and resulted in Franz Mesmer's famous demagnetizing tubs. A number of doctors had identified vital spirits, or the force circulating through the nerves, with electricity. Mesmer began offering his therapy of bathing in tubs that supposedly contained "animal magnetism" in Vienna. Forced out of town, in the 1770s he settled into the capital of the Enlightenment, Paris, and seduced the aristocracy. Though wildly popular, an official committee that included the chemist Antoine Lavoisier, Ben Franklin, and Dr. Ignace-Joseph Guillotin (he of the later guillotine) investigated and concluded that Mesmerism was bogus and Mesmer a fraud.

Confinement in the 18th Century

Enlightened thinking among physicians and social reformers informed a great expansion of asylums—perhaps Foucault's real Great Confinement—and the broadening sense that madness or insanity was a sickness that warranted a therapy. Institutions should not merely house but seek to heal the mentally ill. Reflecting the societal abandonment of spiritual causes for insanity, Lady Mary Wortley Montagu, early proponent of inoculation for smallpox, wrote in 1755 that "madness is as much a corporeal distemper as the gout or asthma . . . Passion may bring on a fit, but the disease is lodged in the blood" (Andrews and Scull 2001, 30).

The French provided a model of combining a workhouse for the indigent with a madhouse, in which the insane would be housed and chained to their work stations. This had the reasonable result of both securing the mad and making them productive and was adopted by many German states. As major urban hospitals appeared in the later 18th century, many included wards or separate facilities for the insane. This both spurred and was spurred by the increasing medicalization of madness, which defined it as a disease and not just a social disability (Vanja 1996, 117–132).

During the 1700s, asylums appeared in the English cities of Manchester, Liverpool, Norwich, York, and Newcastle. The traditional Galenic regimen of carefully controlled diets, exercise, light, good air, clean surroundings, and purgings recommended itself to humane and enlightened managers. In mid-18th century, Bedlam was under the direction of Dr. John Monro, who had replaced his father,

James. In 1751, one of Bedlam's governors, Dr. John Battie, opened St. Luke's in Moorfields near Bedlam as a competing charity hospital. Its simple unadorned lines contrasted with the fancy neoclassical decoration of Bedlam, and they differed in other ways as well.

In 1758, Battie wrote *A Treatise on Madness*, and his competitor, John Monro, immediately rejoined with his scathing *Remarks on Dr. Battie's Treatise*. Both supported their arguments with classical and contemporary authors, but more importantly, they relied on their own experiences. Battie believed that mental illness could be understood and even cured in many cases, since there were many different underlying causes. Some illness was "original," often hereditary, and could not be cured. The rest was "consequential": brought on by drug abuse, physical trauma, or emotional distress, and thus curable if understood. Battie advocated multiple types of therapy and isolating patients from "gawkers." Further, he adhered to the enlightened belief in progress in medical knowledge. Since medical schools still provided no training in treating mental illness, he urged that asylums allow medical students to learn from insane patients as residents in hospitals learned from diseased or wounded patients. He also welcomed constructive public scrutiny of his new institution. Each point was a criticism of Monro and Bedlam, and Monro rejected many of Battie's attitudes and methods. The insane should be managed with humane care, but they are confined because they cannot be cured. Mental illness was a single disease with many manifestations, and thus a single Galenic regimen sufficed to control it. Gawkers were welcome, even physically interacting with the inmates, but medical students had no place, nor did the scrutinizing eyes of the public, at least as long as gentlemen ran the place. In many ways, this was a dispute of Monro's old school against the progressive model championed by Battie (Andrews and Scull 2001, 52–53).

From the later 1600s, London also hosted numerous private madhouses. Some were run as sidelines by physicians, surgeons, or apothecaries, while others were purely business ventures. Though often run-down old manor houses, they were expensive but discreet, and thus useful to the upper classes. And they proved to be very lucrative. "Mad doctors" like Monro and Battie had their own professional private practices, often recommending specific "houses" where they also served as medical consultants. Monro was a business partner in Brooke House, Hackney, a rebuilt 17th-century ruin. The site was waterlogged, but each individual room had its own fireplace. Though most private madhouses hosted fewer than 10, Brooke House managed 50 inmates. It remained to be demolished by the German Luftwaffe in 1940. In 1774, the Royal College of Physicians succeeded in getting passed the first parliamentary act for regulating madhouses, requiring registration and inspection. About 50 passed muster by 1800.

Both Battie and Monro, and many mad doctors in England and elsewhere, kept casebooks with notes on patients, though few of these survive. One of Monro's did and has been published. It is a rare glimpse into the physician's private practice and the life of mentally ill patients in the 18th century.

Late in the 18th century, medical pioneers, of whom Battie was one, set the scene for 19th-century advances in treatment of the insane. In 1788, Florentine physician Vincenzio Chiarugi opened the renovated Bonifazio Hospital for mental patients from the Hospital of Santa Dorotea. Bonifazio was designed as a place of therapy and healing with clear rules for handling the patients in the most humane way possible. During 1793–1794, Chiarugi published his three-volume *On Insanity*, which spread his ideas. In revolutionary Paris, Philippe Pinel adopted Chiarugi's ideas at Bicêtre and Salpêtrière in 1793, striking off their chains (though he later introduced straightjackets) (Shorter 1998, 10–14). In 1796, the Quaker Tuke family of York established a residence for the mentally ill. York Retreat rejected the confinement of residents, based on the Quaker belief that the divine Inner Light each person possessed would be stimulated to heal them (Kilpatrick 1990). Perhaps ironically, many English considered religious "enthusiasts" such as the Quakers and Methodists to be mentally ill simply by virtue of their religious choice.

10

Drugs and Remedies

Between 1500 and 1800, the world became knitted together in ways it had never been before. Europeans were exposed to medical and pharmacological traditions of which they had never dreamed. China, Africa, and Central America exchanged foods, spices, and other health-related substances that remained limited to isolated cultures before 1500. Writing about the new materia medica that was beginning to circulate around the globe was largely a matter for Europeans, though most literate cultures produced new herbals, recipe books, and pharmacopeias that reflected the wide-ranging exchanges. For Europeans at home and abroad as colonists, merchants, or conquerors, the recent innovation of printing provided a revolutionary tool for recording and learning about world cultures and their medical traditions. Through trade and plunder, Europeans acquired the new spices, barks, roots, fruits, and other riches, shipping them home and abroad as the markets demanded (see Schiebinger and Swan 2005). But they also shipped living specimens home to be planted in medicinal and botanical gardens to slake the Renaissance's thirst for new knowledge. Meanwhile, those who retailed herbal simples, compounds, and drugs integrated the new materia medica in with the traditional menu, bringing the world's healing secrets into the most humble lodgings.

TYPES OF MATERIA MEDICA

"Materia medica" is simply the Latin for "medical materials" and refers to the various substances that medical practitioners used in preparing drinks, pills, powders, fumigations, emetics, washes, poultices, clysters, and other remedies. At their simplest, a single ingredient was used, and this was a termed a "simple." A compound consisted of a mixture of two or more simples, perhaps in a pleasing medium such as sugar water, rose water, or wine. In the premodern period, many choices by cultures reflected generations of experience, passed on orally or in writing. Others reflected what we might consider less rational criteria: a root looked like a human limb and could therefore fix that limb; or the red juice of a plant could help with menstrual problems (see Anderson 2005).

Simples

Simples could be animal, vegetable, or mineral, and each culture believed that each simple contained the power to stimulate some positive effect on the human body. Some simples had multiple effects—that intended and those we might call side effects—and the prescriber of these needed to know how much healed and how much could kill. Depending on the culture, animal simples could include blood, claws, feathers, brains or other organs, digestive stones (bezoars), pearls, coral, eyes, horn, tongues, tails, hair, teeth, ground bones, dried cartilage, and even urine and feces. Of course, humans are animals, and human material included the skull of a hanged man, a young boy's urine, "mummy," a virgin's blood, menstrual fluid, sweat, dried placenta, pus, as well as various other parts and waste.

Vegetable simples were often herbs (local) or spices (imported)—many still marketed for a range of assumed medicinal properties—but almost anything edible might be considered medicinal. These constituted the largest category of medical substances in any pharmacopeia, or list of recognized materia medica. Experts in a culture knew when in its life cycle each plant was most effective and what part to use: roots, stems, seeds, leaves, bark, flowers, berries, or other fruits. They knew how and when to harvest them and how to preserve them properly (drying, pickling, sugaring, powdering). They also knew how to prepare them appropriately: bruising, mashing, extracting juice; infusing like tea; boiling to decoct essences; boiling with sugar to make a syrup; mixing with alcohol to make a tincture; distilling in an alembic by boiling and condensing the steam in a separate container; or boiling down to purify or concentrate an essence. Spices and herbs both improved the flavor of foods and most had supposed medicinal properties. Organic theories of health and disease, like the Chinese and the Galenic humoralism of the Muslim and Christian worlds, relied heavily on organic—animal or vegetable—materia medica. One issue during our period of global exploration and discovery was how to categorize newly encountered plants from Asia or the Americas: was a given root or leaf hot or cold, moist or dry? Most worked backward from what effects the materia seemed to have, deducing its qualities (see Elgood 1970, 16–17).

But there was still room for mineral or other inorganic medical ingredients. Certain earths such as clays were thought to be effective as drying agents; semi-precious and precious stones were thought to absorb celestial rays and focus them on the sick person, who either wore them or drank the crushed material. Some metals, especially gold (sun) and silver (moon), were thought to have medicinal value, since their shining surfaces supposedly reflected healing powers best. Sixteenth-century Western alchemists sought two things: the "philosopher's stone" and how to change (transmute) lead into gold. Interestingly, both the "stone" and transmuted gold were considered panaceas, or universal healing mediums, and worth a fortune in the age of plague.

Compounds

The blending of two or more ingredients into a single mixture might achieve any of several desired results. The effect of the main ingredient might be strengthened, or a side effect lessened, or secondary symptoms addressed; or multiple ingredients might make the compound effective against several conditions. Honey or sugar made bitter-tasting herbs palatable, and alcohol helped dissolve certain substances. Materia medica was humorally speaking wet, dry, hot, or cold, and in varying degrees (three in Islamic medicine), and some material was subject to astrological forces. The Western or Chinese herbalist's or apothecary's special skill was the blending of the materials in the correct proportions, and his recipe books were vital for that task. The lore of the African or American herbalists and shamans (medicine men and women) was passed along orally. Some of this was combined as African slaves brought their medical traditions to the Caribbean with its distinctive flora and native medical customs.

EARLY MODERN DISPENSERS OF MEDICINAL MATERIALS AND THEIR SOURCES

The Aztecs

The Native Americans had no equivalent of the West's apothecaries or China's herbalists, but Aztec healers and possibly even mothers commanded an ancient tradition of natural materia medica. The Spaniard Francisco Hernández traveled to Mexico at the order of King Philip II to discover what he could of native medicine and medicinal plants. He catalogued some 3,000 plants, of which 1,200 were considered to have medical value. The Aztecs themselves had a sophisticated categorizing system, some of which found its way into the first Aztec herbal, that was compiled in Nahuatl in 1552 at Tlatelolco by Aztec physician Martín de la Cruz, *Little Book of the Medicinal Herbs* of the Indies (Latinized by Juan Badiano). They organized plants by taste, smell, feel, use, and natural environment. The ruler Moctezuma I is known to have had extensive botanical gardens of some 2,000 specimens cultivated for medicinal and research (often to discover poisons) as well as aesthetic and culinary purposes from 1467. Of course, medicine and supernatural ritual intertwined so that healing included pacifying the spirits and religious ritual included drugs. For example, narcotics such as peyote, jimson weed, marijuana, and psilocybin mushrooms served as medical anesthesia and to dull the senses of human sacrifices. Of course, De la Cruz, Hernández, and other Christian writers filtered out the Aztec spiritual elements, presenting a very one-dimensional view of Aztec healing. Some point out that Spanish preconceptions and beliefs may have influenced even the native-produced medical works.

Healers were not limited to herbal simples or compounds, for they employed a wide range of animal products and minerals. For fevers they used pearls and such cool green stones as turquoise, jade and emeralds; red jasper was good for the kidneys and blood and to stanch hemorrhages. De la Cruz includes wild and domestic animal blood, flesh, urine, and organs in many of his recipes, and others recommend young alligators for scabies and ants for arthritis. When Spanish practitioners interacted with their Aztec counterparts, it was the native materia medica that the invaders best understood and respected. They brought their own apothecaries, and these remained open to discovering the next panacea (see Gates 1939/2000).

Africans and Caribbean Slaves

West African healing utilized a large and varied materia medica whose traditions were millennia in the making. As with the Aztecs, African communities prized their herbalists and healers who had mastered the lore of medicinal plants and their preparation. Likewise, they tended to rely on local plants rather than imported, though since tribal groups were far from stationary, over time they brought important species with them to transplant. The penetration of Islam into Africa's interior and some western regions may have also introduced new plants and practices in some areas. West Africa in many ways had a patchwork of medical traditions. Their differences were evident after their forcible transplantation to the New World (Ransford 1983; Voeks 1993). Sorting them out on Caribbean plantations was essential, since Africans strongly believed that what could heal could also kill.

Ripped from their homelands, the Caribbean slaves were forced to work and live with people from various regions of Africa or native-born Afro-Caribbeans. Unless physicians, whites generally respected the medical traditions of their slaves and usually left them to their own healers. But for many, these people were not *their* healers: these they had left behind in Africa. Medicines, they believed, worked in part because of the rituals that attended their preparation and administering, and who knew the rituals? Where were the familiar African plants? Did similar-looking specimens have the same powers? Were other local varieties better? Black healers had to adapt and empirically create their own pharmacopeias. The English physician Hans Sloane recorded some of this practice on the island of Jamaica in the late 1680s and noted some 800 plant species. He dismissed local healers in the same way his colleagues in London dismissed empirics and midwives: they lacked "philosophy" and Western medical knowledge. Yet for the slaves, establishing a working understanding of the local flora was essential to their very survival (Harrison 2010; Sheridan 1985; Weaver 2006; Sweet 2011).

The Chinese

Chinese materia medica as a medical science is as old as China itself. Shennong's *The Divine Husbandman*, from the first century C.E., was one of the classics of Chinese medicine, listing 365 medical recipes. China's position and trade meant its herbalists and drug preparers had a great materia medica with which to work. From the eighth century C.E., the state established pharmacies with reduced prices of simples and compounds for the poor, and by the ninth century, Chinese materia medica included "precious stones, minerals, trees, fowl, quadrupeds, reptiles/worms, and fish," though herbs topped the list (Unschuld 1986, 13). In 992 C.E., the *Taiping Prescriptions of Sacred Benevolence* contained over 10,000 recipes. Such works contained much but included much redundancy and lacked the organization that would make them useful.

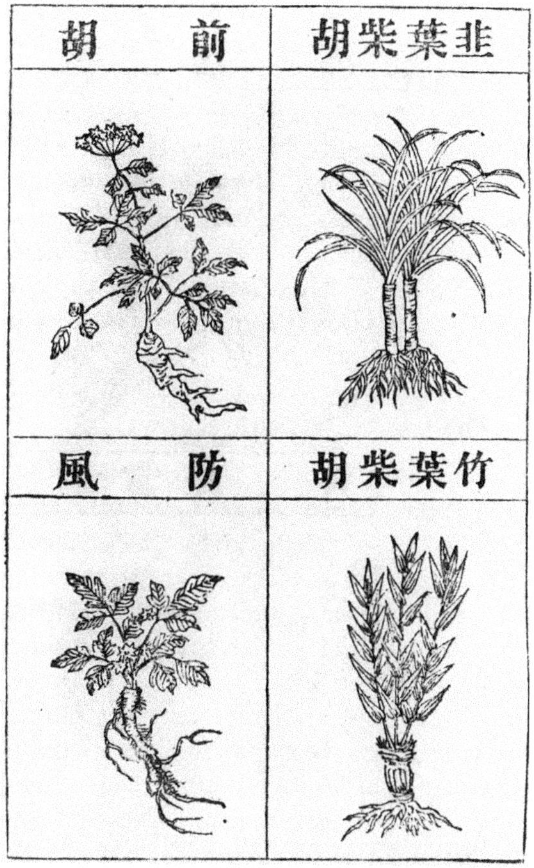

One of 1,160 woodcut illustrations of Chinese medicinal herbs from the enormous *Compendium of Materia Medica* (*Bencao Gangmu*), written by Li Shizhen in the 16th century. His name and image are so famous that they are still used in relation to traditional Chinese medical institutions, companies, and products. (Library of Congress)

The early modern period opens with the imperial project to rationalize the state of Chinese pharmacy. In 1505, Liu Wen-t'ai presented the *Materia Medica Written on Imperial Order, Containing Essential and Important Material Arranged in Systematic Order* to the emperor. It was a compilation containing nothing new, but it reduced the list to 1,786 substances. The emperor died, and the *Materia Medica* was forgotten until about 1700. Several others of varying size and quality followed.

During the second half of the 16th century, Li Shih-chen, who worked in the Imperial Medical Office, produced the magisterial 25-volume *Materia Medica Arranged According to Drug Descriptions and Technical Aspects*, which appeared in 1596. It cut out some of Liu Wen-t'ai's and added 420 new simples for a total of 1,898 substances and 11,096 recipes. For each simple, he included a description, its supposed medicinal qualities, how to prepare it, its uses and how to use it, and his own experiences with it. Huge and expensive, it had little circulation outside of the capital. Five smaller and more practical works between 1624 and 1778 as well as numerous specialized manuals followed it (Unschuld 1986, 140–147; see also Li Shih-chen 1973).

Between 1500 and the later 18th century, little of note moved the field of pharmacy forward in China. Theory and practice remained stable, and writings rehashed what had become tradition. Even the title of a work such as Hsü Ta-ch'un's brilliant *Forgotten Traditions of Ancient Chinese Medicine* (1757) makes this dependence clear (Unschuld 1998). A few new substances, such as American tobacco and Canadian ginseng, entered the pharmacopeia but little changed (Unschuld 1998, 19–23, 146–224). Chinese medicinal products, however, spread worldwide in the bottoms of first Portuguese (1557–1685) and later exclusively British ships (from 1715). Camphor, rhubarb, ginger, cassia, china root (*smilax pseudo-China*), and later tea, were major simples exported from China to the West. Physicians, merchants, and missionaries wrote works on their discoveries in India and China, such as the physician and converted Jew Garcia D'Orta's *Colloquies on Simples and Drugs and Medical Things of India* (Goa, India, 1563) and Cristóvão Acosta's *Treatise on the Drugs and Medicines of the Oriental Indies* (Burgos, Spain, 1582). In 1656, the Jesuit missionary Michael Boym compiled the authoritative *Chinese Flora, or a Treatise on the Flowers, Plants, and Animals Particular to China*, with appropriate medical commentary; and in 1735 Jean-Baptiste du Halde published his encyclopedia of China in four volumes, three of which were taken up with medical matters (see Barnes 2005 and Scheid 2007).

The Islamic World

The Arabs invented the apothecary (from the Greek for "warehouse") and inherited materia medica of both the East and West. Arabia was the linchpin connecting the Mediterranean Sea and Indian Ocean, and their dhows and caravans had carried fragrant cargoes since time immemorial. The markets of Cairo, Baghdad, and Damascus sold culinary and medical herbs and spices from throughout the Islamic world and beyond. Muslim scholars and physicians studied the first-century C.E. Greek *On Medicinal Substances* by Dioscorides, whose 1,000 or so animal, mineral, and especially vegetable simples were known to and written about by Galen a century later (see Riddle 1985). Scholars translated Dioscorides into Arabic in the 10th century. One of the translators, Ibn Juljul of Cordoba in Spain, wrote a work on materials used by Muslim doctors but not in Dioscorides, beginning a tradition of original Islamic works on medicinal materials. The most influential was the 13th-century *Comprehensive Book on Simple Drugs and Foodstuffs* by the Spanish Muslim Ibn al-Baytar, with some 1,400 simples (Pormann and Savage-Smith 2007, 53). Books known as formularies contained the many compounds and specific recipes known to Islamic medicine. Given the many cultures and linguistic groups included in the Islamic world, multilingual synonym books were attempts to provide the many names for simples and compounds. The task proved too daunting, however, and the results were disappointing.

An important healing tool often sold with other materia medica was the talisman. Carried on the person or worn around the neck, the supposed effect of the stone or other object was to focus astral forces or rays down and into the body in such a way as to activate it to respond to the poison or other danger. This was a kind of astrological magic that literally used the skills of a magus, but instructions for creating these were commonly available (Saif 2011).

With the rise of the Savafids in Persia and the Ottoman Turks around the Mediterranean, popular and classic Arabic works were translated but, as in China, little development in theory or practice occurred. Medicine remained Galenic and carefully monitored pharmacists sold their goods—most commonly simples—from market stalls, and dispensaries attached to hospitals distributed cheap or free remedies to the needy. Yet studies of Ottoman gardens, even attached to hospitals, show no interest in growing medicinal herbs or fruits. Among the Ottomans, at least, compounds seem to have been available at court and to elites. There were, however, some inroads of European influence in Istanbul at the Turkish court in the 17th and 18th centuries. Some materia medica from the Western Hemisphere found its way into otherwise traditional formularies, and the new chemical medicine of European Paracelsians (see below) found interested scholars, physicians, and bureaucrats. Yet outside of the Topkapi Palace, Galenic traditions dominated, "with the new only lightly sprinkled here and there" (Pormann and Savage-Smith 2007, 162–171. See also Shefer-Mossensohn 2009, 34–45; Elgood 1970; and Chipman 2010).

The Europeans

During the 12th and 13th centuries, contacts with the Islamic world made numerous Islamic medical works and Islamic versions of classical medical works available to European scholars and physicians. Medieval Europeans likewise borrowed the apothecary and stocked their shelves with spices and other materia medica purchased in Islamic markets (see Freedman 2008, 50–75). By 1500, European apothecaries were on a par with their Muslim contemporaries. Yet the era of the Renaissance, Discovery, and Scientific Revolution saw major advances in European pharmacopeias. Renaissance trends such as the editing, translating, and printing of classical medical works—including Galen and Dioscorides—forced the reconsideration of their Arabic inheritance. Printing helped extend literacy and created markets for medical self-help books and patent medicines advertised in pamphlets. New materia medica of all sorts poured into European markets from the Americas, Asia, and the islands of the Indian and Pacific Oceans, expanding pharmacopeias, both professional and popular. The pseudoscience of alchemy began its long metamorphosis into the science of chemistry with the help of the bombastic 16th-century German empiric Paracelsus. Paracelsus rejected "pagan" Galenic humoralism and laid out a model of human physiology that emphasized the roles of minerals, salts, and metals instead of organic materials (see Moran 2005 and Webster 2008). By the 18th century, biology had been reorganized around the system of Carl Linnaeus, which created a system of relating and labeling all living things, including organic materia medica old and new.

The provision of medical simples and compounds had essentially crystallized by 1500. Officially, local apothecary guilds oversaw the education and operations of their members. One entered the guild after an apprenticeship during which the necessary skills and knowledge were mastered. Only during the 16th century did medical schools begin formally teaching about materia medica (Padua, 1533; Bologna, 1534; Pisa, 1544), but this was for physicians only. Socially, apothecaries were closer to surgeons, who were also trained as apprentices. Apothecaries worked from well-stocked shops, selling to doctors and the public alike. When in need of recipes for specific prescriptions, they referred to formularies, sometimes required by guilds, and created their own blends (see Anderson 2005; Palmer 1985).

Their direct competition was from empirics who lacked formal training and guild membership but provided local herbs and other substances directly to the

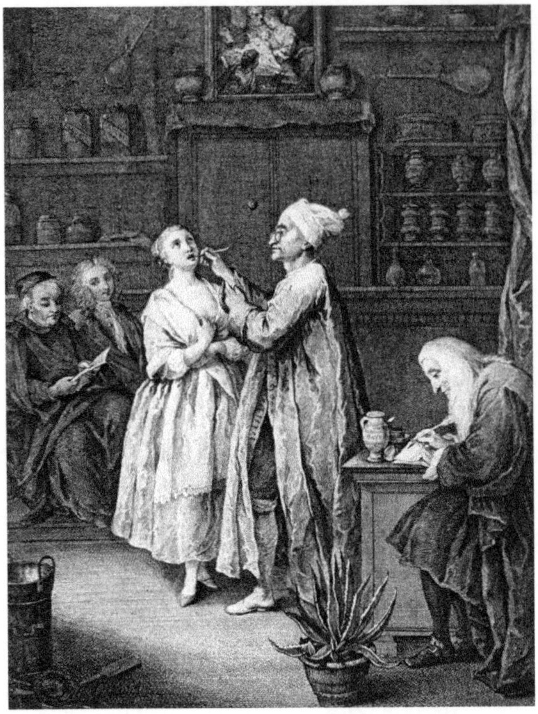

Eighteenth-century depiction of the interior of a European pharmacy with a young woman having her throat examined by the robed and bespectacled apothecary. The walls are lined with jars of herbs and medicines, and an aloe vera plant, still used for healing skin, sits prominently in the foreground. (National Library of Medicine)

suffering. Midwives specialized in women's reproductive problems, while herb-or drug-peddling itinerant charlatans sometimes offered their wares through gaudy and eye-catching "infomercials" performed in town squares from colorful carts or stages ("mountebank" means "to climb on a bench") (see Gentilcore 2006). In England, the so-called patent medicines, advertised in print, played the same role in self-medication from the 1650s (see below). The gardens of monasteries (Strocchia 2011) and old "wisewomen" also produced the herbal simples for remedies demanded by the poor and villagers. Medicinal spices were supposed to be a monopoly of the apothecaries, though spicers and grocers sold many of the same items for cooking. Apothecaries distinguished themselves by displaying a stuffed crocodile representing their exotic wares, or the mortar and pestle in which spices were ground to powder, or signs with images of them.

New treatments appeared for old diseases—tobacco smoke for plague prevention and cinchona bark for malaria—and new treatments for new diseases, such as mercury and guaiacum for syphilis. Books on newly discovered medicines flourished during the 17th and 18th centuries, with exotic titles such as Herman Grimm's *The Medical Treasury of the Island of Ceylon* (1677) and Hendrick van Reede's three-volume *Garden of Malabar* (1678–1682) (see Cook 2007). Women also published recipe books, including the English Countess of Arundel, whose collection of 397 entries was arranged by illness (1606), and French midwife Louise Bourgeois (*Collection of Secrets*, 1626), whose 280 recipes called for almost 300 herbs, 45 animal products, and 27 minerals (see Perkins 1996 and DiMarco 2010). But European medicine was undergoing a movement toward professionalization by around 1650, and society was becoming convinced that only well-educated males should be making medical decisions (see Laroche 2009).

Through their guilds, licensing, royal favors, and increased educational opportunities, surgeons and apothecaries were gaining power and authority over their rivals. Wise women and even midwives were being slaughtered as witches possessed of demonic powers and intents. In England, self-medication took the form of advertised and retailed patent medicines (see below), and across Europe, male medical voices eclipsed those of even the most experienced women practitioners.

THE WORLDWIDE PHARMACOPEIA

Cultures naturally developed their pharmacopeias around the plants, minerals, and animals most readily available. These increased through local discoveries and trade but more dramatically through commerce and other contact with distant cultures.

Tobacco

Tobacco was a New World plant whose active ingredient, nicotine, was rather stronger than in today's varieties. Native Americans used it (*petum*) as a hallucinogen for spirit journeys, as a painkiller for toothache and snakebite, and to treat asthma and curb hunger. Italian Amerigo Vespucci was first to write of it, in 1505, and the Dutchman Rembert Dodoens first included it (*henbane*) in an herbal in 1553. The same year the Portuguese gave the French ambassador, Jean Nicot, some specimens that flourished in his garden, and Europeans have never stopped smoking. The word "tobacco" came from the hollow reed through which Caribbean natives smoked the dried leaf, but it was also chewed and inhaled as snuff and used externally in plasters. Considered healthful, Europeans used tobacco smoke from clay pipes to counteract the "poisoned" air that most thought caused plague. Seventeenth-century English physician Nicholas Culpeper recommended as a cure-all a salve of boiled-down tobacco juice, hog grease, and red wine.

The Portuguese shipped it to Africa and Macao from Brazil, and from Macao to Guangdong in China and Japan from about 1605. Spaniards brought it from Mexico to the Philippines, and from Manila plantations to Fujian, China. Chinese physician Yao Lu believed it helped block malaria, cleared the lungs, and aided digestion, and herbalist Zhang Jiebin included it in his pharmacopeia. India accepted tobacco as a luxury stimulant and not a medicine, and appears to have introduced the water pipe (hookah). These spread to Persia and eventually Turkey, and Chinese women used hookahs to mellow the harsh yang of the smoke through the cooling yin of water (see Gilman and Xun 2004 and Charlton 2004).

Opium and Opiates

Opium is derived from the opium poppy that grows naturally and has long been cultivated in south central Asia (Afghanistan, Iran). An intense relaxant and painkiller, its cultivation spread to the Ganges Valley in India, Iraq, Turkey, and Egypt along Muslim-controlled trade routes. Mongols traded it to China from the 14th century. Indian Ayurvedic medicine considered it hot and dry, but Greeks believed it to be "cold and dry" when used to adjust the humors. Galen claimed it was useful for "venomous bites, headaches, vertigo, deafness, epilepsy, apoplexy, eyesight, bronchitis, asthma, bloody sputum, colic, jaundice, spleen hardening, kidney stones, urinary problems, fever, dropsy, leprosy, menstrual issues, melancholy, pestilences" (Shearing 2004, 15). Muslims noted it intensified sexual pleasure, and the Qur'an did not forbid it, though custom banned its use during the month of Ramadan. It was typically used to calm and control the insane.

Crusaders and Venetian merchants imported small quantities to Europe before 1500, and navigators such as Columbus and Magellan sought its sources. Traditionally taken in the form of a pill, opium was exported from India by the Dutch and spread throughout its trading empire. It seems to have been smoked first in Taiwan, where it was mixed with tobacco to form the very potent *madak*. It was also mixed with Indian hemp (marijuana; *gange* to Arabs), which Robert Hooke both used and recommended for "lunaticks" (Brook 2008; Dikötter, Laamann, and Xum 2004; Shefer-Mossensohn 2009, 39–45; Matthee 2005, 97–116; Elgood 1970, 44–46).

The drug laudanum (from Latin *laudare*, "to praise") was apparently developed by the 16th-century German alchemist and medical practitioner Paracelsus. He found that he could suspend certain opium alkaloids in brandy and deliver the supposed benefits of both. His recipe contained 25 percent opium, along with tobacco juice, crushed pearls, amber, coral, musk, "unicorn" (narwhal) horn, and bezoar stone. In the late 1600s, Dr. Thomas Sydenham, called the English Hippocrates, standardized a formula that consisted of one pint of sherry, two ounces of opium, and one ounce each of saffron, powdered clove, and powdered cinnamon (Dormandy 2006, 130–132). Like many other secret mixtures containing opium, and often alcohol, laudanum was easily marketed as a patent medicine to kill pain and level moods. It had a long life on European and American shelves, well beyond 1800. Opium's addictive quality was well known and regretted, a point made in the first European book about the substance, *Mysteries of Opium Revealed* by Dr. John Jones, himself an addict. This unfortunate quality led to opium's ban from time to time in Safavid Iran and in China in the 1720s and 1790s. The ban on *madak* led to the practice of smoking straight opium purely for the intoxicating effect, and to the infamous opium dens of 19th-century China (see Yangwen 2005).

Alcohol (Spirits)

Unlike tobacco or opium, drinkable alcohol does not occur naturally but needs to be produced through the controlled fermentation of certain carbohydrate-rich fruits, grains, and even roots, such as grapes, rice, and potatoes. Most early modern cultures drank alcoholic beverages such as mead, sake, wine, or beer in place of or along with water, on a daily basis. Of course alcohol was intoxicating and could be addictive, leading to broken lives of lethargy and poverty, or wild mood swings. Islam theoretically banned the use of alcoholic beverages, though both early modern Safavid Iran and the Ottoman Empire struggled to keep its use under control (see Shefer-Mossensohn 2009, 90–92; Elgood 1970, 39–41). Distillation as a chemical process was invented by the Muslim Jabir ibn Hayyan in the eighth century, but German monks were among the first to apply it to wine, creating "burnt wine," or brandy, just before 1500 (Gately 2009, 91–94). Other starchy or sugary foods quickly followed, including grains (whiskey, from *uisge*, Gaelic for "water of life," expanded from monasteries in 16th century; gin from Holland, c. 1650; schnapps, developed in 16th-century Germany), sugar (rum; Barbados, first mentioned in 1651 but much older), and potatoes (vodka; noted in Poland from 15th century). This "spiritous" liquid had concentrated properties of normal beverages, could dissolve many substances, burned very readily, and as aqua vitae (water of life) became a medium for many compounds and drugs, including laudanum (see Moran 2005). Eventually in the West, spirituous liquors became less a calmative or stimulant and more a means of getting drunk quickly, as in the 18th-century stereotypes of gin-swilling London denizens, whiskey-guzzling Irish, or vodka-soaked Russians. In India, alcoholism was treated with an opiate tonic called *filuniya*, much as methadone is used today.

Coffee

The coffee plant's original home was the eastern Indian Ocean. Its bean was harvested and dried or roasted, which dehydrated it out and reduced its weight tremendously. It was ground to a powder and infused—not dissolved—in boiling water to produce the thick, bitter hot drink the West knows as Turkish or Greek coffee, or espresso. After 1500, it spread north through Turkish trade routes to Cairo, Egypt, by 1520, and Damascus, Syria, where the first known coffeehouse appeared in 1530. Constantinople's first opened in 1554, Baghdad's in 1601, and coffee reached India in 1609. Muslims valued the boiled bean as a stimulant where alcoholic drinks were banned, and Sufi poets adopted it as a mild narcotic. Iranian physicians recommended coffee as a remedy for fatigue, "boiling blood," measles, hemorrhoids, nightmares, colic, and "vapors." Like tea, coffee required boiled water, which made the water safe to drink, but the dried beans required grinding, which relegated coffee to the special houses. The buzz stimulated conversation, and in cities, coffeehouses became common gathering places during the day (a trend revived in the 1970s) (Matthee 2005, 144–174; Shefer-Mossensohn 2009, 87; Elgood 1970, 41–44).

Coffee arrived at the French court via Marseille merchant De la Roque in 1644; Venice boasted Europe's oldest coffeehouse, opened in 1645; and in Oxford, a Lebanese named Jacob first served coffee at the Angel in 1652. But coffee was always part beverage and part medicine. European coffeehouses became important meeting places for medical practitioners—especially quacks—and their patients and many establishments sold pills, potions, and other patent medicines. Important in the history of early newspapers, coffeehouses also distributed handbills and other advertisements for medical remedies and services. For the Galenic, coffee was "cold and dry." In his *Sylva sylvarum* of 1627, the English scientist and statesman Francis Bacon insisted "the drink comforteth the brain, the heart, and helpeth digestion," while a printed handbill from London's Pasqua Rosée coffeehouse in 1652—its first year of business—claimed it prevented miscarriages and cured dropsy, gout, and scurvy. Another advertisement praised coffee's value to sexual males: "It collects and settles the spirits, makes the erection more vigorous, the ejaculation more full, adds a spiritual escency [*sic*] to the sperm, and renders it more firm and suitable to the gusto of the womb." Despite such powers, tea replaced coffee in England and elsewhere, while cheap liquor (gin, schnapps, brandy) and cheaper beer kept the masses content (see Ellis 2005; quote from Brandon 2007, 20).

Tea

The delicate leaves of many types of camellia tree have been harvested and dried for later infusion in boiling water to make what the Japanese and Chinese called *chiaa*. Like coffee, it contains caffeine and is a fairly mild stimulant. Green tea is noted for its antioxidants today, and the generally healthful effect may have helped popularize it in East Asia. Though the Japanese developed the famous tea ceremony, they also drank it freely throughout the day. Portuguese and Dutch merchants shipped tea around the Indian Ocean, and it arrived in Portugal about 1650. England's queen from 1660 was Catherine of Braganza, a Portuguese princess, who brought the drink to the island, beginning England's long love affair. The Dutchman Cornelis Bontekoe popularized tea with his 1678 *Treatise on the Excellence of the Herb Called Tea*, which earned him the nickname "The Tea Doctor." He suggested many (up to 50!) daily small cups of weak tea, since when strong it "spoiled" the "stomach, the blood and the brains" (Cook 2007, 293–297). Otherwise, it was considered a panacea, especially good for treating urinary stones and gravel, fevers, and "almost all defects of the blood." Easy to prepare at home, it eclipsed coffee as a stimulating hot drink of choice in many places. Once European merchants wrestled the plants from Canton, they established tea plantations in Ceylon, India, and Java, which reduced the price to the colonial powers and increased its popularity with the lower classes (Matthee 2005, 237–245; Li Shih-chen 1973, 81–87).

Cocoa or Cacao

The Olmec and Mayan peoples first cultivated the *Theobroma cacao* to use for a variety of medical conditions. Its flowers in a bath battled fatigue; the seeds, dried and powdered, helped with digestion, diarrhea, and fever, menstrual issues and conception, as well as the liver. Among the Aztecs, it was the beverage of choice, after water, and the conquistadors were welcomed with the stimulating stuff (it does contain caffeine). Europeans, especially the Dutch, originally drank it in its bitter natural form, but once they discovered what could be accomplished by adding sugar and then milk or cream, hot chocolate took off among women and children (Ortiz de Montellano 1990, 141); Schendel 1968, 116–119; see also Coe and Coe 1996).

Sugar

Sugarcane was produced among the Polynesian peoples and highly valued in the Pacific and Indian Ocean regions for its sweetening properties. Muslim traders circulated sugar north into the Mediterranean, where Muslims and Christians valued it as an ingredient in medicinal syrups, juleps, and electuaries: its sweetness masked the often bitter or otherwise unpleasant tastes of simples and compounds, and it dissolved readily in water and alcohol. In the 15th century, Spanish sugar plantations appeared in the Canary Islands, and Columbus, who stopped there on his second voyage, carried specimens to Santo Domingo in the Caribbean, where planters established the earliest refinery in 1515. Antwerp became the center of European refining, with 19 factories in 1556. Before the 16th century, sugar's rarity and close association with medical formulas meant that in Europe it was handled only by apothecaries. But as its availability spread and its price dropped, it replaced honey in many cuisines and came to be considered a food at least as much as a medicine (see Freedman 2008 and Cook 2007).

Spices

When is cinnamon a spice and when a prophylactic against diabetes? Of course the answer lies in why and how it is used, for it has long been both. The world bordering on the Indian Ocean had had a thriving network of exchange among spice-producing regions and islands long before Muslim ships began supplying the souks and bazaars of Islamic southwest Asia and North Africa. European Christians encountered spices used for flavoring food and as medicines in Spain and Sicily, and while on Crusade. Peppercorns, cinnamon bark, ginger, turmeric, cloves, allspice, saffron, and a literal boatload of other aromatic seeds, barks, stems, roots, and other plant portions sat on apothecary shelves in tightly sealed jars to treat poisonous bites, colic, and poor vision; to prevent epilepsy, digestive problems, and colds; and to promote sweating, urinating, and a sound appetite. The spices that Columbus and others went in search of during the Renaissance were not to make rancid meat taste better but to serve the medicinal needs of those who could afford them, cutting out the Muslim middleman. To shorten supply lines, Europeans often tried to establish plants in distant parts of the world, for example, growing ginger in Mexico (see Freedman 2008, 50–76; Shefer-Mossensohn 2009, 32–39; Cook 2007; Barnes 2005; and Li Shih-chen 1973).

Ginseng

The root of the *panax ginseng* was considered by the Chinese to be so powerful a panacea that only the emperor was supposed to have access to it. During the early modern period, ginseng was one of only two plants to have its own book written (the other was mugwort, used in the important Chinese practice of moxibustion). By the 16th century, it circulated in East Asia, with finer qualities being grown in Manchuria and Korea. A Canadian version of ginseng was discovered in 1715 and exported to Europe and even China at a huge profit. Alvaro de Semedo in 1655 was the first European to mention the plant, calling it "the panacea, and the remedy that dispenses immortality" (Barnes 2005, 104). The Chinese prized it especially as an inducer of "heat," a purifier of blood, a fortifier of the stomach, and an exciter of the pulse. English doctors found it humorally cooling, restoring the appetite and acting against fevers (Li Shih-chen 1973, 301–304; Unschuld 1998, 179–181; Barnes 2005, 100–106, 173–179, 275–279).

Guaiacum

Many early modern Europeans believed that God always provided a remedy in the region where a particular illness was found. When syphilis was first observed in southwestern Europe in the 1490s, it was thought to have been imported from the New World. While many American medicinal imports were tried, including the sudorifics sarsaparilla and sassafras, the resin of the guaiac tree proved to have value. It may have appeared as early as 1508 in Spain and 1517 in Italy. After mocking other attempts, the German author and knight Ulrich von Hutten, himself a sufferer, first mentioned the remedy in 1519, and the Fugger banking family of Augsburg quickly wrestled a monopoly from the cash-strapped Charles, emperor and king of Spain. The guaiacum was decocted and drunk to excite copious sweating, which was believed to cleanse the body of the syphilitic poison. Known as Holy Wood among Catholics and lignum vitae (wood of life) elsewhere, its only real competition was the rather hideous chemical treatment with mercury. From the 1520s, demand for the wood was huge, with a single Roman hospital in a single purchase acquiring 7,287 pounds of the stuff. As household recipe books and herbals show, it remained popular throughout our period for both the pox and other maladies requiring profuse perspiration (Arrizabalaga 1997, Finucci 2008).

Cinchona, or Quinine

Cinchona trees (*kina-kina* to the Peruvians) grew in the Andean highlands and their bark had long been used by locals as a drug against fevers. Jesuit missionaries are thought to have linked its healing properties to malaria, and the Peruvian bark, Jesuit bark, or Jesuit powder arrived in Europe in 1630s. It worked by killing parasites in the blood and reducing fever (except with *vivax*). Its popularity—despite its terribly bitter flavor—led to attempts to transplant it but to no avail. In Europe, apothecaries tended to cut the bark powder with sugar and other substances, reducing its effectiveness. China's introduction seems to have been via Jesuit missionaries who treated the Emperor K'ang Hsi for malaria in 1693. It remained essentially a Spanish monopoly throughout the period, with Colombia alone shipping out 500 tons in 1794 (Rocco 2003; Li Shih-chen 1973, 107. See also Shah 2010 and Webb 2009).

Theriac/Treacle

Galen wrote of theriac, and his Muslim and Christian successors venerated the complex drug. Both taken orally and used as an ointment, theriac was originally believed to counteract poison. With time, its powers expanded to those of a panacea. By the 16th century, Venice produced the best theriac in Europe. Consisting of 70 or 80 ingredients, including viper's flesh, snake venom, and opium, apothecaries prepared it once a year in an open, festival setting, before storing it away in tightly sealed jars to develop its magic. Such a drug was, of course, quite expensive, and in the Ottoman Empire was restricted to the elites. It was a standard remedy and prophylactic in European plague manuals and in household medical books down to the 18th century. In England, it was known as treacle, but after 1700, treacle became synonymous with molasses (for examples see Fabbri 2007; Griffin 2004, and Elgood 1970, 46–48).

Patent Medicines

Medical entrepreneurs who peddled their pills, potions, salves, and creams were found throughout Europe. One of the earliest German producers of a popular proprietary drug was Dr. Caspar Kegler in early-16th-century Leipzig. An alchemist, physician, entrepreneur, and author of popular vernacular works on the plague, he advertised with printed pamphlets and peddled his electuary widely north of the Alps. A generation later, the Italian Leonardo Fioravanti was likewise selling his own medicines directly to consumers (Heinrichs 2012). The English, with a wide self-help streak and relatively few doctors, had developed a ready market by 1650. Apothecaries, bookstores, printers' shops, taverns, and coffee shops offered variously labeled remedies, such as Dr. Lockyer's Pills and Daffy's Elixir Salutis. Lockyer's advertising pamphlets from the 1660s listed 174 different distributors in and around London. English law recognized property rights in inventions (patents), and apothecaries, quacks, and empirics began using the laws to protect their medicinal compounds and their names. The earliest was Anderson's Scots Pills, granted royal letters patent in 1687. The earliest patented compound was Timothy Byfield's 1711 "sal oleosum volatile." Unlike most apothecaries' compounds, these carried distinctive names, brand names, really, that competitors were not allowed to copy: Epsom Salts (1695), Dr. Stoughton's Elixir Magnum Stomachicum (1712), or Turlington's Balsam of Life (1744). Many contained opium, relaxing the user, and most were purgatives that induced sweating, vomiting, or defecating, clear signs to the user that the drugs were working. Daffy's Elixir was the first to be shipped to New England, where it was advertised in newspapers and found a ready market among the colonists. Ships' surgeons, physicians, merchants, hypochondriacs, and a multitude of other Englishmen and women carried these products throughout the world, a world that was rapidly shrinking (see Wallis 2008; Porter 2001; Haydock and Wallis 2005; Issac 1998; and Maehle 1999).

11

War, Health, and Medicine

The early modern world was marked by nearly constant warfare. European kingdoms fought to consolidate their political boundaries, impose dynasties, or expand territories; religious groups battled each other for the sake of Truth; colonial powers waged war with natives and each other over islands, territories, and wealth. Even while Europeans perched nearby like vultures, different factions of Aztecs, Incas, Indians, and African warlords fought among each other. For example, in the 1720s and 1730s, Agaja of Dahomey, Africa, carried out a brutal expansion of his kingdom with a ferocity compared to that of Genghis Khan. Smallpox swept his armies, refugees spread diseases, and the conquered were enslaved locally or sold into European slavery (see Sweet 2011). Revolts, revolutions, and rebellions tore states apart, some leading to the birth of new ones, from the Netherlands to the United States and Haiti.

During the same period and led by Europeans, warfare underwent its own revolution. Firearms and artillery consolidated their roles on the battlefield, ultimately replacing the pike and sword. This required a new form of discipline as ranks of men had to line up shoulder to shoulder to load, fire, and mow each other down on command, and then to withstand the same fire from the other side. This took training, drilling, and professional commitments not seen since the Roman Empire. Armies grew in size as royal budgets did, making the killing fields ever larger and more crowded. The Muslim states of Mughal India and the Safavid and Ottoman Empires became known as the "gunpowder states" because of their adoption of the new weapons. Huge Ottoman cannon had made the conquest of Constantinople possible in 1453. The Turks then rapidly swept through the Near East and Egypt, defeating the less innovative Mamluks who refused to use guns. The technology spread as Asians adopted European tools and methods of warfare; European slavers armed African warlords at the rate of four to six guns per slave; and English colonists in North America traded guns and ammunition with the Indians.

The simple act of building larger and larger national or imperial armies with men from different regions allowed the era's infectious diseases unique opportunities to spread among those with lowered resistance or no immunity. During

European wars, civilians in theaters of war were dragged in as companies of soldiers milled about awaiting their next call to action. But camp life was no picnic, and even between battles, soldiers faced many medical dangers from plague to depression. On the march, soldiers lived with the hapless civilians, and their wounded were left with the nearest community, friend or foe. Lacking the discipline of the battlefield, they often took what they pleased and otherwise brutalized the defenseless populace, inevitably exchanging diseases along the way. Growing cities with improved defenses were besieged for months; swollen with residents, defending soldiers, and refugees and cursed by famine, they became hotbeds for physical suffering of every kind.

At sea, ships became ever-larger platforms for artillery, ready to bombard coasts and port cities as well as one another with devastating fury. Global colonial and trade empires required sailors to serve for months at sea with horrible food and tainted water, as well as limited facilities for recovery when one fell ill, injured, or wounded. Colonial conflicts often pitted men-of-war against canoes and professional soldiers against stone-age warriors in asymmetrical confrontations, usually resulting in massacres.

By the 18th century, political and military leaders came to appreciate the investment they had in each trained soldier. Advanced states such as France and Britain provided unprecedented resources for preserving the soldiers' and sailors' health before and after battle. Surgeons and health officers, field hospitals, and veterans' hospitals appeared in greater numbers to hasten the sick and wounded back onto active-duty lists. They also came to realize the toll that tropical warfare in the Caribbean took, as whole armies melted away from epidemics of imported yellow fever and malaria. Indeed, in every early modern army, disease always took a far greater toll than all the bullets and cannonballs combined. In the long run, military concerns led to important advances in disease control, though before 1800 this was limited to some surgical advances, widespread inoculation for smallpox, and the defeat of scurvy (Grell 2004; Glynn and Glynn 2004; Harvie 2002).

THE AZTEC WAY OF WAR

Aztec society was built on a warrior ethic like those of Homer's heroes, the Japanese Samurai, or Europe's medieval knights. They had established their hegemony by battle and maintained it the same way. Every free male was trained to fight from childhood, with the best forming the elite Jaguar and Eagle units. Negotiations preceded formal conflicts, so a pitched battle was something of a last resort. On both sides men were protected by flimsy hats and padded body armor, and round wooden shields. A battle opened with ritual noise making and the hurling of javelins, arrows, and other missiles. The two sides closed and men fought with flaked obsidian-edged wooden swords, jabbing spears, and obsidian knives. Since obsidian can be flaked to a greater-than-razor sharpness, the knives and slashing swords could cause deep cuts where blows were landed. Arrows were often tipped with obsidian, increasing their ability to penetrate the light armor and skin. The skillfully handled spear could also pierce deeply into the victim's body,

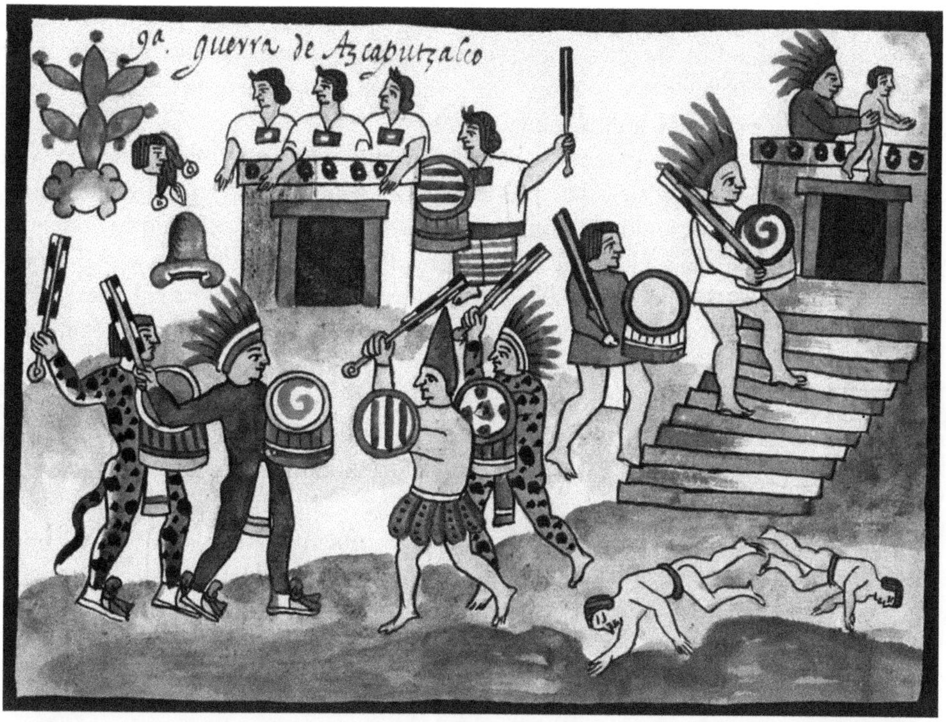

Late-16th-century illustration of the Battle of Azcapotzalco, from the second section of the Tovar (or Ramírez) Codex, attributed to the Mexican Jesuit Juan de Tovar. Soldiers fight with war clubs and shields; at left is a jaguar warrior, one of the elite soldiers of the Aztec, with the glyph of a flowering cactus above him. At right an infant is being sacrificed by a priest at a temple while two victims lie dead on the ground. (Library of Congress)

severing blood vessels, disrupting organs, and causing sepsis if not immediate death.

But the true mark of the warrior was his ability to stun and capture his opponent alive. For this purpose warriors, especially the Jaguars and Eagles, wielded clubs. A vigorous attack could break bones and cause deep bruising, and the flimsy headgear provided little protection for the main target. Once incapacitated, the loser was pulled off the field by lower-level combatants as prisoners. The "flowery war" may seem humanitarian, except that the captives were subsequently sacrificed to the victors' god of war (Uitzilopochtli in the case of the city of Tenochtitlán). Well treated until the appropriate time, the drugged victims had their still-beating hearts removed with a surgical precision made possible by a highly skilled technician and an obsidian blade. The ultimate defeat of a rival city occurred when the victorious warriors invaded and destroyed the temple of its clearly inferior god of war (Soustelle 1961/2002, 203–215).

The Aztec ruler had a general duty to provide for the welfare of his people and a special obligation to his fallen warriors. The wounded received treatment from shamans and healers who accompanied the army in the field. These latter could stanch bleeding wounds, splint broken bones, and apply herbal poultices. Those who were disabled by their wounds were provided light tasks with which to earn their keep. The Aztec state also provided veterans hospitals in the major cities of Tenochtitlán, Texcoco, Cholula, and Colhuacán.

The harming or enslavement of enemy noncombatants was taboo, and likewise the destruction of crops or other property. War was a highly ritualized activity, restrained by mutual understanding and acceptance of the rules. When Hernán Cortés and his 500 Spaniards, 14 cannon, and 16 horses went to war with Tenochtitlán in 1521, they allied themselves with the Tlaxcalans, resentful enemies of Moctezuma II and his Aztec warrior elite. But the Europeans also brought steel, horses, guns, and no respect for—or perhaps understanding—of Aztec warfare. The intention was not to defeat the Aztec god or gain captives for sacrifice but to terrorize, subjugate, and destroy. Men, women, children, old and young fell to the invaders' superior weapons and few were left to tend the wounded. The conquistadors' victory was made all the easier by the destruction of much of the populace by the diseases brought from Europe. Between June and August, it was said that half the city died of smallpox, measles, and other scourges to which the natives had no immunity and little resistance. Thus arrived the European way of war (Schendel 1968, 33).

EUROPEANS AT WAR

During the Seven Years' War (1756–63), the kingdom of Prussia conscripted approximately 25 percent of its young men of military age. Perhaps 180,000 men died while in service. Of those who were in uniform at the war's opening, only 1 of every 15 survived to its end (Parker 1989, 148).

The Early Modern Army

Size of Armies

In 1494, Charles VIII of France invaded Italy and the peninsula cowered in fear before his 18,000 men and 40 cannon. Early modern rulers bankrolled their armies and navies, and with the increasing reliance on firearms and cannon as well as the swelling size of field armies, the cost was huge. In the 1650s, the English Commonwealth spent 90 percent of its budget on its naval war with the Dutch. Around 1700, Louis XIV of France wasted 75 percent of his royal revenues on seemingly endless wars; the upstart Peter the Great of Russia, nearly 85 percent; and Frederick the Great of Prussia, 90 percent (Parker 1989, 62, 148).

In 1632, Swedish King Gustavus Adolphus commanded an army of 183,000 men in Germany, and his was only one among several large armies in the field. By the century's end, Louis XIV's armed forces amounted to some 400,000 troops, and by 1710, Europe was filled with an estimated 1.3 million soldiers. Unlike the annual feudal levies of the Middle Ages, these were men whose lives were dedicated to serve continuously under military discipline. At any one time, however, the majority of European fighting men was in port or garrisoning fortresses or cities, and relatively few were on active campaign. In 1812, Napoleon invaded Russia along a 400-kilometer front with some 600,000 men and 1,500 cannon. In less than a year, an estimated 570,000, or 95 percent, died of wounds, disease, and environmental conditions.

Military Life

When Bernardino Ramazzini wrote his famed work on occupational health and safety in 1700, he included a chapter on the soldier's life. "One cannot imagine a more deplorable kind of existence than a soldier's," he wrote. They suffered from diseases shared in the crowded camps; "unwholesome food and impure water"; "lack of sleep, excessive toil, rain, heat, cold, and sudden alarms"; as well as "filth and neglect of personal cleanliness" (Ramazzini 1940, 359–375). Of course he was far from the first to criticize camp life, but his analysis went deeper than previous observers'. He supported the era's acceptance of miasma, or poisoned air, as a major factor in diseases. Armies camped for too long in one place, and human waste, corpses, and other "corruption" accumulated and tainted the air, causing fevers and other disease. To this simple fact he attributed headaches, delirium, convulsions, and diarrhea. The bad air, he believed, infected wounds, and the heat of late summers made all of this worse.

But Ramazzini also took into account the toll of military service on the human psyche. Having lived briefly among German soldiers in Italy, he noted that they often suffered from what they called *Heimweh* or "homesickness." He quoted their proverb, "Who seeks their Fatherland finds death." Not that homesickness itself kills, but it can become very depressive and distracting and lead to the kind of mistakes that endanger one's life. It can also lead to alcoholism or suicide. Of course the soldier also lives with the constant threat of violent death. Ramazzini records that his informants related how men might get a sense of imminent death: "They would foretell that they would die in the battle that followed," even making their farewells and giving their possessions away to their fellows.

Of course, Ramazzini only scratched the surface. The sex lives of soldiers spread venereal diseases; abuse of alcohol, tobacco, or opiates weakened men's stamina; and new recruits brought with them their own communicable diseases. Diets not only consisted of poor-quality food but often lacked important elements such as vitamins that are necessary for decent health. Careless garbage disposal and food storage invited rats that carried plague fleas. Arguments turned violent cost lives, as did dueling and corporal punishment for infractions of disciplinary rules.

One hero in the battle against senseless military deaths was the 18th-century Englishman John Pringle. As physician-general of the British army from 1742 to 1758, he published his *Observations on the Diseases of the Army* (1752). He and his book advocated a wide range of reforms in military living conditions, from frequent bathing to regular and vigorous exercise, and maintenance of environmental sanitation to avoidance of overcrowding (Smith 2007, 248–250).

Weapons and Wounds

On the battlefields of Europe and around the world, men were subjected to an increasingly dangerous set of conditions. Crossbows were fading out as fired projectiles took their place. Older weapons, eventually carried by officers, included swords that stabbed and slashed, and pole weapons including pikes and halberds that stabbed, slashed, and crushed. The lacerations resulting from the stabbing and slashing were created only with the strength of the human arm and were fairly clear: in and out or across. These, of course, could penetrate vital organs, cause the contents of bowels or stomach to flow into the body cavities and create sepsis, spawn internal hemorrhaging or external bleeding, break bones, or sever tendons and muscles. As long as armies were relatively small, the fallen wounded covered a small area and would often be found and treated rather easily and quickly. Of course, the fewer men fighting the fewer wounded. Wounds could be sutured (sewn) or tourniquets applied; red-hot implements could be used to cauterize wounds; simple fractures could often be splinted. When fighting in the Americas or Asia, Europeans suffered other kinds of wounds, including those caused by war clubs, spears, and arrows. A curious but ineffective treatment for wounds was made popular by a 17th-century Paracelsian: weapon salve. One created the salve and applied it to the wounded person's blood left on the wounding weapon. Sympathetic action at a distance was supposed to make the wound heal. (It of course begs the question how one obtains the offending weapon.) Prominent physician J. B. van Helmont thought it reasonable, though a Jesuit called it the "devil's deceit."

Beside the huge expansion in the size of armies, the so-called military revolution made gunpowder weapons at first rare, then common, then mandated. Both artillery and handheld firearms used the controlled chemical explosion of gunpowder to propel more or less spherical projectiles in the general direction of the enemy. After observing the power of massed Swiss and Spanish pikemen, 17th-century European generals began arranging their firearm-wielding troops in long, straight lines, standing as close together as possible. The inaccuracy of the weapons meant that no one could aim at an individual even 50 yards away and hope to hit him. But a hundred men standing close together and firing simultaneously could hurl a hundred lead balls at a similar mass and certainly hit something. Of course, the closely packed men were just as fine a target as they stood and spent precious seconds—as much as a minute—reloading their weapons. Men were placed several rows deep to allow those in the rear to fire after the front rows did. This created a murderous environment as one mass faced the other and fired away.

Archers could fire much more accurately and with little time between shots, but arrows were relatively clean weapons that penetrated and caused relatively little tissue damage. What Europeans discovered was that once the fired ball entered the body, it could create all kinds of havoc. It moved rather slowly and often lodged in the body. Being made of soft lead, it could change shape upon impact. It could ricochet off bones, splintering them and scattering sharp fragments. It could tear up major organs and break bones. Dead tissue becomes fodder for bacteria, resulting in serious and continuing infections, tetanus, gas gangrene, and painful death. Compared to arrowheads or sharp weapons, musket balls themselves were relatively sterile, but they did carry bits of filthy, germ-laden uniform into the wound and setting infection. In a volley a man could be hit more than once, compounding the internal damage.

Because of the frequency of infection, doctors perceived that the projectiles were poisonous and the wounds needed to be treated accordingly. Pouring hot oil into the wound or cauterizing it with a hot iron was a typical treatment, especially after 1514 when Giovanni da Vigo came out with his *Compendious Practice of the Art of Surgery*. It was translated across Europe and saw 40 editions. An important figure who challenged this orthodoxy was the French surgeon Ambroise Paré. Over his career, he served four French kings on 17 military campaigns in the mid-16th century. At the siege of Turin in 1537, he ran out of boiling oil and replaced it with a mixture of turpentine, egg yolks, and rose oil. This far gentler approach worked much better and revolutionized gunshot treatment through its inclusion in his *Method of Treating Gunshot Wounds* of 1545. Paré pioneered numerous means of increasing battlefield victims' survival rates. He created new medical instruments; he used sour wine as a form of antiseptic; he performed amputation on the battlefield before infection set in and ligatured blood vessels afterward; and he created workable prosthetic devices for amputees (Ellis 2009, 125; Gabriel and Metz 1992, 59–60).

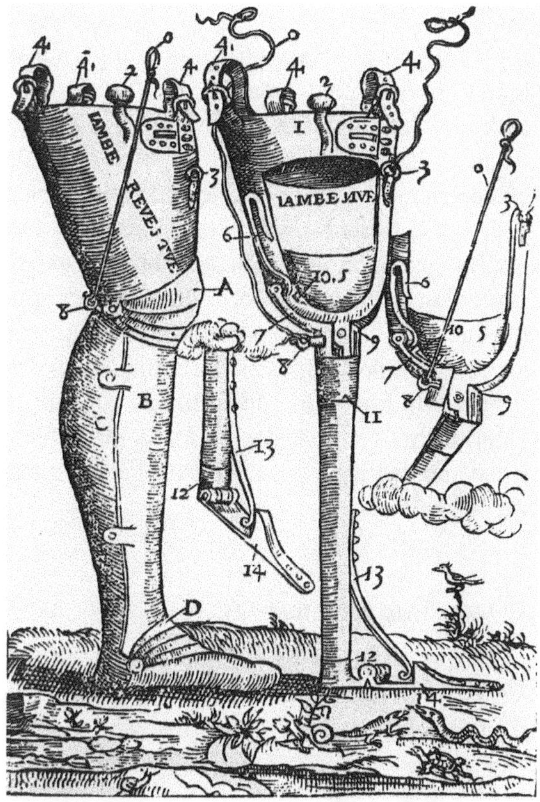

Full and cutaway views of an artificial leg with joints at the knee and ankle, invented by the French military surgeon Ambroise Paré. This is from a 1575 edition of his works. (National Library of Medicine)

One of the major sources of leg wounds requiring amputation was the cannonball. This was usually a solid sphere of iron varying in size with the diameter of the cannon's barrel. Obviously, these did not explode but rather acted like low-flying, or even rolling, bowling balls, tearing through the massed infantry ranks, hitting not one man but potentially many before coming to a stop. These were also used against fortifications, making venerable medieval walls and towers obsolete. When striking masonry, they sent an explosion of brick, stone, and mortar fragments that could lacerate and blind. Other types of ordnance were also developed, including several types of antipersonnel shrapnel designed to hurl a wave of small metal projectiles at infantry at close range, and at sea chains that were fired into the enemy's rigging to shred sails and mangle masts. Early cannon suffered from poor metallurgy, poorly formulated or stored powder, ill-fitting projectiles, and a general lack of standardization among guns in a given unit. Over time, industry provided weapons and ammunition that were more reliable, more accurate, more mobile, standardized into predictable and interchangeable sizes, and overall more deadly.

Finally, this new battlefield paradigm meant many burns of different types. Poorly cast cannon overheated or even exploded; powder could be very unstable and either not work or do so unpredictably; gunners made errors in pouring powder into hot barrels and causing premature flashes; firing mechanisms misfired, especially a problem with early matchlock firearms that had to be lit with a burning fuse-like match. Faces, hands, and fingers were the most common victims. Deep burns could fester and become infected and even small explosions could blind and deafen. For such burns, Paré suggested a folk remedy of salt and crushed onions.

War and Disease

In the midst of the Enlightenment, in the 1750s and 1760s during the Seven Years' War, European armies in Europe, Asia, and North America lost 88 men to death by disease for every 1 man who died of battle wounds.

Camp Diseases

As we have seen, camp life could hold many dangers, but the most immediate was disease. Thousands of men living densely together, in far from sanitary and hygienic conditions, eating and drinking whatever came their way: this was the perfect milieu for many diseases. Dysentery was caused by protozoa or bacteria consumed in tainted drinking water. Once passed out of the body in feces or urine, where there are poor hygiene and sanitation, the cycle continues. While it might not kill one directly, it did dehydrate the victim and weaken his immune responses, making it easier for him to catch other illnesses. Very similar in spread was the bacterial disease typhoid fever, an intestinal disease that could reach epidemic levels if general food or water supplies were affected.

Typhus was caused by a bacterial organism that is carried by human body lice. These thrived where clothing was heavy and rarely laundered, and the body rarely bathed. Flu-like chills, fever, and nausea usually did not lead to prostration and death, but they can and did. Typhus's first appearance in history was among the Spanish besieging Granada, Spain, in 1489–1490. Seventeen thousand died in their camps. Only a few years later perhaps 30,000 French soldiers succumbed during their siege of Spanish-held Naples. Mosquitoes carried and spread malaria, and local epidemics were known as far north as England. Since mosquitoes fed on humans, they simply passed the protozoa from infected carrier to new victim. Since the insects preferred marshy environments, it is not surprising to find outbreaks in low-lying ground where troops had landed or besieged port cities.

Overcrowding in camps allowed tuberculosis, scarlet fever, influenza, and measles to spread quickly among the nonimmune members of the army. Since the medical cultures of the day had no knowledge of the diseases' causes, means of spreading, and ways to control them, army officials had no medical reason for taking the steps that would have made military service much safer.

The Spread of Disease Due to War

The spread of disease due to war did not require that an army on the move be diseased from the beginning. As the men marched and countermarched across the countryside, they interacted with populations that harbored unfamiliar diseases—especially true outside of Europe—and like a saturated and dripping sponge developed the diseases themselves and spread them in their wake. Armies and local populations exchanged all manner of diseases, from plague to venereal diseases. Wounded soldiers were routinely left to suffer with local villagers or towns; stragglers and deserters could carry disease far and wide, as could refugees fleeing from approaching troops. Poor locals often stripped clothing from fallen soldiers, providing fresh meals for hungry lice, and troops often stole bedding and spare clothing from unlucky and disease-ridden villagers.

Men also passed through civilian populations as they gathered for war before an offensive or to defend the frontiers of a state. Fortified towns and cities were strongholds in which soldiers lived alongside residents, sharing food, water, insects, and even beds. After a loss or unsuccessful campaign, deserters multiplied and scattered across the countryside, living off whatever came their way. Weakened by hunger, fatigue, and the shock of battle, with nothing in the way of medical aid or other resources, they were easy targets for many diseases even hundreds of miles from their camps.

War in the Tropics

European colonialism came at a tremendous military cost. Ever-larger ships whose sides were lined with an ever-larger number of cannon and manned by ever-larger skilled crews (650–950 men per ship of the line in the later 18th century) transported tens of thousands of infantry across rough seas to disease-ridden ports whose climates were like sauna baths. The British, French, and Spanish, and to a lesser extent the Dutch and Portuguese, wrestled for control of small islands in the Caribbean Sea and Indian Ocean with both elements of their national armies and battalions of mercenaries who worked for commercial organizations such as the Dutch East India Company and the English East India Company (see Harrison 2007, 87–120). (During the French Revolution, the British East India Company controlled a force of between 115,000 and 155,000 mercenaries and sepoys, making it one of the largest armies in the world.) They fought with each other, with the natives, and with local competitors for bases, influence, and control of resources. Far more costly than any pitched battles or duels at sea were the losses due to tropical diseases, including yellow fever and malaria, and environmental illnesses such as heat stroke.

For example, in 1741 the British sent a force of 22,000 troops to seize Cartagena (Colombia); it was the largest known amphibious landing of troops until World War II. Already weakened by bad food shipboard and the other discomforts of the crossing, fully half of the force fell to yellow fever during the unsuccessful three-month campaign. In the same year, half of a force sent to capture Santiago, Cuba, fell ill to malaria and yellow fever and the attack was aborted. The British captured Havana, Cuba, in 1762, but disease eliminated about 8,000 of their 15,000-man force. In 1782, the British sent 7,000 troops to Jamaica. As reported by physician John Hunter, soon after landing, only 2,000 were fit for duty; fully 25 percent died of disease. During the wars of the French Revolution, the British tried unsuccessfully to seize French holdings in the Caribbean. They won victories on several islands in 1793, but they abandoned them all as disease destroyed their occupying armies. An estimated 80,000 British troops died on Martinique, St. Lucia, and Guadeloupe, with perhaps 50,000 killed on St. Domingue alone. On their part, the French sent 35,000 men, of whom only 6,000 lived to return to France.

Africa would soon become known as the white man's graveyard, and most colonial ventures date from after our period. Europeans did, of course, have slaving colonies along the west coast. Yellow fever was endemic among native populations in many regions, but in what is today Senegal, the disease was unknown. When a ship brought slaves carrying the disease into the British fort of St. Louis, the result was what is considered Africa's first yellow fever epidemic, as mortality rates reached 60 percent.

The major problem was what the British called lack of "seasoning." Residents who had lived in tropical regions for some time often acquired immunity from light initial infections of certain diseases, especially yellow fever. When a large influx of "unseasoned" Europeans set up camp, the result was an epidemic and the weakening or destruction of the force. The British had the correct idea in creating 12 West Indian regiments of black soldiers to protect their Caribbean colonies.

Malaria and yellow fever were not alone in crippling colonial armies. Typhus took its toll, as did dysentery and other enteric (bowel) illnesses. These were accompanied by dehydration and fever, which could quickly weaken and kill sufferers. A study of the 1820s and 1830s in the British Caribbean indicated that these cases were second only to yellow and malarial fevers as causes for death, and 20 percent of cases were fatal. Other potentially fatal conditions that were common included venereal diseases, alcohol abuse, lung problems, vitamin deficiencies, skin conditions and abscesses, and wounds of various types. Britain's black soldiers may have been naturally protected from yellow fever and malaria, but they were subject to smallpox, respiratory problems, dysentery and other bowel conditions (Sheridan 1985, 13–16).

CARE FOR THE WOUNDED AND VETERANS

Care in the Field

We noted above that the Aztec state provided care for those of their warriors who were wounded and disabled in battle. These facilities were the closest things to hospitals that their culture had, since most sick and injured people were treated in their homes. Though Europeans had had hospitals for centuries, they played virtually no role in medieval military health care. This changed during the early modern period. As the 17th-century French leader Cardinal Richelieu claimed, "2,000 men leaving hospital cured, and in some sense broken into the profession, are far more valuable than even 6,000 new recruits." A century earlier, the English army surgeon Thomas Gale attacked the "cobblers, horse-gelders, and tinkers" who treated soldiers, and established six rules for the military surgeon: he should be paid decently; he should do no harm; he should work quickly lest the wound worsen; he should give a truthful prognosis; he should be aware of the pain he is inflicting; and he should accept no cash from the wounded (Friedenberg 2009, 160). Battlefield surgeons appeared first among the Swiss in the 16th century, and German armies borrowed the practice. The 16th-century Spanish armies quickly created the most responsive field facilities, but few advances followed. By 1600, standardized kits with instruments, bandages, and useful drugs were being issued to medics, and by 1700, barber-surgeons served at the company level. Books helped surgeons prepare for the terrible conditions they would face (but only 34 titles appeared across 18th-century Europe), while 18th-century France (1731), Saxony (1748), Austria (1784), and Prussia (1795) established military surgical schools (see Wright 2011).

Hospitals for the Wounded

The Spanish commander the Duke of Alva in 1567 established the earliest recognized military hospital at Mechelen (Malines) in the Netherlands, though it had a rocky start. It was made a permanent facility in 1585 and given a staff of 49 and 330 beds. From 1596, fines on rowdy soldiers supported the hospital. For almost 100 years, it was the only such permanent facility in Europe (Parker 1989, 72–73, 94, 185–186). In 1629, French military authorities required every French fortress to provide an infirmary for the sick and injured, and a surgeon to attend them. The project took 80 years to complete. London provided wounded Englishmen with some 350 dedicated beds in two large hospitals, and from the early 17th century, countries were expected to care for wounded soldiers, especially during the Civil War (Harrison 2004, 66; Gruber von Ami 2006).

Britain's naval authority was the Admiralty, and it formed a "Sick and Hurt Board" to see to medical facilities for the ill and injured. From the 1740s permanent hospitals were established in Portsmouth (Haslar) and Plymouth (Stonehouse), England's two busiest naval ports. Here one could get the oversight, care, and discipline lacking in inns or private houses. Staff were prepared to treat every type of condition from depression to serious wounds to venereal disease. A study of Haslar Hospital for 1753–1757 indicates that of 14,418 patients, 9,862 were discharged as cured, a rate of 68 percent. The other third died, remained, or were moved to a longer-term care facility (Harrison 2004, 66; Crimmin 2007).

Care for Veteran Soldiers

Facilities to provide long-term care for invalid veterans were rather later in coming. Since these were not men who were being recycled to the battlefield, there was less of an incentive for authorities to provide medical care or even a residence. Nonetheless, such provision was at least a sign of good faith on the part of governments. When founded in kingdoms, they were also a form of royal charity. French king Henry IV built the House of Christian Charity in 1605 to house disabled veterans. Another of the earliest was "Our Lady of Hals," created as a charity for crippled Spanish veterans serving in the Netherlands. In 1640, it housed 346 residents. Nearby, the Dutch established the Soldatengasthuis (lit. "Soldier Guest House") in Amsterdam, which was set up in the 1640s near the end of the Thirty Years' War. In 1670, Louis XIV established the famous Hôtel des Invalides in Paris, where Napoleon is buried today; and in Dublin, the English founded Kilmainham Royal Hospital a decade later. The Royal Hospital at Chelsea appeared in 1682 and that for ex-sailors at Greenwich near London in 1694, both designed by the great architect Christopher Wren. Most disabled veterans in England were cared for in county facilities, with quality of care differing widely across the island (Stevenson 2007).

Historian Geoffrey Hudson studied Greenwich Hospital and noted that these huge facilities were effective controlling the residents and their activities. They wanted their freedom to move about as much as they were able, come and go as they pleased, have sex, fight, use vulgar language, abuse alcohol, and otherwise live as military men did. Since the hospital staff were far more interested in maintaining a disciplined living environment than providing much in the way of medical help, confinement was the rule. This changed over time, however, as the institution became more medicalized, and practitioners replaced shipboard discipline with more therapeutic policies. This included better food and environmental conditions such as ventilation and light (Hudson 2007; Hudson 2000).

Both the hospitals for the wounded and veterans' facilities proved to be the perfect places for medical training and for experimentation with untried techniques and drugs such as patent medicines. The military had a stake in quick and inexpensive answers to medical problems. With only a thin veil of ethics, doctors and surgeons could follow the courses of a wide variety of therapies to determine when and how well they worked. On the one hand, many new orthopedic and surgical methods emerged from such experimentation. On the other hand, 18th-century patent medicines saturated with opiates, alcohol, or both were given countless trials. An army or navy contract for providing some proprietary remedy could earn a man a fortune.

WAR WITHIN THE HOUSE OF ISLAM

Despite their nickname, the "gunpowder states" lagged behind Europeans in the adoption and development of firearms. Ottoman heavy artillery, most effective in sieges of walled fortifications, put the Turks ahead of their Safavid and Mughal rivals. But the Ottoman Empire fought on at least two fronts, in the east against India and Persia and in the Balkans and Central Europe against the Holy Roman Empire and its allies. Traditional weapons such as swords, polearms, and arrows continued in use alongside matchlocks and later muskets. Turkish armies were well organized and highly disciplined by comparison with those of European states. Training and punishment were brutal and effective. Camp life was far healthier for the Turks, whose leaders saw that ample food was supplied, provisions made for the sick and wounded, and a standard of sanitation established. Nonetheless, maintaining tens of thousands of men in the confines of an encampment or siege setting invited disease. The rule of thumb was when mustering troops to double the number of men needed to be battle-ready.

Turkish commanders limited campaign stops to 30 to 40 days, even when besieging a city or fortress. Their siege of Safavid Baghdad in 1638 lasted just 39 days. As in Europe, both besiegers and besieged suffered from crowded conditions, deteriorating sanitation, and dwindling supplies. Diseases that included dysentery, dropsy, influenza, and—perhaps most common—typhus (*huma-i muharrika*) took an enormous toll. In 1630, between 8,000 and 9,000 Ottoman soldiers died in battle at Hillah fighting the Safavids. During the previous two-year campaign, disease took an estimated 30,000 lives. When defeat was the order of the day, retreat could mean a trek of hundreds of desert miles with the scourges of wounds, heat, hunger, thirst, and disease. In 1626, an English observer with a retreating Ottoman army noted that in a single day some 12,000 men perished.

Soldiers who suffered serious battle wounds were provided stipends known as "wounded injury money" from imperial coffers; families of dead soldiers received pensions. Among the Turks, battlefield surgeons were at least as common as among early modern European forces, and sultans took pride in staffing mobile medical detachments (Murphey 1999, 130–131). Turkish commanders and the sultan himself were aware of European advances in dealing with the wounded, and many innovations were readily adopted. Safavid Persian surgeons also utilized both traditional and newly developed methods of dealing with battle wounds. An arrow was either left in place until pus provided a lubricant for its removal, or it was wiggled back and forth to loosen and remove it, or a special knife was employed to penetrate the wound to where the tip of the arrow was lodged. In the case of poisoned arrows, the surrounding flesh was cut away to halt the progress of the toxin. To remove bullets, during the rule of Shah Abbas (d. 1629), surgeons developed an extractor with a spoon-shaped tip (Elgood 1970, 156–159). As always, necessity was the mother of invention.

CONCLUSION

Impressed by the successes of the European way of waging war, the Islamic gunpowder states, the Chinese and Japanese empires, and even North American natives adopted some of its tools and methods. Yet the costs in lives and treasure of creating and maintaining huge and continuously serving armies were enormous. Newer weapons were expensive, complicated, and of questionable reliability but offered much greater killing and maiming power. Yet the calculus of the germ was every early modern army's greatest foe. Military health care developed around the need to recycle the wounded so they could fight and bleed another day.

12

Medical Institutions

For most of human history, most people lived most of their lives within a few miles of where they had been born. The family has always been the primary institution of health care in every known society. As communities developed greater specialization, epidemics of infectious diseases became more common, and individuals traveled and relocated more, societies developed a wider and wider range of health-related authorities and facilities. The bulk of this chapter is taken up with Western institutions, since Western societies developed a very wide range of types and institutions, and transplanted many of these across the globe between 1500 and 1800. In the centuries that followed, most of the rest of the world borrowed and adapted them for themselves. Several important facilities, such as insane asylums and military hospitals, are dealt with in detail in other chapters.

THE CHINESE

Chinese Medical Authorities

China had a highly hierarchical society, with the emperor and his court in Peking (Beijing) at the apex of the pyramid. Though possessed of theoretically unlimited power, China's ancient religious culture mandated that imperial benevolence flow from the top down. Seeing that his people—especially the poor—had adequate provision for their health when needed was an important part of this mandate. For example, state storehouses had long supplied medicinal herbs and other necessities, and state infirmaries tended the acutely ill or injured. Medical education was both a part of and a specialty within the preparation for service in the state bureaus, and there was often a matter of preference as to whether one was a bureaucrat or physician. Medical specialists served to organize medical provision and practice at every level from prefecture to county, and formal medical bureaus dated back to the early 14th century. At times of extraordinary need, the state provided special medical bureaus with expanded duties and powers. The Chinese were no strangers to droughts, floods, famines, and epidemics, especially in the 1580s and 1640s. Were special bureaus motivated by benevolence? Perhaps in part, but the overriding factors were control of the people and maintenance of order.

Order was above all the responsibility of the Imperial Medical Bureau (*taiyiju*). Located in the imperial palace, it had responsibility for the health and well-being of the imperial family and household and for overseeing all of the emperor's benevolence that flowed down to the towns and villages. The bureau was the principle repository and copying center for Chinese medical classics and the national center for medical education and professional testing (as the Imperial Medical Institute [*taiyi yuan*] from the fifth century C.E.). It established the official curriculum and canon of recognized medical classics for the nation, and oversaw the provision of medical officers and bureaucrats throughout China (Wang 1999, 162–167).

Chinese Medical Facilities

The multigenerational Chinese family remained the keystone of society, and whenever possible, problems of health or illness were confined to its quarters. While Chinese culture provided for the local poor in donation-supported settlements called *yangji yuan*, and for travelers who became sick or injured, the old, infirm, insane, or diseased were their families' responsibility. In addition, since many diseases and conditions were thought to result from angry spiritual forces, there was an important element of avoiding shame or "keeping face" when a family member fell ill. Additionally, the belief in troublesome spirits or demons made Buddhist and Daoist monasteries and shrines natural places of reconciliation and healing. Monks were often very adept not only at spiritual healing but at herbal and manipulative therapies as well. State-supported infirmaries tended the needy as outpatients or by providing limited live-in arrangements, but these did not evolve into hospitals in the Western sense. Benevolence was also an individual's responsibility, and many wealthy Chinese supported charity dispensaries that distributed medicines and had salaried physicians on staff. In short, the Chinese provided a high level of health care for its people but not by developing the kinds of institutions associated with the West. One exception would be the leper asylum.

Chinese Leper Houses

Hansen's disease, commonly called leprosy, takes a terrible toll on the human body. The bacteria attack the skin and nerves causing physical deformation, especially of the face. As the condition progresses, the sufferer will reek from the disease and is likely to lose bits of his or her body. Though it is only mildly contagious, the fearsomeness and unpleasantness of leprosy, and the belief that the cause was supernatural punishment, led the ancient Chinese to exclude lepers from society, forcing them to beg along the roads.

This policy shifted in the 16th century, and leprosy became the only chronic disease for which people were institutionalized in early modern China. In 1518, the first asylum for sufferers of *mafeng* appeared in Fujian Province. Many other *mafeng yuan* followed across Qing China. Local civil authorities established these as a matter of public order, funneling some financial support from the state. Usually these were small, walled villages of huts located well outside cities, yet close enough so that the lepers could beg for their subsistence. Supporting lepers was good charity, so donations provided some relief and may have kept begging lepers out of the public eye. But the *mafeng yuan* was not a religious establishment, and trustees of the asylum rather than monks or others kept order and tended the suffering. It was rather a place of isolation where the incurable went to die. Though there was no set imperial policy or central direction, the 1724 imperial edict to provide official communal facilities for the poor and the acutely insane included leper asylums (Leung 2009, 96–109).

THE ISLAMIC WORLD

The *Bimaristan*

Like the Chinese, Muslims valued aid to the needy as a religious and cultural benefit. But "needy" had a broader context for Islam. Along with the physically and economically disadvantaged, scholars, some religious authorities, and people on the *hajj*, or pilgrimage to Mecca, were worthy of charitable support from individuals, including women and society's political leaders. Since the Prophet Muhammad's time, such giving has been formalized as one of the four pillars of Islam. The characteristic Muslim institution for the provision of health care was the *bimaristan*. Scholars argue about the *bimaristan's* early history, but it is clear that Islam had adapted ancient Greek, Christian, and Persian hospitals to their own purposes in Baghdad by the ninth century C.E., even earlier elsewhere. A city such as Baghdad, Cairo, Damascus, or Istanbul might have dozens of these facilities, built across generations by individual patrons—including caliphs and sultans—or donations from many. *Bimaristans* provided care for the poor, travelers, and those who needed special treatments such as cataract removals. In 1284, a magnificent example, the Mansuri, was constructed in Cairo. It admitted men and women, excluding no one (some places did exclude slaves and soldiers, for example), and is said to have had accommodations for 8,000. Certain cases were relegated to special wards to isolate them from others, and a wide variety of physicians and specialist healers were available. Teaching was carried out, often utilizing patients as examples, long before the practice appeared in Christian Europe. A pharmacy was on site, as were a dispensary, medical library, and prayer room. An ex-palace, the grounds were graced by restful gardens, streams, and fountains (Shefer-Mossensohn 2009, 160–165). Provision of water was for both hygienic and therapeutic reasons. The sound of flowing water was good for the spirit, and bathing in water was a form of treatment for certain conditions (Shefer-Mossensohn 2009,83–84, 152–155). It seems that the high quality of accommodations, food, and care of these places drew the lazy and shiftless, which led to careful screening for admissions (Pormann and Savage-Smith 2007, 99–100; Shefer-Mossensohn 2009, 99).

The Ottoman Empire

Muslim Turks had their own facilities for the poor, sick, and travelers, the *imareti*, which is often translated as "soup kitchen" (Shefer-Mossensohn 2009, 20). As they collected new territories, they constructed more of these, adopted the *bimaristan* (*bimarhane* in Turkish), and continued supporting many of the existing hospitals from Istanbul to Mecca. The conquerors were making their mark in the tradition of the Muslim dynasties that preceded them. As with Christian charitable foundations, for Muslims the act of founding or supporting a *bimaristan* was spiritually beneficial, part of the benevolence expected of one on his way to paradise. These hospitals were usually named for the founder and supported with endowments of agricultural land that provided rents (Shefer-Mossensohn 2009). All classes could find treatment, foreigners included, and all services were rendered without any compensation or expectation of donations. The patient, however, had to be Muslim and in need of medical help. Non-Muslims were not welcome and in larger cities could usually find their own medical help. The standard endowment agreement stipulated that only "the sick, the wounded, and those who suffer injuries and aches" could be admitted. Ottoman hospitals even housed the mentally and emotionally ill, unlike most European hospitals. Like Londoners and Aztecs, Turks visited the grounds during spring to be entertained by the mad (Shefer-Mossensohn 2009, 135, 169–170. Also see Dols 1992). Women, on the other hand, might have their own quarters either within the *bimarhane* or in a

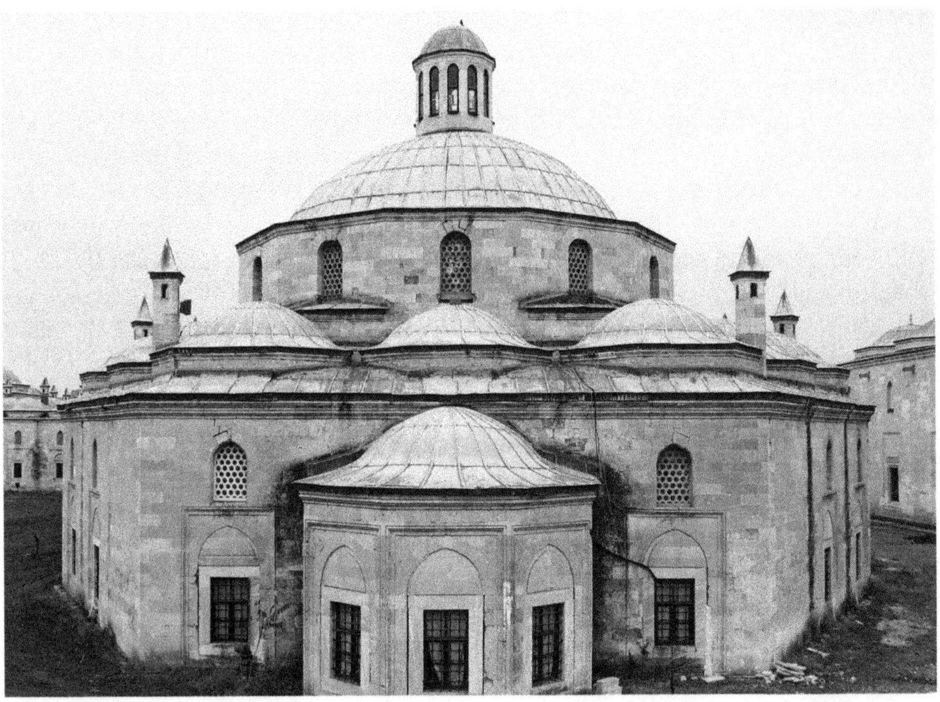

The Ikinu Beyazit Kulliyesi (welfare complex) on the grounds of the Sultan Bayezid II Mosque in Edirne, Turkey. Dating from the 15th century, the institution included a medical school and hospital. The complex now houses a museum dedicated to the history of medicine in Turkey. (Valery Shanin/Dreamstime.com)

separate facility, or they would be denied treatment. When possible, women healers rather than male physicians were employed to deal with female patients (Shefer-Mossensohn 2009, 117–137).

Though within the hospital certain spaces were functionally separate, such as women's quarters and the prayer room, regardless of complaint, pairs of patients randomly shared small rooms. The Galenic notion of miasma—poisoned air as the cause of disease—trumped physicians' recognition of contagion (Shefer-Mossensohn 2009, 172–179; see also Stearns 2011). This differed from, for example, Cairo's Mansuri Hospital, in which patients were segregated by ailment into wards. Also, Ottoman hospitals were not so much themselves the all-purpose complexes that they had been earlier but rather one part of a site that contained a bathhouse, imaret, madrassa (religious school), mosque, and other facilities that were typical objects of the charity of the wealthy.

Yet given the size of the major cities, the numbers of facilities and beds available were small. Istanbul, Cairo, and Aleppo each had only a half dozen major foundations in the 16th century. A few new major medical facilities graced the growing cities of the 17th century, but there were not many, and their traditional layout and patterns of use began to change (Shefer-Mossensohn 2009, 115, 198). As the sultans edged westward, adopting a wider and wider range of European medical ideas and practices during the 18th century, the hospitals that were founded reflected the latest in European medicine.

The Safavids

Next door to the Turks, the picture was very different. In the vast region dominated from Persia, the *bimaristan* had been in decline since even before the Mongol destruction of the 13th century. Unlike the Ottoman sultans, the Safavid shahs spent virtually nothing on repairing medical facilities or building new ones. Both travelers' accounts and native records describe once proud structures reduced to holding a few madmen, serving as prisons, or being used as warehouses for food to be given to the poor. Those that still functioned were described as being overcrowded with the sick poor and with none of the amenities traditionally associated with the venerable institution (Elgood 1970, 27, 107).

THE EUROPEANS

As early modern states gained more authority over their citizens or subjects, they exercised more power over health care providers and facilities through public officials and boards. Royal and municipal hospitals replaced church hospitals in both Protestant and Catholic countries, though in Catholic lands, they remained staffed by dedicated men and women religious. Over time, new and more specialized facilities emerged with new needs: general hospitals, veterans' and sailors' hospitals, lunatic asylums, pest (plague) houses, clinics, and teaching hospitals.

European Health Authorities

About the time of the Black Death (1347–1352), most European urban areas had two types of health-related authorities. One was the guild or guilds that regulated the organization, qualifications, and practices of physicians, surgeons, and apothecaries. The second was various sets of local laws that set standards for those who sold food, for the location of loud or noxious businesses such as smiths, tanneries, or butcher shops, and for the cleanliness of public streets and byways. Central governments, such as the English or French monarchs, tended to have little to say outside of London or Paris. In large part, this was due to the lack of any effective bureaucracy that would have been able to carry into effect the royal writ. During and in the wake of the plague, a few self-governing Italian city-states—Venice, Milan, Florence—experimented with special emergency boards consisting of a few important men (but not physicians) who created extraordinary rules for handling the epidemic or aftermath. In 1485, Venice established a permanent health magistracy; Milan followed quickly, and Florence did so in 1527. Being permanent, these magistracies expanded their oversight and legislative authority to include a very wide range of concerns, including prostitution, sanitation, medical care, trade during times of epidemic, and control of the poor and itinerant tramps. During plague time, these magistracies had extensive powers to round up plague victims who could or would not be cared for at home and compel them to enter pest houses, to restrict the movements of anyone suspected of having the plague, and even to enter the homes of victims and destroy all of their belongings in the name of public safety (Byrne 2006).

In the 16th century, the Spanish crown developed the office of *protomedicato*, a regional board of respected physicians (*protomédicos*), usually crown-appointed, that was given responsibility for health and medical matters. England relied on Parliament to make most public health decisions, with local jurisdictions reliant on parish officials and sheriffs. As epidemics swept through the islands in the 16th and 17th centuries, Parliament and local officials dusted off the regulations and plans from the past episodes and reinstated them. There was one clear evolutionary trend, though, and that was toward the ever-greater use of coercion, from forced closures of theaters and other meeting places to quarantine of suspected people and goods, to mandatory isolation of victims in the local pest house or with one's entire family in one's own house. France followed Milan in developing health commissions across the country by 1600. These had broad powers in normal times and expansive ones during an emergency. During 1720–1721, Western Europe's last major plague epidemic ravaged France's Mediterranean coast around Marseille. The royal government took control and utilized the army to create and man a cordon sanitaire, or health blockade, to keep potentially infected people from moving outside the stricken region. It was a tool used by the Habsburg government along its long border with the Turks, and in both cases it appears to have helped keep the plague at bay (Slack 1988; Cook and Cook 2009). In 1772, Louis XVI established the Royal Society of Medicine whose real function was to investigate medical practitioners and medicinal suppliers to ensure that all were meeting the society-approved levels of quality (Porter 1996, 7, 47).

It seems clear that in 1500 only a few attempts at any sort of public health organization of policy were to be found in Europe, whereas by 1800 organizational infrastructures existed across much of the continent. Countermeasures against plague played a large, if not determining, role in developing these organizations

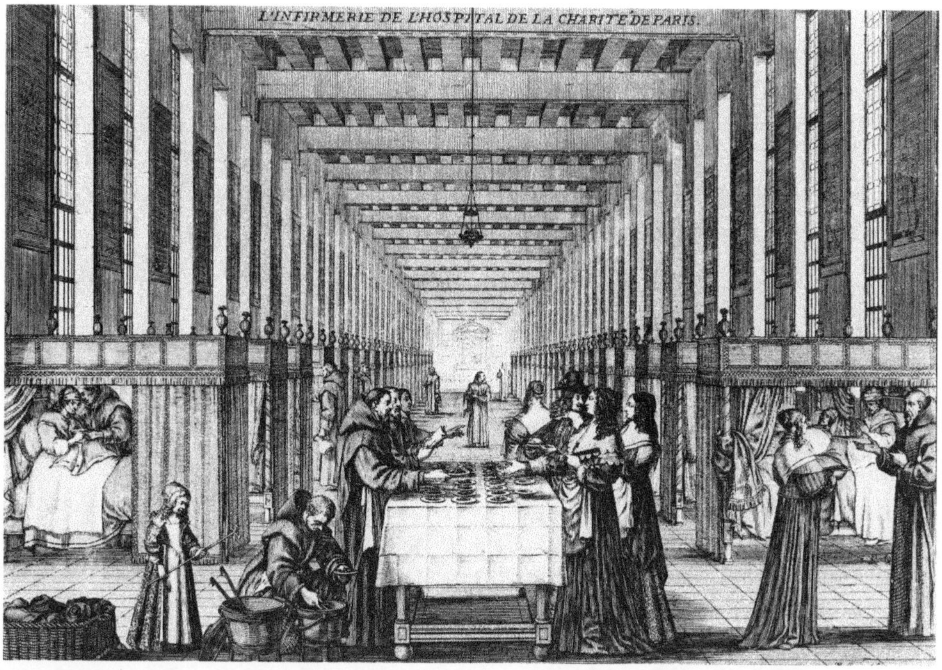

Engraving by 17th-century artist Abraham Bosse, "The Infirmary of the Sisters of Charity (La Charité) during a Visit of [French Queen] Anne of Austria, ca. 1640." The Parisian hospital has high ceilings and tall windows that allow good light and ventilation, and the patients have beds in curtained-off cubicles. (Hulton Archive/Getty Images)

and policies. But there were other considerations. Europe's authoritarian governments extended their tentacles of power down to the village levels with bureaucrats, commissioners, and health officers—in Prussia literally health police—to ensure that their greatest resource, people, was kept in reasonably sound health and the exploding populations in good order. In the long run, controlling health is the surest way to control a society (Porter 1996, 5–8).

European Health Facilities

Before 1500, Europe's most advanced nations and city-states had developed only a handful of types of health care facilities. Monasteries and convents had infirmaries for sick religious and in rural areas for local folk and travelers who fell ill. Leprosaria were in decline as the dreadful Hansen's disease faded from Europe, but lazarettos or "houses" in which plague victims were placed were just being developed. Hospitals had evolved little from their medieval ancestors, housing the elderly, crippled, pregnant, sick, diseased, and exhausted. Unlike the Islamic *bimaristan*, the later medieval hospital was strictly for the economically needy. Larger cities might also have an orphans' home and one for foundlings (abandoned children), and perhaps a facility specifically for sick or pregnant prostitutes (often named after Saint Mary Magdalen, traditionally the prostitute Jesus converted). No one really expected cures to take place in hospitals, as they were essentially warehouses of the incapable. A babe might be born, a fracture knit, or a fever break, but these charitable institutions, almost always connected to the Catholic Church, were only secondarily places of healing (Jones 1996). For cures there were religious shrines, from local holy wells or churches with relics to major pilgrimage destinations, such as Rome, Compostela, or Canterbury. When, out of Christian love for God and one's neighbor, the wealthy provided hospices or any health-related facility, the act was considered an aid for one's eternal destination after death. Doing such a good deed helped balance the bad or evil actions in one's life and increased the odds of joining God in paradise.

Between 1500 and 1800, a flurry of new types of care facilities changed the landscape of institutional health care. Even before the Reformation (from 1517), the Catholic king of France secularized hospitals, though nuns and religious brothers still provided much of the staffing. Protestant Henry VIII of England shut down the Catholic hospitals when he closed the kingdom's monasteries, and they revived only slowly under subsequent civil control. While a few major hospitals remained "general" hospitals, many more specialized centers emerged. Some of these were for infectious diseases, others for elder care or pregnant women. Kings, city governments, and wealthy patrons created smaller and arguably more effective places where healing of the body trumped that of the spirit. This trend toward creating specific spaces where medicine was practiced in the hope of healing is sometimes called the medicalization of health care institutions.

Continuing Problems

The Leprosarium

Medieval leprosaria were charitable houses located outside towns to house the sufferers from this terrible disease. By the 13th century, perhaps 19,000 of these hospices were scattered from Russia to Ireland. By the early modern period, however, most of these had been closed as the disease all but disappeared from Europe south of Scandinavia. Still, even in the 17th century, Dutch towns usually had a leper house. This may have been made necessary by the Dutch commercial contacts with areas of Scandinavia and the Indian Ocean where leprosy was still very active (Bruijn 2009, 108; Zumthor 1994, 155).

The Pest House, or Lazaretto

The pest house, or lazaretto, for plague victims grew out of the leprosarium, and even the name "lazaretto" and its variations derive from Saint Lazarus, the patron of lepers. Formal medicine blamed bubonic plague on poisoned air, or miasma, yet there was a clear popular notion that plague was contagious. If indeed contagious, then victims needed to be isolated to prevent plague's spread, whether within or beyond a given community. Sometimes called a plague hospital, the pest house was normally a temporary feature on the landscape, since unlike leprosy the plague was acute—the patient either dying or recovering within a short time.

Epidemics generally lasted four or five months, centering on August, and returned on average at 10- or 15-year intervals. Though some Dutch and northern French cities had permanent lazarettos, most accommodations were temporary collections of huts or requisitioned monasteries or hospitals. Major, permanent facilities were famously located in Venice from the later 15th century and in Milan from 1524. Milan's later facility had an enormous courtyard for temporary shelters as well as 288 surrounding rooms, and Venice's held an estimated 7,000 sufferers at one time in 1630. To the extent possible with such numbers, paid personnel nursed victims with the hope of their recovery. Smaller institutions had fairly high recovery rates, as high as 50 percent in 17th-century Tuscany. Quarantine facilities were related to pest houses, except that people were placed in quarantine for a set period—traditionally 40 (Italian *quaranta*) days—to see if they developed the illness. In the 18th century, many of these permanent facilities found new life in the battle against such diseases as yellow fever, smallpox, and, later, cholera (Byrne 2006).

Orphanages and Foundling Hospitals

In Catholic Europe, female monasteries and convents and parish rectories were the dropping-off point for abandoned children and most unfostered orphans. In the wake of plague, there were inevitable spikes of both orphaning and abandonment, and these spurred the foundations of facilities dedicated to caring for and raising both types of unfortunate children. Foundlings differed somewhat in that they had been "thrown away" by a parent or parents, and there was the possibility that the mother might return to retrieve the child. In his 1410 will, the Tuscan merchant Francisco Datini founded two, a foundation for foundlings in Prato and the famous Ospedale degli Innocenti in Florence. Having been orphaned as a child and having fathered an illegitimate child, he understood the societal need (see Gavitt 1991). With the Reformation, the need did not disappear in Protestant countries, but the monasteries and nuns did. New arrangements had to be made, as discussed in chapter 5.

General Hospitals and Hôtels Dieu

General hospitals and *hôtels dieu* were medieval institutions that served a wide variety of needs: hospice for the dying or sick travelers, orphanage, maternity hospital (usually for unwed mothers), and old folks' home. The great example was in Paris, but London's St. Thomas and St. Bartholomew, Granada's King's Hospital, and the Royal Hospital in Santiago di Compostela followed similar lines. In Catholic countries, Augustinian and Franciscan women religious provided most of the caregiving staff, but the French began secularizing the administration of its *hôpitaux généraux* even before 1500. This was in part because the French crown did not trust the institutional Church, and also because of the perception that women's religious orders had decayed since the 14th century. Increasingly, these hospitals were medicalized by the emphasis on permanent medical staff (surgeons, physicians, apothecaries) and the exclusion of many long-term residents. During the late 17th and early 18th centuries, France boasted some 200 new general hospitals and 2,000 other medical foundations, many staffed by new Catholic nursing orders. Henry VIII closed London's hospitals but reinstated St. Thomas and St. Bart's, which remained London's only general hospitals until the mid-18th century.

The 1700s witnessed a great growth in hospital numbers and sophistication. Patients now slept in separate beds, only the sick were admitted, wards for various conditions minimized cross-infection, and record keeping allowed for administrators and authorities to see patterns in illnesses and the effectiveness of treatments. Not only did educational anatomical dissections increase in line with Europe's Enlightenment, but pathology emerged as a branch of medicine. In London, five new hospitals appeared between 1720 and 1745, each with a special emphasis, and by 1800, London hospitals could serve 20,000 patients annually. The remainder of Britain had no general hospitals before 1700, but by 1750, Edinburgh (1729), Winchester and Bristol (1737), York (1740), Exeter (1741), Bath (1742), and Northampton (1743) were supplied, as were all sizeable towns by 1800 (Porter 2006, 184–185). In the Netherlands, Scotland, London, Vienna, and elsewhere, medical teaching was increasingly linked to major hospitals. The Enlightened Habsburgs in Austria adopted the idea of medical police and secularized much of their health care provision, including the creation of the *Allgemeines Krankenhaus* (General Hospital) in 1784. It had four surgical wards, and 86 beds for clinical teaching out of a total of 1,600 beds. The Habsburg Empire added new hospitals in Olmütz (1787), Linz (1788), and Prague (1789). By the outbreak of the French Revolution, the French could count 177 general hospitals, and Paris alone had 48 hospitals with 20,000 beds for the city of 700,000 people. Even Catherine the Great's Russia had a new (if backward by Western standards) facility in the Obukhov Hospital (Jones 1996; Risse 1996).

New Needs Met

Syphilis, or Pox, Hospitals

Syphilis or pox hospitals emerged in the 16th century with the horrific spread of the new disease syphilis, or the pox, which suddenly struck Europe in the mid-1490s. Hospital authorities across Europe were loath to mix these new patients, carrying the obvious blight of their sexual misconduct, with their other patients, and the troubling possibility of contagion led to isolation. First, separate wards appeared in some hospitals, and this led to separate structures when symptoms were found to be chronic. In Germany, dozens of small, publicly funded facilities—usually about a dozen beds, though Augsburg had 122—sprang up. In Italy, these were the Incurable Hospitals. Naples's held 600 patients in 1535; Rome's San Giacomo served 1,400 men and 330 women in 1569. Despite the Italian label, people were here to be cured by extreme sessions of sweating to purge the "humoral" poison. Mercury and/or a native American tree wood known as guaiac were used to induce perspiration, a regimen that could last up to 30 days, making the "cure" almost as bad as the disease. In Germany, between 16 and 24 percent of patients died as a result of treatment. The need for treatment and care continued through the early modern period, though the religious or moral prejudice against the venereal component of venereal disease (sexual misconduct) tended to fade. Older hospitals expanded, and new ones, such as Lock Hospital in London (1746), were established to meet the ongoing need (Jütte 1996).

Insane Asylums

Insane asylums also appeared in the 16th century for the first time. The insane had traditionally been allowed to wander at will, with the dangerously insane locked away in jails, cellars, attics, or prisons. As chapter 9 discusses, from the 16th through 18th century cities and individual patrons created new facilities called hospitals, asylums, or residences for those emotionally or mentally disturbed people who had no family to care for them. As with other illness and institutions, insanity and the asylum were gradually medicalized so that by the later 18th century the asylum became a place of therapy as well as human storage.

Eighteenth-Century Innovations

The professionalization of medical practitioners, the Enlightened belief in science, progress, and humanity, and the growth of state self-interest in preserving its population in good health combined to make the 18th century a watershed in the institutionalization of medicine. Growing populations meant more of every type of illness, and medical specialization among practitioners led to even more specialized spaces for treatment. Between 1749 and 1765, London's pregnant poor got beds in four new lying-in or maternity hospitals. Originally only for married women, the administrators soon learned to ask no questions. These quickly became excellent training facilities for midwives, both male and female.

Londoners also pioneered dispensaries—what Americans might call walk-in clinics—for the poor. Physician George Armstrong set up the first in Red Lion Square in 1769 to help the mothers of sick infants with advice and medicine. A second was founded by the Quaker John Lettsom to serve any poor person. His General Dispensary became the model for another 11: set up in a rented space, offering neither beds nor surgery, just drugs and counsel. Subscribers who made regular contributions were called governors, and each was allowed to send one patient per guinea donated. In 1770, it had 100 governors; eight years later, it had 1,400 (Kilpatrick 1990).

The nearly constant drumbeat of war in Europe and its colonies led to the fielding of armies of unprecedented size. Training was time consuming, and the veteran soldier or sailor was not easily replaced. As discussed in chapter 11, the Enlightened self-interest of rulers and their military advisers led to the foundation of dozens of military hospitals that cared for the wounded and ill, and to veterans' hospitals in which those permanently damaged by service might be cared for. The experimentally inclined of the age found that these facilities were perfect forums for testing new methods of treatment and drugs, for clinical teaching and training of military surgeons, and for conducting autopsies and the study of pathology.

EUROPEAN INSTITUTIONS ABROAD

An 18th-century scholar remarked that by the mid-17th century, Europe and its colonies "around the world" could boast of some 563 medical facilities (Graves 2001, 152). Some of these in "colonies" served the merchants, soldiers, sailors, and other resident whites, while some served the natives with European medicine or a mix of European and local medical traditions. In many cases, European medicine abroad both influenced local healing and was in turn influenced by it.

Mexico

The Aztecs provided a few hints of their pre-Columbian institutions. The importance of the warrior in society was underlined by the existence of institutions for both the recuperating wounded and the permanently disabled. They were provided by the ruler and were located in Tenochtitlán, Cholula, Colhuacán, and Texcoco. The Aztec state also used these places as centers for the distribution of food to the poor. In Tenochtitlán, the state also provided for people with disfiguring characteristics that kept them from being considered normal members of Aztec society. These unfortunates with withered limbs, clubfeet, harelips, skin diseases, or other deformities were housed near the royal zoo and gawked at by visitors, much as Londoners visited the insane asylum at Bedlam for amusement. Those with serious diseases had long been sacrificed to the gods, their maladies understood as signs of divine displeasure. Under the later kings, however, they were isolated away from society and treated with a salve known as *teocotl* in Nahuatl. One final health-related institution was the royal botanical garden established by Moctezuma I. Sources claimed it was five miles in circumference and contained medical specimens from throughout southern North and Central America. It allowed Aztec healers to study the growth and healing properties of plants but also supplied the needed materia medica for the court (Ortiz de Montellano 1990).

The Spanish brought the institutions of European medicine with both colonists and natives in mind. Every mission was a medical station that sought to heal the native body as well as spirit. As many Mexicans discovered, however, the robed and bearded men brought death—by contagion—at least as often as health. San Nicolás in Santo Domingo, the first hospital for poor Spaniards, was founded in the New World (1503). In 1517, the *protomedicato*, with oversight on all aspects of formal health care provision, was appointed to Santo Domingo.

The city government rather than the crown appointed the first *protomedicato* for Mexico City, in 1525. The first order of business was regulation of all practitioners who were neither physicians nor surgeons, including both natives and colonists .The year before, Hernán Cortés founded the first general hospital in the New World, the *Hospital de la Concepción de Nuestra Señora.* Known simply as the

Hospital de Jesús, it was the headquarters for the *protomedicato*. Cortés provided estates to support his foundation, which welcomed poor Spaniards and Indians. He also set up the hemisphere's first leprosarium, in 1526/28 at Tlaxplana on his estate near Mexico City (see Schendel 1968, 89, 90, 92, 105). Shortly after, Vasco Quiroga set up a series of Christian missionary pueblos with hospitals in the province of Michoacán. In the early 1530s, Pedro de Gante founded the Hospital Real de Indios exclusively for natives in Mexico City. After expansion it had eight wards and beds for 200 patients. In 1534, the Royal Hospital of St. Joseph for Natives was set up by the Franciscans with the patronage of King Charles I. In the mid-1530s, the first Archbishop of Mexico City created the Hospital of St. John the Divine for syphilitic Spaniards. A second appeared in the 1539, the *Hospital del Amor di Dios*, also with episcopal support and a staff of 18. A second leprosarium was also founded in 16th-century Mexico City: San Lazaro by Dr. Pedro Lopéz in 1572. In 1541, Charles decreed that every town have at least one hospital for poor Spaniards and natives. These would be staffed by both Spanish and Indian physicians, surgeons, and apothecaries.

In Mexico City, one might say that the earliest medical education institution was the barber-surgeon Francisco Soto, who was licensed to take both Spanish and native apprentices to learn his craft. The National University of Mexico was founded in 1551, and the faculty of medicine was in place by 1575. In 1628, the *protomedicato* was formalized, reorganized, and became the ex officio head of the medical faculty, which operated until 1832. Its members were appointed by the crown and absorbed all remaining health care authority in New Spain. The office of the *protomedicato* now licensed all practitioners, prosecuted malpractice cases, and oversaw medical education, midwives, public sanitation, apothecaries, and the sales of food (Schendel 1968, 99–100). Since many missionaries were practitioners, and the Catholic Church ran so many Mexican hospitals (128 by the early 1600s), this was also a power play by the government against the Church (Fields 2008, 76–80; Schendel 1968).

Colonial Mexico's needs for health care facilities remained great because the shocks of the initial importation of new germs and diseases by colonists continued to reverberate, and the Spanish invaders suffered from native diseases and from the conditions of the transatlantic voyage. Epidemics swept Mexico through the 18th century, and in 1770 King Charles III of Spain even established the Mexican National Lottery to help fund treatment for sufferers from smallpox and syphilis (see Cook and Lovell 1992; Cooper 1965; Schendel 1968, 119–120).

Caribbean Slaves

Institutional care for slaves, who were considered little more than chattel property, was no matter of benevolence or even humanistic obligation but of the maintenance of human tools. To its owner, keeping a slave well enough to function was the equivalent of maintaining a plow horse in good health. Provision of health care was a matter of self-interest, and the humanity of the slave was at best a second thought. As property, the slave was expected to remain on the master's property even when desperately ill, so public or church-run facilities had no place. The typical plantation did have some accommodation for the sick and injured, but these differed radically from one to the next. "Infirmaries," "hothouses," "hospitals," or "sick houses" were often permanent but simple one-room buildings, sometimes segregating the sexes by a wall. A trustee caregiver oversaw the place, which would have been supplied with simple instruments and drugs characteristic for the environment and season. If a slave needed a white physician or surgeon, the practitioner would meet the patient in these quarters, so practitioners saw their conditions firsthand. But these facilities were as much prisons as hospitals, and the overseer had to ensure that no one was taking advantage of the rest they afforded. Even critics accepted the need for barred windows, locked doors, and shackles inside (Sheridan 1985, 268–290).

One might think these dated back to the earliest slave presence, but until the Enlightenment and abolition movement of the 18th century, many owners paid little attention to slave health since they could be so cheaply replaced. Now, wars and laws threatened the traffic in enslaved Africans, and both slave health and reproduction became matters of concern. In the British West Indies, the earliest mention of a slave hospital is from about 1750, and Cuban records postdate 1800. Visiting and resident physicians wrote recommending hospitals for slaves, and Dr. James Grainger in 1769 urged they be well ventilated and provided with a fireplace, toilet, bathing facility, and an herb garden for medicinal plants. As slave hospitals appeared, the owners defended them, but both slaves and medical practitioners decried the awful conditions. Critics pointed to the minimal concern for hygiene and resulting infection, the food that was poor even by standards of slavery, and the lack of adequate personnel. The slave caregivers were untrained and unmotivated, and white practitioners made all too rare an appearance. Slaves themselves resented the facilities, as they separated them from their families and friends; they stunk and their people, even if black, forced nasty medicines and painful treatments on them; and they were houses of death from which too many never returned.

From 1784, French authorities in Haiti required plantation hospitals built well on good, well-drained ground, with good ventilation and paved floors. The *hôpitalière* was to run the facility and live in a room in it, alongside male and female wards (Weaver 2006). In 1798, the Leeward Islands mandated the provision of plantation hospitals, and two years later the governor of Trinidad required access to each plantation's facilities and personnel and an annual summary of activity.

Asia and the Indian Ocean

Provision of European-style health care in Asian and Indian Ocean colonies, trading colonies, and open ports was not a matter of sharing European medicine with the natives, except where Roman Catholic missions established the Church's presence. Most infirmaries, clinics, hospitals, and other institutions arose from the need to treat white sailors, merchants, colonists, soldiers, and emissaries who were far from their Portuguese, Spanish, Dutch, French, or English homes. These varied in size from small infirmaries to the 1,500-patient Portuguese Royal Hospital of the Holy Spirit in Goa. In 1569, the hospital of Saint Raphael was founded in Macao and quickly became a major Jesuit establishment. Unusually, its staff used both Western Galenic medicine and Chinese healing techniques, such as acupuncture and moxibustion. It was also unusual in that it had a ward for sufferers from Hansen's disease (leprosy) (Barnes 2005, 46).

Traditional leper hospitals were often founded by Europeans, ostensibly to serve (or incarcerate) native victims. In Goa, the Portuguese established Saint Lazarus hospital as early as 1529. In 1578, the Franciscan friars were operating a leprosarium at Naga in Japan, and later the Spanish invited them to establish one in Manila (see Newson 2009). Dutch Calvinists also founded leper hospitals, as at Batavia, where two were situated onshore and a third at Purmevend. The ideal was to have lepers cared for at home under mandatory isolation, but when doctors found them without supervision, they were locked up. In 1690, 171 inmates were resident, of whom 164 were natives and 7 were European or mixed ancestry (Cook 2007, 375; Bruijn 2009, 108–109).

13

Disease and Healing in the Arts

The various literary, visual, and performance arts are means by which a culture expresses its shared hopes and fears, likes and dislikes, joys and frustrations. They may be a matter of pure entertainment or contain important messages. They can be used to teach, warn, celebrate, vent, mock, or merely record. During the early modern period poets, painters, playwrights, physicians, satirists, illustrators, historians, and other creative folk produced works of art, literature, and drama that did all of these. What follows is a sampling of some of these cultural responses to human health, illness, drugs, and healing.

THE VISUAL ARTS

The Physician Portrayed

In matters of health and wellness, there was no more typical icon than the physician. In the visual art of China, Europe, and the Islamic world, he stands out quite literally from his sick patients: teacher, healer, philosopher. In later medieval European illustrations, he stands taking a pulse or holding up a urine flask or lecturing from a podium over a cadaver. His fine robes and headgear set him apart from those around him. Pulse taking was an iconic activity when depicting a physician, since all of the learned traditions of medicine utilized it. Chinese and Muslim artists used the image in paintings and illustrations ranging from books of occupations to medical classics. Among Europeans, it was the Dutch genre artists of the 17th century who presented well-dressed doctors gently holding the wrist of their—usually female—patient (Anderson, Barnes, and Shackleton 2011, 100–101). Doctors also appeared at hospital bedsides and deathbeds. While European artists generally stayed away from depicting doctors engaged in much beyond consulting with a patient or diagnostic pulse taking, Ottoman, Safavid, Mughal, and Chinese artists often depicted other medical procedures. This may have been due to the fact that European physicians were very jealous of their social role as the practitioners who diagnosed and prescribed while surgeons or others performed the messy tasks.

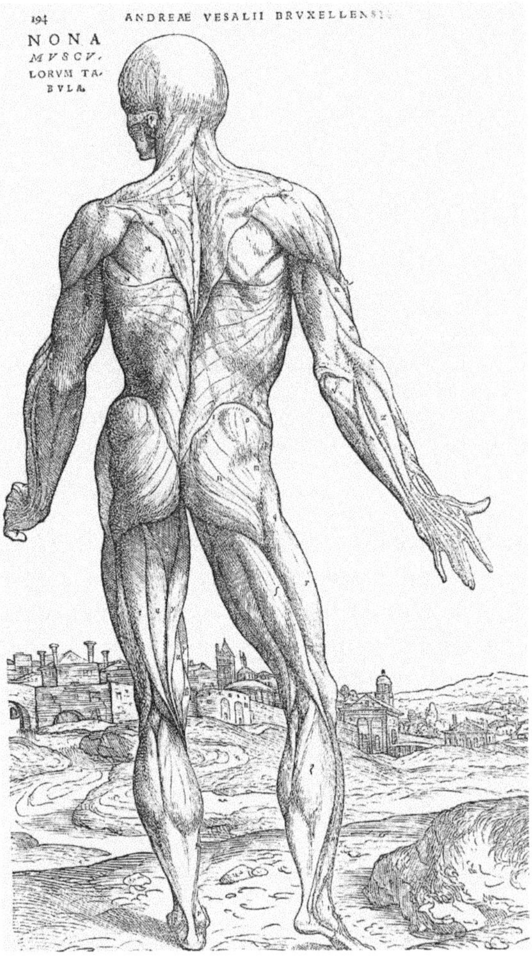

Image of the musculature of the human body from Andreas Vesalius's *On the Fabric of the Human Body*, 1543. (National Library of Medicine)

While most of these pictures were meant to be merely illustrative and their doctors generic, the Renaissance also developed the personal portrait. Throughout the early modern period, many European physicians had themselves painted as members of their society's elite. Most European physician portraits depict the subject in an intellectual setting, surrounded by books, art, and other symbols of good taste and learning. Perhaps the most famous painting of a physician, however, is that by Rembrandt of the Amsterdam doctor Nicolas Tulp. Surrounded by eager and well-dressed students, he sits over a cadaver dissecting it and explaining what they all see. He is shown as expert and teacher, not only a healer but also one who hands his experience and knowledge to others (Loudon 1997, 18–22).

Not all portraits of medical men were flattering, however. A well-documented type was the quack hawking his wares from a stage. Another was the physician's caricature. The artists sought to demean traits of certain doctors or of generic members in a variety of ways. Some were shown as animals such as blood-sucking leeches or ignorant donkeys; others had distorted physical features or carried moneybags or terrifying medical instruments. The doctor often appeared as greedy, as killer no less than curer, as one thankful for the outbreak of disease, as fawning sycophant, or as incompetent boob (Anderson, Barnes, and Shackleton 2011, 109–110, 113–118).

Vesalius and Anatomical Illustration

Andreas Vesalius of Brussels studied and taught medicine in Padua, Italy. Trained as a Galenist, he found by conducting his own dissections that the old Greek was wrong on many counts. He produced a massive and beautifully illustrated guide to anatomy titled *On the Fabric of the Human Body* (1543) that revolutionized anatomical depiction. Though he wrote the text, a true artist working in Venice, perhaps with Titian, produced the many masterful engravings. The frontispiece shows Vesalius in a dissection theater in direct contact with the cadaver while a great crowd swirls in an arc around him. He is in charge because he is the expert, and according to Vesalius, the expert gets his hands dirty.

The illustrations are of the human body variously posed from bare skeleton to fully covered in skin. Their naturalism was right in step with the tastes of the age and the attention to detail made them very useful as tools for medical training. Both his criticisms of Galen and the extraordinary quality of the images were the gold standard for those who would produce books of anatomy (Sawday 1996; Rifkin, Ackerman, and Folkenberg 2006, 68–81, 83–227; Anderson, Barnes, and Shackleton 2011, 34–35).

Hogarth and the Ills of London Society

William Hogarth was a painter and engraver who worked in 18th-century London. He is most noted for his several series of engraved scenes that depict the downfall of contemporary unfortunates. They are at the same time tragic, amusing, and serious social commentary. The earliest was a series of five scenes called the *Harlot's Progress* of 1732. Instead of taking an honest job, young Moll Hackabout enters a brothel and dedicates her life to the sex trade. At first a comfortable

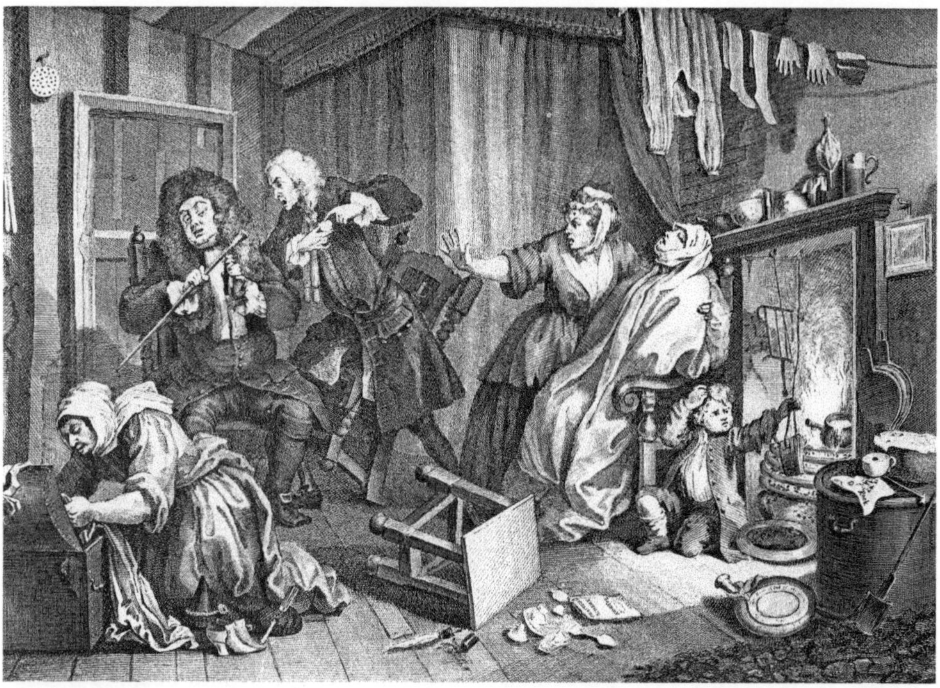

In this plate from William Hogarth's *A Harlot's Progress* (1732), Moll sits in a chair dying while two doctors argue over their cures. (National Library of Medicine)

mistress, she declines into becoming a streetwalker who contracts venereal disease (sexually transmitted disease). In the fifth and final scene, she lays dying as two identifiable physicians with their backs to her argue over which remedy will save her. A year later, the very popular *Rake's Progress* featured a young man-about-town who lives a life of dissolute self-indulgence. In the eighth and last panel, we find the antihero ruined and a patient in Bedlam, London's notorious madhouse. In *Marriage A-la Mode* (1745), Hogarth depicted the rise and fall of another young woman. She married a nobleman and then found a lover, who killed her husband and was in turn hanged for the crime. In the last scene, her child is held up to her as she sinks into eternal slumber, empty by her side the bottle of laudanum that she drained to kill herself.

Hogarth's undated "Damn the Doctor" features a miserable man with a bandaged head sitting on the side of his bed vomiting into a basin. Above him on the bed curtains is the phrase "Damn the Doctor," which is no doubt a commentary on the labeled bottle of physician-provided "Gargle" sitting on the nearby shelf. In 1726, he visually commented on a contemporary news item: a woman gave birth to a score of rabbits! In *Cuniculari or The Wise Men of Godliman in Consultation*, three physicians from London stand by the birth bed seriously considering the phenomenon as rabbits frolic about the room. Here Hogarth lampoons the gullibility of the doctors (and society in general) for taking the hoax at face value. Finally, one might point to the famous "Beer Lane and Gin Alley" in which Hogarth attacks the contemporary lower-class love of high-proof distilled gin over the less intoxicating beer preferred by the middling classes. Beer Lane is a place of order, peace, and prosperity, while the poverty-stricken drunkards of Gin Alley loll about inebriated, a mother letting fall a baby from her ample lap as she reels in laughter (see Anderson, Barnes, and Shackleton 2011, 188–119). As the Chinese used to say: a picture is worth a thousand words.

DOCTORS IN DRAMAS AND NOVELS

Among progressive later 18th-century Hebrew and Yiddish-speaking European Jews, the *maskil* was a heroic figure. He was the man of science and medicine, icon of the Haskalah, the Jewish Enlightenment. He was rational and thus effective. As a healer, he sought to reform the older approaches to healing that were embedded in Jewish communities. He was secular and European and stood in contrast to rabbinical and traditional Jewish folk healers. His popularity as a figure was expressed in such comedies as Isaac Euchel's 1793 *Rabbi Henekh or What One Does with It* (Efron 2001, 66).

Tobias Smollett and the Royal Navy

In 1748, English novelist Tobias Smollett published *The Adventures of Roderick Random*. He had been trained as a surgeon in Glasgow and became a ship's surgeon on one of the ships that sailed British troops to Cartagena in the ill-fated 1740 invasion. Thousands died as yellow fever swept the soldiers and sailors, and commanding officers did little to save the expedition. Smollett constructed a portion of his novel around a second surgeon's mate who had to deal with the fruitless orders he was given and the utter chaos of the doomed effort. The picture of both naval and medical incompetence that cost the lives of so many shocked contemporary society (Smollet 2012). His description of his own first posting to the sick bay on *The Thunderer* reflects his horror and revulsion at conditions of the ill at sea:

> Here I saw about 50 miserable distempered wretches suspended [in hammocks] in rows, so huddled upon one another that not more than 14 inches of space was allotted for each with his bed and bedding; and deprived of the light of the day, as well as of fresh air; breathing nothing but a noisome atmosphere of the morbid steams exhaling from their own excrements and diseased bodies, devoured with vermin hatched in the filth that surrounded them.

In *Roderick*, the captain is an unreasonable disciplinarian who states that there should be no sick men on his ship and that all 60 of those on sick call were faking to avoid duty. The ship's doctor is no more than a toady who confirms in turn that each is indeed a fraud. As all undergo discipline rather than rest and care, many of the 60 die of their medical conditions and the floggings. *Roderick* was fiction, but it revealed to the English reading public the dark underside of the famed naval service that was building and protecting the British Empire (quotations from Harper 1930).

Chinese Dramas

Theater was a rather new art form in China during the Ming period. Most playwrights were scholars who would have studied medicine to some extent and may have practiced as physicians. Revered historical or divine physicians sometimes appear as characters, and they are dressed in priests' robes and treated very respectfully. Various sorts of medical practitioners also appear in many period plays or operas. As a stock type, these figures were usually either "painted face characters" played as "humorous, proud and exaggerative" or as outright jesters in the guise of country hicks with very ugly faces. The characters' Chinese names often reflect their clown-like status: Dr. Sending People to Their Death-Bed or Dr. Stupid Worm. Often appearing in romantic comedies, they are called on to "heal a broken heart" or advance some scheme on the lovers' parts. They bumble through diagnoses and confuse medical terms, prescribe ridiculous treatments, or otherwise display a total lack of common sense. Some are quite open about their incompetence. In the play *Tan Kuei's Bracelet Box*, the title character's mother hires the doctor Si Chuan, who came from three generations of doctors and introduces himself as follows:

> I know well how to feel people's pulse and remember well the characteristics of medicine. How can I guess what disease that people get? Spells are my only prescriptions. I don't know what's cold or fever, leprosy or insane. To the consumptive [lung] cases, I give purgative drugs and to the digestive disturbances, I give cardiatonics [heart medicine]. I tell the adult he gets children's disease, and the gentleman

> that he gets woman's ailment. I make people cry and weep all around me. Yesterday I was compelled to attend a funeral service in which I offered my apology, and this morning I was beaten like hell for having made a wrong treatment. I am the messenger of the king of Hades as well as the assistant of the coffin shops. Several times I've decided to give up my job, but then I've nothing to make a living (Lee 1950, 36–37).

Not exactly confidence inspiring but then it is farce.

Often the plays have fun with cultural norms, such as the unwillingness of women to be examined by a male doctor and specific diagnostic techniques such as pulse taking. In the work *Lung Kao Chi*, a sick girl's father has his servants hire a doctor. The man of medicine mocks the practice of diagnosis: "Your excellency! What do the doctors know about pulse feeling in this day? A good doctor is a doctor who guesses right." He goes on to explain that he plans to experiment on the girl: "Sir, is there a doctor who does not treat his patient as an experimental object?" Finally, the father calls out: "Attendants, I have told you to get a good doctor, and why do you get a fellow like him? Get him out of here!" (Lee 1950, 38–39). Like the father, the playwright knows that there are both good and poor physicians. Chinese theatrical pieces did not take aim at the medical profession itself as much as mock and perhaps criticize the practitioners who had little to offer and yet were allowed to peddle their services.

Not all stage doctors were clowns, however. In tragic operas they could be anything from mischievous to evil, depending on the librettist's needs. Since doctors determined life and death for their patients, if gain were to be had from killing a patient, it took little motivation to tip the scale. Doctors knew drugs that healed and those that killed, and often the most helpless were in their care. Poisoned medicine was a favorite means. But doctors could also be heroic, though they were usually in stories of the gods of medicine or appeared in contemporary stories in the guise of good, knowledgeable physicians (Lee 1950, 34–48).

Molière's French Doctors

The great 16th-century French playwright known as Molière wrote his comedies for the royal court. His audiences were not common folk but the age's aristocracy, including King Louis XIV himself. Above all else, the playwright hated hypocrisy and mercilessly lampooned the false and self-righteous. He also had little use for physicians and featured them in several of his plays: *The Flying Doctor, Love Is the Doctor, The Doctor in Spite of Himself,* and *The Imaginary Invalid.*

The Doctor in Spite of Himself is Sganarelle the woodcutter (originally played by Molière himself) mistaken for a physician. Despite having neither knowledge nor skills, he decides to play the role to the hilt and adopts the costume, behaviors, and even vocabulary of a man of medicine. His cynical side comes out in lines such as "payment comes whether we kill or cure," and "dead men, of all people the most discreet, tell no tales of the doctor who has sent them to their long account." Sganarelle's fraudulence is that of many stock characters in European fiction, but like many others, Molière harbored and displayed a true disgust with the pretensions of the medical professionals. Where the Chinese playwright might recognize that there were honorable physicians, one senses that everyone in Molière's world was a Sganarelle.

In act 2 of *Love Is the Doctor*, no fewer than five physicians are called upon to cure the depressed female lead. The result is a cacophony of theories and recommendations meant by the playwright to undermine any faith that there is a science behind medicine. Though Dr. Filerin counsels getting along, it is only for the sake of not making the profession look bad, not to reassure or aid the patient. In the end, her lover, feigning to be a doctor, reveals her disease to be love sickness and himself to be the cure. *The Flying Doctor* has no wings but is in fact the lead's valet who jumps in and out of a window pretending to be both the physician and the physician's twin brother.

The *Imaginary Invalid* (1673) was Molière's final work and is a complicated farce in three acts. The title character was the hypochondriac Argan, whose daughter he hoped to marry off to the spindly son of his physician, Dr. Purgeon. The daughter, of course, loves another. The faithful and feisty maid, Toinette, pretends to be a second doctor who undermines Argan's faith in all doctors by prescribing that his eye and arm be removed since they are sucking up all his body's nutrients. After ridding himself of Purgeon and the son, Argan himself is made a physician in a ritual performed by the ethnic group called the Roma. Molière played Argan the hypochondriac during a performance of which he died of a very real hemorrhage brought on by his tuberculosis (Brockliss and Jones 1997, 336–344).

MEDICINE IN POETRY

In antiquity, poets were believed to possess special gifts from the gods, their creative spirits touched by the divine. By the early modern period that notion had faded, though poets continued to thrive through the relevance and beauty of their works. Printing was revivified in China and introduced into Europe, stimulating demand for new and popular works and supplying a relatively inexpensive way to fill demand. Matters medical, from printed acupuncture charts to treatises on childhood diseases to multivolume studies of tropical medicinal plants, enjoyed a steady demand. Poetic literature offered everything medical from nutritional advice to deep social criticism clothed in biological terms.

Syphilus

Girolamo Fracastoro was an early-16th-century Italian physician and poet. He was born in Verona and trained in medicine at Padua. He is noted as a scientist for his study *On Contagion* (1546), a pioneering work on infectious diseases that imagined them as caused by tiny seeds. In 1530, Fracastoro published his Latin poem *Syphilus, or Three Books on the French Disease*. He had begun the work 20 years earlier during a retreat to the countryside during a plague epidemic. The ravages of the new venereal scourge were at the center of the medical world's attention. Poetic treatment of diseases and other medical problems was neither new nor rare. Book 1 follows the standard model in describing the symptoms of the French disease (or Neapolitan if you were French). In book 2, Fracastoro poetically lays out the current treatments, concentrating on the use of mercury, both poison and healing agent. Book 3 is the popularization of the newly discovered South American natural remedy called guaiacum. He wraps this in a fable about a South American shepherd boy named Syphilus. One day the youngster inadvertently cursed the sun, and the sun god responded by inflicting the lad with a horrible disease. After repenting for his blasphemy, Syphilus discovered the remedy guaiacum and was cured in body and spirit. The poem presents a medical message promoting guaiacum wrapped in a typical Renaissance pastoral form, with a deeper message of the connections between immorality and disease, and repentance and cure (Fracastoro 2007; Arrizabalaga, Henderson, and French 1997, 245–251).

Medical Illness and Societal Illness

As the Chinese Ming dynasty came to an end in its failing struggle with the Manchu in 1637, poet Zhang Dai compared the Ming defeat to an epidemic:

> Dead soldiers, dead bandits, death spread everywhere.
> The defeat of Liaodong is like a piece of rotting flesh.
> The poison spread by hostile spears more powerful than the plague (Spence 2007, 187–188).

Poets in Europe as well as China saw their societies as metaphorical human bodies writ large. Like the body, society could be healthy or unhealthy, harming itself or under attack by external forces. It was an old theme that found favor in early modern times. The sick society needed to be strengthened and healed, lest it died. But who was the doctor? And what was the proper treatment?

During epidemics, the trope of the sick society became most evident. When plague struck, literally the entire population was affected. Like a plague, political corruption and incompetence, immorality, poverty and shiftlessness, toleration of the wrong religion, and a host of other ills undermined the health of societies. Poet-critics such as Englishman Thomas Dekker called out for change. In Dekker's eyes, the plague was God's way of punishing the many sins of human—and especially London—society. When Queen Elizabeth died and James I came to the throne (1603), the plague raged in London. Dekker claimed that God was punishing England for glorifying Elizabeth and called on the new ruler (personified as the healing god Apollo) to make England well again. The idea that illness is a divine punishment for immoral behavior was quite ancient, but writers like Dekker used the moralizing in a particularly effective way: repent and stop sinning, or we will all be punished with plague again and again. The sins Dekker denounced were not individual failings as much as social ones: the harming of the poor and disadvantaged; the flight of political leaders, doctors, priests, and the rich from London during epidemics; shutting the plague-stricken poor in their houses; and placing faith in medicine rather than God (Healy 2002). In the mid-17th century, Thomas Hobbes also wrote of the sick English political body of his day. For him, the disease was the antiroyalist radicalism of many members of Parliament and those who supported them; the cure was the surrender to royal absolutism.

In 18th-century France, the sickness poets tried to cure was the absolutist royal court with all of its indolence, corruption, wars, and lack of concern for the people. The aristocrats that populated it were "tapeworms" who sucked the life from the rest of the body politic. Revolution would serve as a purgative, ridding the social body of the worm and return the body to health. In another metaphor, the king himself was the gangrenous limb infecting the rest of the body. Execution of the king was merely amputation of the infected limb. Critics of Caribbean slavery varied the theme: slavery was a sickness that infected the island societies. Every act of violence against the workers was a wound. Abolition was the cure, and the physician was either the mother countries' leaders or the islands' own revolutionaries (see Weaver 2006).

Medical Poetry among the Safavids

From its Near Eastern roots, Islam developed two particularly indigenous art forms, calligraphy and poetry. In the Safavid Empire, poised between the Mughals to the east in India and the Ottoman Turks to the West, there continued a form of "common person's medical guide," or what we might call a medical self-help literature. This is interesting more for its form than its content, as it was composed in verse not prose. The huge infusion of Greek prose scientific literature during the Middle Ages, and its translation into Arabic, set the tone for Islamic medical writing throughout our period. When writing for the commoner, however, some physicians utilized easily memorized poetry to convey fundamentals of health and healing when a physician or surgeon was not at hand. Best known was *The Poem on Medicine* by the 11th-century Persian philosopher and physician Avicenna (Ibn Sina). The qasida is a poem of undetermined length that maintains a consistent rhyme pattern, and a ruba'i consists of four lines, the first, second, and fourth of which rhyme. A rubaiyat is a set of many four-line poems that are related.

The best and most prolific of these medical poets was Yusuf of Herat, a physician and son of a physician, writing in the 16th century. He wrote only in Persian verse and usually on medical subjects. Perhaps his earliest work in qasida is a 128-line poem on drugs ("Selected Benefits") penned in 1507. By 1530, he had entered the service of the first Mughal emperor in India, for whom he wrote his qasida "Elegy on the Protection of Health." Two short works of qasida, "Evidence from the Urine" and "Evidence from the Pulse," appeared in 1535. His most famous rubaiyat were "The Medicine of Yusuf" and "Collection of Benefits," the latter of which remained a popular guide down to the 20th century. Advice for good health includes the lines,

> To keep your brain clear each day eat some meat,
> But avoid all foods which increase body heat.
> Stay not awake in the hours of the night
> And to sleep much by day is also not mete.

His advice for the corpulent rings true today:

If you are obese, I mean covered with fat,
I will tell you a cure that will remedy that.
Avoid foods that give pleasure, shun comfort and sloth,
And you'll soon have a shape that you like to look at.

On the other hand, we do have better remedies for venereal diseases today:

Oh you who suffer from Foreigners' Pox,
This treatment, I am sure, health's door soon unlocks.
First an ointment of mercury wisely prepare,
For daily applied paths of spreading it blocks (Elgood 1979, 106–115).

Shorter poetic medical fragments appear in other Safavid works across the period. In the 18th century, there was a revival among Arab speakers of poetic works that discuss the same themes of self-help, diet, and herbal remedies (Pormann and Savage-Smith 2007, 68, 171). Though embedded in a centuries-old tradition, these may have been influenced by 17th-century popular medical literature in English and other vernaculars, though these were rarely versified.

Laudanum and Romanticism

In the 1960s, American Dr. Timothy Leary personally experimented with and advocated the recreational use of LSD. It was a drug that supposedly "expanded the mind" and increased the vision and creativity of artists and musicians. The medicine laudanum played something of the same role among poets and writers of the later 18th century. Laudanum was a blend of opium derivative and strong alcohol. Medically used to curb pain, it was addictive and when used in moderation induced a pleasant high that released one from inhibitions. Romanticism was a European cultural movement that abandoned the emphasis on rationality and intellect that shaped the Enlightenment and its Age of Reason. For the Romantic poet or painter, the natural world was not something to dominate and harness but to experience and to which one should succumb. An emphasis on subjective feelings replaced the search for objective knowledge among these artists. The pharmacy provided the drug that seemed to induce artificially the introspection and spontaneity of the poet; it was believed to loosen the bonds people had on their passions, releasing them to explore the world, intensify their feelings, and express themselves on the page.

The list of notable Romantic poets who experimented with or became addicted to laudanum is long and impressive. In France, it included the creative circle around Chateaubriand. Among German Romantics who used laudanum were Johann Wolfgang Goethe, Friedrich Schiller, and Friedrich Schlegel; and English poets included Samuel Taylor Coleridge, Sir Walter Scott, William Wordsworth, Percy Bysshe Shelley, John Keats, and Lord Byron. For his part, Coleridge had suffered several diseases when young, was given laudanum, and early on became addicted to opiates. Shelley on the other hand took the drug as a means of calming his nerves. He became dependent and was rarely without a bottle. He admitted the negative side effects of using laudanum, including uncontrollable muscle spasms, memory lapses, and bizarre dreams. Knowing it to be a poison, he came close to killing himself with the drug that supposedly enhanced poetic genius (Dormandy 2012, 76–84; Dormandy 2006, 134–136).

GLOSSARY

alembic
A setup for distilling liquids.

amulet
An object worn by a person that is believed to protect him or her from harm.

aseptic
Free of disease-causing germs.

asymptomatic
Not displaying symptoms.

cachexy
General physical weakness caused by malnutrition.

chrysome
Cloth in which a newborn is wrapped.

clyster
Enema.

cupping
Western medical technique of heating a cup whose mouth was pressed against the skin creating suction and supposedly drawing out illness-causing substances in the body.

decoct
To extract by boiling.

emetic
Substance that induces vomiting.

endemic
Disease or condition that is continually present among a population.

enteric
Related to the intestines.

feral
Usually of an animal: undomesticated or wild.

guild
European civic organization of masters in a single occupation or profession; included physicians, surgeons, and apothecaries.

invasive
A medical procedure that affects internal organs or structures by breaking through the skin or entering through an orifice.

jinn
In Islam a spirit, often troublesome or malevolent.

lithotomy
Surgical procedure to remove kidney, gall bladder, or bladder stones.

lochia
Postpartum vaginal discharge of blood, mucus, and placental material.

miasma
Poisoned air that causes disease.

motile
Able to move by its own power.

Nahuatl
The language of the Aztecs.

natalism
Set of attitudes or policies that promote high rates of birth in a population.

opiate
Derivative of opium poppies.

panacea
Substance that is claimed to cure all ills.

pandemic
Outbreak of a disease across a large geographic area and for a long time.

pathogen
Disease-causing agent.

phlebotomy (also bloodletting, bleeding)
Medical procedure that opens a blood vessel to release what a practitioner considered excess blood.

podagra
Gout or inflammation of the big toe.

poultice
A soft mixture of ingredients smeared on the body to induce healing.

purgative
Substance that causes the body to evacuate or purge a particular substance; laxative is an example.

sepsis
Blood poisoning.

souk
Middle Eastern market.

sudorific
Drug that induces perspiration.

suppurate
To produce and discharge pus.

talisman
Object handled or worn to bring good luck, heal, or protect one from sickness or evil.

thoracic
Related to the human chest area.

BIBLIOGRAPHY

Aberth, John, ed. *The Black Death: The Great Mortality of 1348–1350: A Brief History with Documents.* Boston: Bedford/St. Martin's, 2005.

Alchon, Suzanne Austin. *A Pest in the Land: New World Epidemics in a Global Perspective.* Albuquerque: University of New Mexico Press, 2003.

Allen, Robert C., Tommy Bengtsson, and Martin Dribe, eds. *Living Standards in the Past: New Perspectives on Well-Being in Asia and Europe.* New York: Oxford University Press, 2005.

Anderson, Julie, Emm Barnes, and Emma Shackleton. *The Art of Medicine: Over 2000 Years of Images and Imagination.* Chicago: University of Chicago Press, 2011.

Anderson, Stuart. *Making Medicines: A Brief History of Pharmacy and Pharmaceuticals.* London: Pharmaceutical Press, 2005.

Andrews, Jonathan, and Andrew Scull. *Customers and Patrons of the Mad-Trade: The Management of Lunacy in Eighteenth-Century London, with the Complete Text of John Monro's 1766 Case Book.* Berkeley: University of California Press, 2002.

Andrews, Jonathan, and Andrew Scull. *Undertaker of the Mind: John Monro and Mad-Doctoring in Eighteenth-Century England.* Berkeley: University of California Press, 2001.

Arnold, Catharine. *Bedlam: London and Its Mad.* New York: Pocket Books, 2008.

Arnold, David. *Warm Climates and Western Medicine: The Emergence of Tropical Medicine, 1500–1900.* Atlanta, GA: Rodopi, 1996.

Arrizabalaga, Jon, John Henderson, and Roger French, eds. *The Great Pox: The French Disease in Renaissance Europe.* New Haven, CT: Yale University Press, 1997.

Ballard, Martha. *A Midwife's Tale: The Life of Martha Ballard Based on Her Diary, 1785–1812.* Edited by Laurel Ulrich. New York: Knopf, 1990.

Barnes, Linda L. *Needles, Herbs, Gods, and Ghosts: China, Healing, and the West to 1848.* Cambridge, MA: Harvard University Press, 2005.

Bell, Rudolph. *How to Do It: Guides to Good Living for Renaissance Italians.* Chicago: University of Chicago Press, 1999.

Bengtsson, Tommy, Cameron Campbell, and James Lee, eds. *Life under Pressure: Mortality and Living Standards in Europe and Asia, 1700–1900.* Cambridge, MA: MIT Press, 2004.

Berinstain, Valerie. *India and the Mughal Dynasty.* Translated by Paul G. Bahn. New York: Abrams, 2001.

Bollet, Alfred Jay. *Plagues and Poxes: The Impact of Human History on Epidemic Disease.* New York: Demos, 2004.

Borsch, Stuart J. *The Black Death in Egypt and England: A Comparative Study.* Austin: University of Texas Press, 2005.

Brandon, David. *Life in a 17th Century Coffee Shop.* Stroud, UK: Sutton, 2007.

Brentjes, Sonja. *Travelers from Europe in the Ottoman and Safavid Empires, 16th–17th Centuries: Seeking, Transforming, Discarding Knowledge.* Aldershot, UK: Ashgate, 2010.

Brockliss, Laurence, and Colin Jones. *The Medical World of Early Modern France.* New York: Oxford University Press, 1997.

Brockliss, Laurence, and Heather Montgomery, eds. *Childhood and Violence in the Western Tradition.* Woodbridge, CT: Oxbow Books, 2010.

Broman, Thomas H. *The Transformation of German Academic Medicine, 1750–1820.* New York: Cambridge University Press, 1996.

Brook, Timothy. *Vermeer's Hat: The Seventeenth Century and the Dawn of the Global World.* London: Bloomsbury Press, 2008.

Broomhall, Susan. *Women's Medical Work in Early Modern France*. New York: Manchester University Press, 2004.

Bruijn, Iris. *Ship's Surgeons of the Dutch East India Company: Commerce and the Progress of Medicine in the Eighteenth Century*. Leiden, Netherlands: Leiden University Press, 2009.

Burke, Michael E. *The Royal College of San Carlos: Surgery and Spanish Medical Reform in the Late Eighteenth Century*. Durham, NC: Duke University Press, 1977.

Burton, Robert. *Some Anatomies of Melancholy* (1621). New York: Penguin Books, 2008.

Byrne, Joseph P. *Daily Life during the Black Death*. Westport, CT: Greenwood Press, 2006.

Byrne, Joseph P., ed. *Encyclopedia of Pestilence, Pandemics, and Plagues*. Westport, CT: Greenwood Press, 2008.

Carlin, Claire L. *Imagining Contagion in Early Modern Europe*. New York: Palgrave, 2005.

Carrell, Jennifer Lee. *The Speckled Monster: A Historical Tale of Battling Smallpox*. New York: Dutton, 2003.

Chakravarti, Paromita. "Natural Fools and the Historiography of Renaissance Folly." *Renaissance Studies* 25 (2011): 208–227.

Charlton, A. "Medical Uses of Tobacco in History." *Journal of the Royal Society of Medicine* 97 (2004): 292–296.

Chipman, Leigh. *The World of Pharmacy and Pharmacists in Mamluk Cairo*. Boston: Brill, 2010.

Cipolla, Carlo. *Faith, Reason, and the Plague in Seventeenth-Century Tuscany*. New York: Norton, 1981.

Coe, Sophie D., and Michael D. Coe. *The True History of Chocolate*. New York: Thames and Hudson, 1996.

Cook, Alexandra Parma, and Noble David Cook. *The Plague Files: Crisis Management in Sixteenth-Century Seville*. Baton Rouge: University of Louisiana Press, 2009.

Cook, Harold J. *Matters of Exchange: Commerce, Medicine, and Science in the Dutch Golden Age*. New Haven, CT: Yale University Press, 2007.

Cook, Noble David. *Born to Die: Disease and New World Conquest, 1492–1650*. New York: Cambridge University Press, 1998.

Cook, Noble David, and W. George Lovell, eds. *"Secret Judgments of God": Old World Disease in Colonial Spanish America*. Norman: University of Oklahoma Press, 1992.

Cooper, Donald B. *Epidemic Disease in Mexico City, 1761–1813*. Austin: University of Texas Press, 1965.

Crimmin, Patricia. "British Naval Health, 1700–1800: Improvement over Time?" In *British Military British Military and Naval Medicine, 1600–1830*, edited by Geoffrey L. Hudson, 183–200. New York: Rodopi, 2007.

Crosby, Alfred W. *The Columbian Exchange: Biological Consequences of 1492*. Westport, CT: Greenwood Press, 1972.

Crosby, Alfred W. *Ecological Imperialism: The Biological Expansion of Europe, 900–1900*. New York: Cambridge University Press, 1986.

Cunningham, Andrew, and Ole Peter Grell. *The Four Horsemen of the Apocalypse: Religion, War, Famine and Death in Reformation Europe*. New York: Cambridge University Press, 2000.

Dean, Carolyn. "Sketches of Childhood." In *Minor Omissions: Children in Latin American History and Society*, edited by Tobias Hecht, 21–51. Madison: University of Wisconsin Press, 2002.

Dikötter, Frank, Lars Laamann, and Zhou Xun. *Narcotic Culture: A History of Drugs in China*. Chicago: University of Chicago Press, 2004.

DiMarco, Vincent. *It Has Helped to Admiration: Eighteenth-Century Medical Cures from the Kitchen Book of Bridget Lane, 1737.* New York: iUniverse, 2010.
Dols, Michael W. *The Black Death in the Middle East.* Princeton, NJ: Princeton University Press, 1977.
Dols, Michael W. *Majnun: The Madman in Medieval Islamic Society.* Oxford: Clarendon Press, 1992.
Dormandy, Thomas. *Opium: Reality's Dark Dream.* New Haven, CT: Yale University Press, 2012.
Dormandy, Thomas. *The Worst of Evils: The Fight against Pain.* New Haven, CT: Yale University Press, 2006.
Duffin, Jacalyn. *Medical Miracles: Doctors, Saints and Healing in the Modern World.* New York: Cambridge University Press, 2009.
Dunlap, Barbara. "The Problems of Syphilitic Children in Eighteenth-Century France and England." In *The Secret Malady: Venereal Disease in Eighteenth-Century Britain and France*, edited by Linda Evi Meriens, 114–127. Lexington: University Press of Kentucky, 1997.
Eckman, Peter. *In the Footsteps of the Yellow Emperor: Tracing the History of Traditional Acupuncture.* San Francisco: Long River Press, 2007.
Efron, John M. *Medicine and the German Jews: A History.* New Haven, CT: Yale University Press, 2001.
Elgood, Cyril. *Safavid Medical Practice: The Practice of Medicine, Surgery, and Gynecology in Persia between 1500 and 1750.* London: Luzac, 1970.
Ellis, Harold. *The Cambridge Illustrated History of Surgery.* New York: Cambridge University Press, 2009.
Ellis, Markman. *The Coffee House: A Cultural History.* London: Orion, 2005.
Equiano, Olaudah. *The Life of Olaudah Equiano.* Mineola: Dover Books, 1995.
Evenden, Doreen. *The Midwives of Seventeenth-Century London.* New York: Cambridge University Press, 2006.
Fabbri, Christiane Nockels. "Treating Medieval Plague: The Wonderful Virtues of Theriac." *Early Science and Medicine* 12 (2007): 247–283.
Ficino, Marsilio. *Three Books on Life.* Translated by Carol Kaske and John Clark. Tempe, AZ: Medieval and Renaissance Texts and Studies, 1998.
Fields, Sherry. *Pestilence and Headcolds: Encountering Illness in Colonial Mexico.* New York: Columbia University Press, 2008.
Finucci, Valeria. "'There's the Rub': Searching for Sexual Remedies in the New World." *Journal of Medieval and Early Modern Studies* 38 (2008): 523–557.
Finzsch, Norbert, and Robert Jütte, eds. *Institutions of Confinement: Hospitals, Asylums, and Prisons in Western Europe and North America: 1500–1950.* New York: Cambridge University Press, 1996.
Fissell, Mary E. *Vernacular Bodies: The Politics of Reproduction in Early Modern England.* New York: Oxford University Press, 2004.
Foucault, Michel. *Discipline and Punish: The Birth of the Prison.* Translated by Alan Sheridan. New York: Pantheon, 1977.
Foucault, Michel. *Madness and Civilization: A History of Insanity during the Age of Reason.* Translated by Richard Howard. New York: Pantheon, 1965.
Fracastoro, Girolamo. *The Sinister Shepherd: A Translation of Girolamo Fracastoro's Syphilidis sive de morbo libri tres.* Translated by William van Wyck. Whitefish, MT: Kessinger, 2007.
Franco, G., F. Franco, and L. Paita. "Focusing Bernardino Ramazzini's Preventive View in Health Protection." In *Contributions to the History of Occupational and Environmental Prevention*, edited by Antonio Grieco, Sergio Iavicoli, and Giovanni Berlinguer, 31–41. New York: Elsevier, 1999.

Freedman, Paul. *Out of the East: Spices and the Medieval Imagination.* New Haven, CT: Yale University Press, 2008.

French, Roger. *Dissection and Vivisection in the European Renaissance.* Burlington, VT: Ashgate, 1999.

Friedenberg, Zachary B. *Surgery over the Centuries.* London: Janus, 2009.

Furst, Lillian R., ed. *Women Healers and Physicians: Climbing a Long Hill.* Lexington: University Press of Kentucky, 1997.

Furth, Charlotte. *A Flourishing Yin: Gender in China's Medical History, 960–1665.* Berkeley: University of California Press, 1999.

Gabriel, Richard A., and Karen Metz. *A History of Military Medicine.* Vol. 2, *From the Renaissance through Modern Times.* Westport, CT: Greenwood Press, 1992.

Gately, Iain. *Drink: A Cultural History of Alcohol.* New York: Gotham Books, 2009.

Gates, William. *An Aztec Herbal: The Classic Codex of 1552.* Mineola, NY: Dover, 1939/2000.

Gavitt, Philip. *Charity and Children in Renaissance Florence: The Ospedale degli Innocenti, 1410–1536.* Ann Arbor: University of Michigan Press, 1991.

Gavitt, Philip. *Gender, Honor, and Charity in Late Renaissance Florence.* New York: Cambridge University Press, 2011.

Gelfand, Toby. *Professionalizing Modern Medicine: Paris Surgeons and Medical Science and Institutions in the Eighteenth Century.* Westport, CT: Greenwood Press, 1980.

Gélis, Jacques. *History of Childbirth: Fertility, Pregnancy, and Birth in Early Modern Europe.* Translated by Rosemary Morris. Cambridge: Polity Press, 1991.

Gentilcore, David. *Medical Charlatanism in Early Modern Italy.* New York: Oxford University Press, 2006.

Gilman, Sander, and Zhou Xun. *Smoke: A Global History of Smoking.* London: Reaktion Books, 2004.

Glynn, Ian, and Jenifer Glynn. *The Life and Death of Smallpox.* New York: Cambridge University Press, 2004.

González, Ondina E. "Down and Out in Havana: Foundlings in Eighteenth-Century Cuba." In *Minor Omissions: Children in Latin American History and Society,* edited by Tobias Hecht, 102–113. Madison: University of Wisconsin Press, 2002.

González, Ondina E., and Bianca Premo, eds. *Raising an Empire: Children in Early Modern Iberia and Colonial Latin America.* Albuquerque: University of New Mexico Press, 2007.

Gorbach, Sherwood L., John G. Bartlett, and Neil R. Blacklow, eds. *Infectious Diseases.* Philadelphia: Lippincott, 2003.

Graves, Rolande. *Born to Procreate: Women and Childbirth in France from the Middle Ages to the Eighteenth Century.* New York: Peter Lang, 2001.

Green, Monica. *Making Women's Medicine Masculine: The Rise of Male Authority in Pre-modern Gynaecology.* New York: Oxford University Press, 2008.

Grehan, James. "Smoking and 'Early Modern' Sociability: The Great Tobacco Debate in the Ottoman Middle East." *American Historical Review* 111 (2006): 152–177.

Grell, Ole Peter. *Paracelsus: The Man and His Reputation, His Ideas and Their Transformation.* Leiden, Netherlands: Brill, 1998.

Grell, Ole Peter. "War, Medicine and the Military Revolution." In *The Healing Arts: Health, Disease, and Society in Europe, 1500–1800,* 257–283. Manchester, UK: Open University Press, 2004.

Griffin, J. P. "Venetian Treacle and the Foundation of Medicines Regulation." *British Journal of Clinical Pharmacology* 58 (2004): 317–325.

Gruber von Arni, Eric. *Hospital Care and the British Standing Army, 1660–1714.* Burlington, VT: Ashgate, 2006.

Hanson, Marta. *Speaking of Epidemics in Chinese Medicine: Disease and the Geographic Imagination in Late Imperial China.* New York: Routledge, 2011.

Hargreaves, A. S. "Toothdrawers in English Popular Literature." *Bulletin of the History of Dentistry* 41 (1993): 51–57.

Hargreaves, A. S. *White as Whales Bone: Dental Services in Early Modern England.* Leeds, UK: Northern Universities Press, 1998.

Harper, Paul. "Tobias Smollett and the Practice of Medicine." *Yale Journal of Biology and Medicine* 2 (1930): 409–416.

Harrison, Mark. "Disease and Medicine in the Armies of British India, 1750–1830." In *British Military and Naval Medicine, 1600–1830*, edited by Geoffrey L. Hudson, 87–120. New York: Rodopi, 2007.

Harrison, Mark. *Disease and the Modern World: 1500 to the Present.* Malden, MA: Polity Press, 2004.

Harrison, Mark. *Medicine in an Age of Commerce and Empire: Britain and Its Tropical Colonies, 1660–1830.* New York: Oxford University Press, 2010.

Harvie, David I. *Limeys: The Conquest of Scurvy.* Stroud, UK: Sutton, 2002.

Hayden, Deborah. *Pox: Genius, Madness, and the Mysteries of Syphilis.* New York: Basic Books, 2004.

Haydock, David Boyd, and Patrick Wallis. *Quackery and Commerce in Seventeenth-Century London: The Proprietary Medicine Business of Anthony Daffy.* London: Wellcome Trust, 2005.

Healy, Margaret. *Fictions of Disease in Early Modern England: Bodies, Plagues and Politics.* New York: Palgrave, 2002.

Hecht, Tobias. *Minor Omissions: Children in Latin American History and Society.* Madison: University of Wisconsin Press, 2002.

Heinrichs, Erik Anton. "The Plague Cures of Caspar Kegler: Print, Alchemy, and Medical Marketing in Sixteenth-Century Germany." *Sixteenth Century Journal* 43 (2012): 417–440.

Hopkins, Donald R. *The Greatest Killer: Smallpox in History.* Chicago: University of Chicago, 2002.

Hudson, Geoffrey. "Disabled Veterans and the State in Early Modern England." In *Disabled Veterans in History*, edited by D. A. Gerber, 117–144. Ann Arbor: University of Michigan Press, 2000.

Hudson, Geoffrey. "Internal Influences in the Making of the English Military Hospital: The Early-Eighteenth-Century Greenwich." In *British Military and Naval Medicine, 1600–1830,* edited by Geoffrey L. Hudson, 253–272. New York: Rodopi, 2007.

Hunter, Paul. *Waterborne Disease: Epidemiology and Ecology.* New York: Wiley, 1997.

Issac, Peter. "Pills and Print." In *Medicine, Morality and the Book Trade*, edited by Robin Myers and Michael Harris, 25–48. New Castle, DE: Oak Knoll Press, 1998.

Jannetta, Ann Bowman. *Epidemics and Mortality in Early Modern Japan.* Princeton, NJ: Princeton University Press, 1987.

Jenner, Edward. *Vaccination against Smallpox.* Amherst, MA: Prometheus, 1996.

Jones, Colin. "The Construction of the Hospital Patient in Early Modern France." In *Institutions of Confinement: Hospitals, Asylums, and Prisons in Western Europe and North America*, edited by Norbert Finzsch and Robert Jütte, 55–74. New York: Cambridge University Press, 1996.

Jones, Colin. "Pulling Teeth in Eighteenth-Century Paris." *Past and Present* 166 (2000): 100–145.

Jones, Susan D. *Death in a Small Package: A Short History of Anthrax.* Baltimore: Johns Hopkins University Press, 2010.

Jütte, Robert. "Syphilis and Confinement: Hospitals in Early Modern Germany." In *Institutions of Confinement: Hospitals, Asylums, and Prisons in Western Europe and North America*, edited by Norbert Finzsch and Robert Jütte, 97–115. New York: Cambridge University Press, 1996.
Kidwell, Clara Sue. "Aztec and European Medicine in the New World, 1521–1600." In *The Anthropology of Medicine: From Culture to Method*, edited by Lola Romanacci-Ross, Daniel E. Moerman, and Laurence R. Tancredi, 19–30. Westport, CT: Bergin and Garvey, 1997.
Kilpatrick, Robert. "'Living in the Light': Dispensaries, Philanthropy, and Medical Reform in Late Eighteenth-Century London." In *The Medical Enlightenment of the Eighteenth Century*, edited by Andrew Cunningham and Roger French, 254–280. New York: Cambridge University Press, 1990.
King, Helen. *Midwifery, Obstetrics and the Rise of Gynaecology: The Uses of the Sixteenth-Century Compendium*. Burlington, VT: Ashgate, 2007.
King, Roger. *The Making of the "Dentiste," c. 1650–1760*. Aldershot, UK: Ashgate, 1998.
Kiple, Kenneth F., ed. *Cambridge Historical Dictionary of Disease*. New York: Cambridge University Press, 2003.
Kiple, Kenneth F., and Stephen Beck. *Biological Consequences of the European Expansion, 1450–1800*. Aldershot, UK: Ashgate, 1997.
Klairmont-Lingo, A. "Women Healers and the Medical Marketplace of Sixteenth-Century Lyon." *Dynamis* 19 (1999): 79–94.
Knight, Katherine. *How Shakespeare Cleaned His Teeth and Cromwell Treated His Warts: Secrets of the Seventeenth-Century Medicine Cabinet*. Stroud, UK: Tempus, 2006.
Kusukawa, Sachiko. "The Medical Renaissance of the Sixteenth Century: Vesalius, Medical Humanism, and Bloodletting." In *The Healing Arts, 1500–1800*, edited by Peter Elmer, 58–83. Manchester, UK: Manchester University Press, 2004.
Laroche, Rebecca. *Medical Authority and Englishwomen's Herbal Texts, 1550–1650*. Burlington, VT: Ashgate, 2009.
Lawlor, Clark. *From Melancholia to Prozac: A History of Depression*. New York: Oxford University Press, 2012.
Laws, Bill. *Spade, Skirret, and Parsnip: The Curious History of Vegetables*. Stroud, UK: Sutton, 2004.
Lee, T'ao. "The Doctor in Chinese Drama." *Chinese Medical Journal* 68 (1950): 34–48.
Leiby, John S. "San Hipólito's Treatment of the Mentally Ill in Mexico City, 1589–1650." *The Historian* 54 (1992): 491–498.
Leti, Geneviève. *Santé et société esclavagiste à la Martinique*. Paris: Editions L'Harmattan, 1998.
Leung, Angela Ki Che. *Leprosy in China: A History*. New York: Columbia University Press, 2009.
Lindemann, Mary. *Medicine and Society in Early Modern Europe*. New York: Cambridge University Press, 1996.
Lipsett-Rivera, Sonya. "Model Children and Models for Children in Early Mexico." In *Minor Omissions: Children in Latin American History and Society*, edited by Tobias Hecht, 52–71. Madison: University of Wisconsin Press, 2002.
Li Shih-Chen. *Chinese Medical Herbs: A Modern Edition of a Classic Sixteenth-Century Manual*. Mineola, NY: Dover, 1973.
Liu, Xinru. *The Silk Road in World History*. New York: Oxford University Press, 2010.
Loudon, Irvine, ed. *Western Medicine: An Illustrated History*. New York: Oxford University Press, 1997.
Maehle, Andreas-Holger. *Drugs on Trial: Experimental Pharmacology and Therapeutic Innovation in the Eighteenth Century*. Atlanta, GA: Rodopi, 1999.

Mantovani, A., et al. "A historical Overview of Occupational Diseases Connected with Animals." In *Contributions to the History of Occupational and Environmental Prevention*, edited by Antonio Grieco, Sergio Iavicoli, and Giovanni Berlinguer, 239–246. New York: Elsevier, 1999.

Marland, Hilary, ed. *The Art of Midwifery: Early Modern Midwives in Europe*. New York: Routledge, 1993.

Marland, Hilary, and Margaret Pelling. *The Task of Healing: Medicine, Religion, and Gender in England and the Netherlands, 1450–1800*. Rotterdam: Erasmus, 1996.

Martensen, R. L. *The Brain Takes Shape: An Early History*. New York: Oxford University Press, 2004.

Martin, A. Lynn. *Alcohol, Violence, and Disorder in Traditional Europe*. Kirksville, MO: Truman State University Press, 2009.

Matossian, Mary K. *Poisons of the Past: Molds, Epidemics, and History*. New Haven, CT: Yale University Press, 1989.

Matthee, Rudi. *The Pursuit of Pleasure: Drugs and Stimulants in Iranian History, 1500–1900*. Princeton, NJ: Princeton University Press, 2005.

McCaa, Robert. "Spanish and Nahuatl Views on Smallpox and Demographic Catastrophe in Mexico." *Journal of Interdisciplinary History* 25 (1995): 397–431.

McClure, Margaret. *Coram's Children: The London Foundling Hospital in the Eighteenth Century*. New Haven, CT: Yale University Press, 1981.

McNeill, J. R. *Mosquito Empires: Ecology and War in the Greater Caribbean, 1620–1914*. New York: Cambridge University Press, 2010.

Meriens, Linda Evi. *The Secret Malady: Venereal Disease in Eighteenth-Century Britain and France*. Lexington: University Press of Kentucky, 1997.

Monahan, W. Gregory. *Year of Sorrows: The Great Famine of 1709 in Lyon*. Columbus: Ohio State University Press, 1993.

Moran, Bruce T. *Distilling Knowledge: Alchemy, Chemistry, and the Scientific Revolution*. Cambridge, MA: Harvard University Press, 2005.

Morens, David. "Characterizing a 'New' Disease: Epizootic and Epidemic Anthrax, 1769–1780." *Journal of Public Health* 93 (2003): 886–893.

Murphey, Rhoades. *Ottoman Warfare, 1500–1700*. New Brunswick, NJ: Rutgers University Press, 1999.

Nappi, Carla. *The Monkey and the Inkpot: Natural History and Its Transformation in Early Modern China*. Cambridge, MA: Harvard University Press, 2009.

Needham, Joseph. *Science and Civilisation in China*. Vol. 6, *Biology and Biological Technology*, Part 6, *Medicine*. Edited by Nathan Sivin. New York: Cambridge University Press, 2000.

Newson, Linda. *Conquest and Pestilence in the Early Spanish Philippines*. Honolulu: University of Hawaii Press, 2009.

Ng, Vivian W. *Madness in Late Imperial China: From Illness to Deviance*. Norman: University of Oklahoma Press, 1990.

Numbers, Ronald, ed. *Medicine in the New World: New Spain, New France, and New England*. Knoxville: University of Tennessee Press, 1987.

Nutton, Vivian. "The Fortunes of Galen." In *The Cambridge Companion to Galen*, edited by R. J. Hankinson, 355–390. New York: Cambridge University Press, 2008.

Ortiz de Montellano, Bernard R. *Aztec Medicine, Health, and Nutrition*. New Brunswick, NJ: Rutgers University Press, 1990.

Osterfeld, Richard S., Felicia Keesing, and Valerie T. Eviner, eds. *Infectious Disease Ecology*. Princeton, NJ: Princeton University Press, 2008.

Osterhammel, Jürgen, and Niels Petersson. *Globalization: A Short History*. Princeton, NJ: Princeton University Press, 2005.

Packard, Randall M. *The Making of a Tropical Disease: A Short History of Malaria*. Baltimore: Johns Hopkins University Press, 2007.

Paice, Edward. *Wrath of God: The Great Lisbon Earthquake of 1755*. Waltham, MA: Quercus, 2010.

Palmer, Richard. "Pharmacy in the Republic of Venice in the Sixteenth Century." In *The Medical Renaissance of the Sixteenth Century*, edited by Andrew Wear, R. K. French, and I. M. Lonie, 100–117. New York: Cambridge University Press, 1985.

Paré, Ambroise. *The Apologie and Treatise of Ambroise Paré Containing the Voyages Made into Divers Places with Many of His Writings upon Surgery*. Edited by G. Keynes. Mineola: Dover Books, 1968.

Parker, Geoffrey. *The Military Revolution: Military Innovation and the Rise of the West, 1500–1800*. New York: Cambridge University Press, 1989.

Patterson, K. David. *Pandemic Influenza, 1700–1900*. Totowa, NJ: Rowman and Littlefield, 1986.

Pelling, Margaret. *The Common Lot: Sickness, Medical Occupations and the Urban Poor in Early Modern England*. New York: Longman, 1998.

Perkins, Wendy. *Midwifery and Medicine in Early Modern France: Louise Bourgeois*. Exeter, UK: University of Exeter Press, 1996.

Peterson, Kaara L. *Popular Medicine, Hysterical Disease, and Social Controversy in Shakespeare's England*. Burlington, VT: Ashgate, 2010.

Phillips, Derek. *Well-Being in Amsterdam's Golden Age*. Amsterdam: Pallas, 2008.

Piekarski, C. "Some Aspects of Early Developments in Occupational Health Care in the German Mining Industry." In *Contributions to the History of Occupational and Environmental Prevention*, edited by Antonio Grieco, Sergio Iavicoli, and Giovanni Berlinguer, 187–193.New York: Elsevier, 1999.

Pierce, John R., and Jim Writer. *Yellow Jack*. Hoboken, NJ: Wiley, 2005.

Ping, Chen, ed. *History and Development of Traditional Medicine*. Beijing: Science Press, 1999.

Pollock, Linda. *With Faith and Physic: The Life of a Tudor Gentlewoman, Lady Grace Mildmay, 1552–1620*. London: Collins and Brown, 1993.

Pormann, Peter E., and Emilie Savage-Smith. *Medieval Islamic Medicine*. Washington, DC: Georgetown University Press, 2007.

Porter, Dorothy, ed. *The History of Public Health and the Modern State*. Amsterdam: Rodopi, 1996.

Porter, Roy, ed. *Cambridge History of Medicine*. New York: Cambridge University Press, 2006.

Porter, Roy. *Quacks: Fakers and Charlatans in Medicine*. Stroud, UK: Tempus, 2001.

Porter, Roy, and Mikulas Teich. *Drugs and Narcotics in History*. New York: Cambridge University Press, 1997.

Pretel, A., and M. Ruiz Bremón. "Social and Medical Protection for the Working Population in the Age of Philip II." In *Contributions to the History of Occupational and Environmental Prevention*, edited by Antonio Grieco, Sergio Iavicoli, and Giovanni Berlinguer, 159–170. New York: Elsevier, 1999.

Quinn, Tom. *Flu: A Social History of Influenza*. London: New Holland, 2008.

Radden, Jennifer, ed. *The Nature of Melancholy: From Aristotle to Kristeva*. New York: Oxford University Press, 2000.

Ramazzini, Bernardino. *The Diseases of Workers*. Translated by Wilmer C. Wright. Chicago: University of Chicago Press, 1940.

Ransford, Oliver. *Bid the Sickness Cease: Disease in the History of Black Africa*. London: John Murray, 1983.

Rawcliffe, Carole. *Leprosy in Medieval England.* Rochester, NY: Boydell, 2006.

Read, Kirk D. *Birthing Bodies in Early Modern France.* Burlington, VT: Ashgate, 2011.

Riddle, John. *Dioscorides on Pharmacy and Medicine.* Austin: University of Texas Press, 1985.

Riddle, John. *Eve's Herbs: A History of Contraception and Abortion in the West.* Cambridge, MA: Harvard University Press, 1997.

Rifkin, Benjamin A., Michael J. Ackerman, and Judith Folkenberg, eds. *Human Anatomy: A Visual History from the Renaissance to the Digital Age.* New York: Abrams, 2006.

Risse, Gunter B. "Before the Clinic Was 'Born': Methodological Perspectives in Hospital History." In *Institutions of Confinement: Hospitals, Asylums, and Prisons in Western Europe and North America,* edited by Norbert Finzsch and Robert Jütte, 75–96. New York: Cambridge University Press, 1996.

Rocco, Fiammetta. *Quinine, Malaria and the Quest for a Cure That Changed the World.* New York: HarperCollins, 2003.

Ruff, Julius R. *Violence in Early Modern Europe, 1500–1800.* New York: Cambridge University Press, 2001.

Saif, Liana. "The Arabic Theory of Astral Influence in Early Modern Medicine." *Renaissance Studies* 25 (2011): 609–626.

Sawday, Jonathan. *The Body Emblazoned: Dissection and the Human Body in Renaissance Culture.* New York: Routledge, 1996.

Scheid, Volker. *Currents of Tradition in Chinese Medicine, 1626–2006.* Seattle, WA: Eastland Press, 2007.

Schendel, Gordon. *Medicine in Mexico: From Aztec Herbs to Betatrons.* Austin: University of Texas Press, 1968.

Schiebinger, Londa. *Plants and Empire: Colonial Bioprospecting in the Atlantic World.* Cambridge, MA: Harvard University Press, 2004.

Schiebinger, Londa, and Claudia Swan, eds. *Colonial Botany: Science, Commerce, and Politics in the Early Modern World.* Philadelphia: University of Pennsylvania Press, 2005.

Schmidt, Jeremy. *Melancholy and the Care of the Soul: Religion, Moral Philosophy and Madness in Early Modern England.* Burlington, VT: Ashgate, 2007.

Schrader, Catharina. *"Mother and Child Were Saved": The Memoirs (1693–1740) of the Frisian Midwife Catharina Schrader.* Translated by Hilary Marland. Amsterdam: Rodopi, 1987.

Scull, Andrew. *The Disturbing History of Hysteria.* New York: Oxford University Press, 2009.

Shah, Saria. *The Fever: How Malaria Has Ruled Mankind for 500,000 Years.* New York: Farrar, Straus, Giroux, 2010.

Shahar, Shulamith. *Childhood in the Middle Ages.* New York: Routledge, 1992.

Sharp, Jane. *The Midwives' Book: Or The Whole Art of Midwifery Discovered* (1621). New York: Garland, 1985.

Shearing, Colin R. *Opium: A Journey through Time.* London: Mercury Books, 2004.

Shefer-Mossensohn, Miri. *Ottoman Medicine: Healing and Medical Institutions, 1500–1700.* Albany: State University of New York Press, 2009.

Sheridan, Richard. *Doctors and Slaves: A Medical and Demographic History of Slavery in the British West Indies, 1680–1834.* New York: Cambridge University Press, 1985.

Sherman, Irwin W. *The Power of Plague.* Washington, DC: American Society for Microbiology, 2006.

Shorter, Edward. *A History of Psychiatry: From the Era of the Asylum*. New York: Wiley, 1998.

Shoshan, Boaz. "The State and Madness in Medieval Islam." *International Journal of Middle East Studies* 35 (2003): 329–340.

Shrady, Nicholas. *The Last Day: Wrath, Ruin, and Reason in the Great Lisbon Earthquake of 1755*. New York: Viking, 2008.

Slack, Paul. "Responses to Plague in Early Modern Europe: The Implications of Public Health." *Social Research* 55 (1988): 433–453.

Smith, Leonard. *Lunatic Hospitals in Georgian England, 1750–1830*. London: Routledge, 2007.

Smith, Virginia. *Clean: A History of Personal Hygiene and Purity*. New York: Palgrave Macmillan, 2007.

Smollett, Tobias. *The Adventures of Roderick Random*. Athens: University of Georgia Press, 2012.

Soustelle, Jacques. *Daily Life of the Aztecs*. London: Phoenix Press, 1961/2002.

Spence, Jonathan D. *Return to Dragon Mountain: Memories of a Late Ming Man*. New York: Viking, 2007.

Stannard, Jerry. *Herbs and Herbalism in the Middle Ages and Renaissance*. Edited by Richard Kay and Katherine E. Stannard. Burlington, VT: Ashgate Variorum, 1999.

Stearns, Justin. *Infectious Ideas: Contagion in Premodern Islamic and Christian Thought in the Western Mediterranean*. Baltimore: Johns Hopkins University Press, 2011.

Stein, Claudia. *Negotiating the French Pox in Early Modern Germany*. Burlington, VT: Ashgate, 2009.

Stevenson, Christine. "From Palace to Hut: The Architecture of Military and Naval Medicine." In *British Military and Naval Medicine, 1600–1830*, edited by Geoffrey L. Hudson, 227–252. New York: Rodopi, 2007.

Strocchia, Sharon. "The Nun Apothecaries of Renaissance Florence: Marketing Medicines in the Convent." *Renaissance Studies* 25 (2011): 627–647.

Sweet, James H. *Domingos Álvares, African Healing, and the Intellectual History of the Atlantic World*. Chapel Hill: University of North Carolina Press, 2011.

Swiderski, Richard. *Anthrax: A History*. Jefferson, NC: McFarland, 2004.

Terpstra, Nicholas. *Lost Girls: Sex and Death in Renaissance Florence*. Baltimore: Johns Hopkins University Press, 2010.

Unschuld, Paul U. *Forgotten Treasures of Ancient Chinese Medicine: The I-hsüeh Yüan Liu Lun of 1757, by Hsü Ta-ch'un*. Brookline, MA: Paradigm, 1998.

Unschuld, Paul U. *Medical Ethics in Imperial China: A Study in Historical Anthropology*. Berkeley: University of California Press, 1979.

Unschuld, Paul U. *Medicine in China: A History of Ideas*. 2nd ed. Berkeley: University of California Press, 2010.

Unschuld, Paul U. *Medicine in China: A History of Pharmaceutics*. Berkeley: University of California Press, 1986.

Unschuld, Paul U. *What Is Medicine? Western and Eastern Approaches to Healing*. Translated by Karen Reimers. Berkeley: University of California Press, 2009.

van de Pol, Lotte. *The Burgher and the Whore: Prostitution in Early Modern Amsterdam*. New York: Oxford University Press, 2011.

Vanja, Christina. "Madhouses, Children's Wards, and Clinics: The Development of Insane Asylums in Germany." In *Institutions of Confinement: Hospitals, Asylums, and Prisons in Western Europe and North America*, edited by Norbert Finzsch and Robert Jütte, 117–132. New York: Cambridge University Press, 1996.

Veith, Ilza, trans. *The Yellow Emperor's Classic of Internal Medicine*. Berkeley: University of California Press, 2002.

Vesalius, Andreas. *On the Fabric of the Human Body* (1543). 5 vols. Translated by William Frank Richardson. Novato, CA: Norman, 2003–2009.

Vila, Anne C. *Enlightenment and Pathology: Sensibility in the Literature and Medicine of Eighteenth-Century France*. Baltimore: Johns Hopkins University Press, 1998.

Voeks, Robert. "African Medicine and Magic." *Geographical Reviews* 83 (1993): 66–79.

Waite, Gloria M. *A History of Traditional Medicine and Health Care in Pre-colonial East-Central Africa*. Lewiston, NY: Edwin Mellen, 1993.

Wallis, Patrick. "Consumption, Retailing, and Medicine in Early Modern London." *Economic History Review* 61 (2008): 26–53.

Wang, Zhenguo. *History and Development of Traditional Chinese Medicine*. Beijing: Science Press, 1999.

Watts, Sheldon. *Disease and Medicine in World History*. New York: Routledge, 2003.

Weaver, Karol K. *Medical Revolutionaries: The Enslaved Healers of Eighteenth-Century Saint Domingue*. Chicago: University of Illinois Press, 2006.

Webb, James L. A., Jr. *Humanity's Burden: A Global History of Malaria*. New York: Cambridge University Press, 2009.

Webster, Charles. *Paracelsus: Medicine, Magic, and Mission at the End of Time*. New Haven, CT: Yale University Press, 2008.

Whaley, Leigh. *Women and the Practice of Medical Care in Early Modern Europe, 1400–1800*. New York: Palgrave Macmillan, 2011.

Wilbert, Johannes. *Tobacco and Shamanism in South America*. New Haven, CT: Yale University Press, 1987.

Will, Pierre-Etienne. *Bureaucracy and Famine in Eighteenth-Century China*. Stanford, CA: Stanford University Press, 1990.

Will, Pierre-Etienne, and R. Bin Wong, eds. *Nourish the People: The State Civilian Granary System in China, 1650–1850*. Ann Arbor: University of Michigan, 1991.

Wilson, Lindsay. *Women and Medicine in the French Enlightenment: The Debate over Maladies des Femmes*. Baltimore: Johns Hopkins University Press, 1993.

Withey, Alun. "'Persons That Live Remote from London': Apothecaries and the Medical Marketplace in Seventeenth-and Eighteenth-Century Wales." *Bulletin of the History of Medicine* 85 (2011): 222–247.

Woods, Robert. *Death before Birth: Fetal Health and Mortality in Historical Perspective*. New York: Oxford University Press, 2009.

Wooley, Benjamin. *Heal Thyself: Nicholas Culpeper and the Seventeenth-Century Struggle to Bring Medicine to the People*. New York: HarperCollins, 2004.

Woolley, Hannah. *The Gentlewoman's Companion; or, A Guide to the Female Sex: The Complete Text of 1675*. Totnes, UK: Prospect Books, 2001.

Wright, John. *A History of War Surgery*. Stroud, UK: Amberley, 2011.

Wu, Yi-Li. *Reproducing Women: Medicine, Metaphor, and Childbirth in Late Imperial China*. Berkeley: University of California Press, 2010.

Yangwen, Zheng. *The Social Life of Opium in China*. New York: Cambridge University Press, 2005.

Yuan-Ling, Chao. *Medicine and Society in Late Imperial China*. New York: Peter Lang, 2009.

Zinsser, Hans. *Fleas, Rats and History*. Boston: Little, Brown, 1963.

Zumthor, Paul. *Daily Life in Rembrandt's Holland*. Stanford, CA: Stanford University Press, 1994.

About the Editor and Contributors

Editor

Ruth Clifford Engs, PhD, is Professor Emerita, School of Public Health, Indiana University, Bloomington, Indiana. Her research has focused upon student drinking patterns in addition to social reform movements of the early 20th century. Her many works include *The Field Hospital That Never Was* (2015), *Unseen Upton Sinclair* (2009), *The Eugenics Movement* (2005), *The Progressive Era's Health Reform Movement* (2003), and *Clean Living Movements: American Cycles of Health Reform* (2000). Other major works include two oral histories, *Conversations in the Abbey: Senior Monks of Saint Meinrad Archabbey Reflect on their Lives* (2008) and *Conversations in the Abbey, Volume 2* (2016).

Contributors

Deborah Brunton was awarded a doctorate from the University of Pennsylvania in 1990 and was, until recently, senior lecturer in the history of medicine at the Open University in Milton Keynes in Britain. She has researched extensively on public health, particularly smallpox prevention. She is author of *The Politics of Vaccination: Practice and Policy in England, Wales, Ireland and Scotland, 1800–1874* and of *Medicine in Modern Britain: 1780–1950.*

Joseph P. Byrne, PhD, is a historian and professor of humanities in the honors program at Belmont University in Nashville, Tennessee. He has written *The Black Death* (Greenwood, 2004), *Daily Life during the Black Death* (Greenwood, 2006), the *Encyclopedia of the Black Death* (ABC-CLIO, 2012), and *The World of Renaissance Italy: A Daily Life Encyclopedia* (Greenwood, 2017). He has also edited the *Encyclopedia of Pestilence, Pandemics, and Plagues* (Greenwood, 2008).

William H. York, PhD, earned his doctorate in the history of science, medicine, and technology from the Johns Hopkins University with a focus on medieval and early modern European history. He is a member of the faculty in the Honors College at Portland State University, where he teaches courses on the history of science and medicine, environmental history, and the history of animals. He is currently serving as the president of Medica: The Society for the Study of Healing in the Middle Ages.

Index

Boldface numbers refer to volume numbers.